Health Issues in Indigenous Children: An Evidence-Based Approach for the General Pediatrician

Guest Editors

ANNE B. CHANG, MBBS, MPHTM, PhD, FRACP
ROSALYN SINGLETON, MD, MPH

PEDIATRIC CLINICS OF NORTH AMERICA

www.pediatric.theclinics.com

December 2009 • Volume 56 • Number 6

SAUNDERS an imprint of ELSEVIER, Inc.

W.B. SAUNDERS COMPANY
A Division of Elsevier Inc.

1600 John F. Kennedy Boulevard • Suite 1800 • Philadelphia, Pennsylvania 19103-2899

http://www.theclinics.com

THE PEDIATRIC CLINICS OF NORTH AMERICA Volume 56, Number 6
December 2009 ISSN 0031-3955, ISBN-13: 978-1-4377-1258-2, ISBN-10: 1-4377-1258-4

Editor: Carla Holloway
Developmental Editor: Theresa Collier

The Pediatric Clinics of North America (ISSN 0031-3955) is published bimonthly by Elsevier Inc., 360 Park Avenue South, New York, NY 10010-1710. Months of issue are February, April, June, August, October, and December. Periodicals postage paid at New York, NY and additional mailing offices. Subscription prices are $167.00 per year (US individuals), $378.00 per year (US institutions), $227.00 per year (Canadian individuals), $503.00 per year (Canadian institutions), $270.00 per year (international individuals), $503.00 per year (international institutions), $83.00 per year (US students and residents), and $142.00 per year (international and Canadian residents and students). To receive students/resident rare, orders must be accompanied by name of affiliated institution, date of term, and the signature of program/residency coordinator on institution letterhead. Orders will be billed at individual rate until proof of status is received. Foreign air speed delivery is included in all *Clinics* subscription prices. All prices are subject to change without notice. **POSTMASTER:** Send address changes to *The Pediatric Clinics of North America*, Elsevier Health Sciences Division, Subscription Customer Service, 3251 Riverport Lane, Maryland Heights, MO 63043. **Customer Service: 1-800-654-2452 (US and Canada). From outside of the US and Canada: 1-314-447-8871. Fax: 1-314-447-8029. For print support, E-mail: JournalsCustomerService-usa@elsevier.com. For online support, E-mail: JournalsOnlineSupport-usa@elsevier.com.**

Reprints. For copies of 100 or more, of articles in this publication, please contact the Commercial Reprints Department, Elsevier Inc., 360 Park Avenue South, New York, NY 10010-1710. Tel.: 212-633-3812; Fax: 212-462-1935; E-mail: reprints@elsevier.com.

The Pediatric Clinics of North America is also published in Spanish by McGraw-Hill Inter-americana Editores S.A., Mexico City, Mexico; in Portuguese by Riechmann and Affonso Editores, Rua Comandante Coelho 1085, CEP 21250, Rio de Janeiro, Brazil; and in Greek by Althayia SA, Athens, Greece.

The Pediatric Clinics of North America is covered in *MEDLINE/PubMed (Index Medicus)*, *Excerpta Medica*, *Current Contents*, *Current Contents/Clinical Medicine*, *Science Citation Index*, *ASCA*, *ISI/BIOMED*, and *BIOSIS*.

Printed and bound by CPI Group (UK) Ltd, Croydon, CR0 4YY

Transferred to Digital Print 2011

GOAL STATEMENT

The goal of the *Pediatric Clinics of North America* is to keep practicing physicians and residents up to date with current clinical practice in pediatrics by providing timely articles reviewing the state-of-the-art in patient care.

ACCREDITATION

The *Pediatric Clinics of North America* is planned and implemented in accordance with the Essential Areas and Policies of the Accreditation Council for Continuing Medical Education (ACCME) through the joint sponsorship of the University Of Virginia School Of Medicine and Elsevier. The University Of Virginia School of Medicine is accredited by the ACCME to provide continuing medical education for physicians.

The University of Virginia School of Medicine designates this educational activity for a maximum of 15 *AMA PRA Category 1 Credits*™ for each issue, 90 credits per year. Physicians should only claim credit commensurate with the extent of their participation in the activity.

The American Medical Association has determined that physicians not licensed in the US who participate in this CME activity are eligible for a maximum of 15 *AMA PRA Category 1 Credits*™ for each issue, 90 credits per year.

Credit can be earned by reading the text material, taking the CME examination online at http://www.theclinics.com/home/cme, and completing the evaluation. After taking the test, you will be required to review any and all incorrect answers. Following completion of the test and evaluation, your credit will be awarded and you may print your certificate.

FACULTY DISCLOSURE/CONFLICT OF INTEREST

The University of Virginia School of Medicine, as an ACCME accredited provider, endorses and strives to comply with the Accreditation Council for Continuing Medical Education (ACCME) Standards of Commercial Support, Commonwealth of Virginia statutes, University of Virginia policies and procedures, and associated federal and private regulations and guidelines on the need for disclosure and monitoring of proprietary and financial interests that may affect the scientific integrity and balance of content delivered in continuing medical education activities under our auspices.

The University of Virginia School of Medicine requires that all CME activities accredited through this institution be developed independently and be scientifically rigorous, balanced and objective in the presentation/discussion of its content, theories and practices.

All authors/editors participating in an accredited CME activity are expected to disclose to the readers relevant financial relationships with commercial entities occurring within the past 12 months (such as grants or research support, employee, consultant, stock holder, member of speakers bureau, etc.). The University of Virginia School of Medicine will employ appropriate mechanisms to resolve potential conflicts of interest to maintain the standards of fair and balanced education to the reader. Questions about specific strategies can be directed to the Office of Continuing Medical Education, University of Virginia School of Medicine, Charlottesville, Virginia.

The faculty and staff of the University of Virginia Office of Continuing Medical Education have no financial affiliations to disclose.

The authors/editors listed below have identified no financial or professional relationships for themselves or their spouse/partner:

Timothy Beal, MD, MPH; Lawrence R. Berger, MD, MPH; Nancy M. Bill, MPH, CHES; George Brenneman, MD; Ngiare Brown, BM, MPHTM, FRACGP; Catherine A. Byrnes, MBChB, FRACP, GCCE; Matthew M. Cappiello, BA; Jonathan R. Carapetis, MBBS, B Med Sc, PhD, FRACP, FAFPHM; Anne B. Chang, MBBS, MPHTM, PhD (Guest Editor); CC Chang, MBBS, FRACP; Lance Chilton, MD; Bart J. Currie, FRACP, FAFPHM, DTM+H; Heather J. Dean, MD; Sheila Gahagan, MD, MPH; Keith Grimwood, MBChB, FRACP, MD; Rosamund L. Harrison, DMD, MSc, MRCD(C); Carla Holloway (Acquisitions Editor); Malcolm King, PhD; Amanda J. Leach, PhD; James McCarthy, MD, FRACP; Robert I. Menzies, MPH; Michael EK Moffatt, MD, MSc, FRCPC; Kelly Moore, MD; Peter S. Morris, MBBS, FRACP, PhD; Polly Olsen, BA; Karen Rheuban, MD (Test Author); Everett Rhoades, MD; Susan M. Sayers, MBBS, DCH, FAAP, FRACP, PhD; Elizabeth AC Sellers, MD, MSc; Robert J. Schroth, DMD, MSc; Gurmeet R. Singh, MBBS, DCH, DGO, MD, DNB, MPH & TM, FRACP, PhD; Andrew C. Steer, MBBS, BMedSc, FRACP; Michael Storck, MD; Judith Thierry, DO, FAAP, MPH; P.J. Torzillo, MBBS, FRACP, FJFICM; and LJ David Wallace, MSEH.

The authors/editors listed below identified the following professional or financial affiliations for themselves or their spouse/partner:

Ross M. Andrews, PhD, M App Epid, MPH, Dip App Sci (Env Hlth) is an industry funded research/investigator for GlaxoSmithKline Australia.

David A. Forbes, MBBS, FRACP received supplies from Dako and Axoid.

Jan Garver Bacon, MSW, PhD is a consultant and sole proprietor for the company Jan G. Bacon, PhD.

Kerry-Ann O'Grady, PhD is an industry funded research/investigator for GlaxoSmithKline.

Gregory J. Redding, MD serves on the Speakers Bureau for Merck and is a consultant for Astra-Zeneca.

Alan R. Ruben, MBBS, M Appl Epid, FRACP, FAFPHM is an industry funded research/investigator for Wyeth Pharmaceuticals (financial relationship ended in 2006.)

Rosalyn Singleton, MD, MPH (Guest Editor) is an industry funded research/investigator for Wyeth.

Disclosure of Discussion of Non-FDA Approved Uses for Pharmaceutical Products and/or Medical Devices

The University of Virginia School of Medicine, as an ACCME provider, requires that all faculty presenters identify and disclose any off-label uses for pharmaceutical and medical device products. The University of Virginia School of Medicine recommends that each physician fully review all the available data on new products or procedures prior to clinical use.

TO ENROLL

To enroll in the Pediatric Clinics of North America Continuing Medical Education program, call customer service at 1-800-654-2452 or visit us online at www.theclinics.com/home/cme. The CME program is available to subscribers for an additional fee of $195.00

Contributors

GUEST EDITORS

ANNE B. CHANG, MBBS, MPHTM, PhD, FRACP
Professor, Child Health Division, Menzies School of Health Research, Charles Darwin University, Darwin, Northern Territory; Queensland Children's Respiratory Centre, Queensland Children's Medical Research Institute, Royal Children's Hospital, Brisbane, Queensland; Poche Centre for Indigenous Health, University of Sydney, Sydney, New South Wales, Australia

ROSALYN J. SINGLETON, MD, MPH
Director, Immunization Program, Alaska Native Tribal Health Consortium; Arctic Investigations Program, National Center for Preparedness, Detection, and Control of Infectious Diseases, Coordinating Center for Infectious Diseases, Centers for Disease Control and Prevention, Anchorage, Alaska

AUTHORS

ROSS M. ANDREWS, PhD, MApp Epid, MPH, Dip App Sci (Env Hlth)
Associate Professor, Menzies School of Health Research, Charles Darwin University, Darwin, Northern Territory, Australia

JAN GARVER BACON, MSW, PhD
Clinical Instructor, Department of Psychiatry and Behavioral Sciences, University of Washington, Seattle; Program Director-Psychologist, Ketron Cottage - Child Study and Treatment Center, Department of Social and Health Service, State of Washington, Lakewood, Washington

TIMOTHY BEAL, MD
(Cherokee Tribe), Fellow in Child Forensic Psychiatry, Instructor in Psychiatry, Department of Psychiatry, Strong Memorial Hospital, University of Rochester School of Medicine and Dentistry, Rochester, New York

LAWRENCE R. BERGER, MD, MPH
Clinical Assistant Professor of Pediatrics, Department of Pediatrics, University of New Mexico School of Medicine, Albuquerque, New Mexico; Injury Prevention Program, Indian Health Service, Rockville, Maryland

NANCY M. BILL, MPH, CHES
Program Manager, Certified Health Education Specialist, Injury Prevention Program, Indian Health Service, Rockville, Maryland

GEORGE BRENNEMAN, MD, FAAP
Catonsville, Maryland

NGIARE BROWN, BM, MPHTM, FRACGP
Associate Professor, Director, Bullana, the Poche Centre for Indigenous Health, The University of Sydney, Sydney, New South Wales, Australia

CATHERINE A. BYRNES, MBChB, FRACP, GCCE
Senior Lecturer and Honorary Consultant, Department of Paediatrics, Starship Children's
Hospital, Auckland University, Auckland, New Zealand

MATTHEW M. CAPPIELLO, BA
Research Assistant, Division of Child Development and Community Health, University
of California at San Diego, La Jolla, California

JONATHAN R. CARAPETIS, MBBS, BMedSc, PhD, FRACP, FAFPHM
Director and Professor, Menzies School of Health Research, Charles Darwin University,
Darwin, Northern Territory, Australia

ANNE B. CHANG, MBBS, FRACP, PhD
Professor, Child Health Division, Menzies School of Health Research, Charles Darwin
University, Darwin, Northern Territory; Queensland Children's Respiratory Centre,
Queensland Children's Medical Research Institute, Royal Children's Hospital, Brisbane,
Queensland; Poche Centre for Indigenous Health, University of Sydney, Sydney, New
South Wales, Australia

CHRISTINA C. CHANG, MBBS, FRACP
Department of Infectious Diseases, Alfred Hospital, Monash University, Melbourne, New
South Wales, Australia

LANCE CHILTON, MD
Associate Professor, Department of Pediatrics, Young Children's Health Center,
University of New Mexico, Albuquerque, New Mexico

BART J. CURRIE, FRACP, FAFPHM, DTM+H
Professor, Menzies School of Health Research, Charles Darwin University, Darwin,
Northern Territory, Australia

HEATHER J. DEAN, MD, FRCPC
Professor, Department of Pediatrics and Child Health, University of Manitoba, Winnipeg,
Manitoba, Canada

DAVID A. FORBES, MBBS, FRACP
Professor, School of Paediatrics and Child Health, University of Western Australia; Chair,
Paediatric Medicine Clinical Care Unit, Paediatric Gastroenterologist Princess Margaret
Hospital, Perth, Western Australia, Australia

SHEILA GAHAGAN, MD, MPH
Professor and Martin T. Stein Endowed Chair in Developmental-Behavioral Pediatrics;
Chief, Division of Child Development and Community Health, Department of Pediatrics,
University of California at San Diego, La Jolla, California

KEITH GRIMWOOD, MBChB, FRACP, MD
Professor, Queensland Paediatric Infectious Diseases Laboratory, Queensland Children's
Medical Research Institute; Conjoint Professor, Discipline of Paediatrics and Child Health,
University of Queensland; Paediatric Infectious Diseases Physician, Royal Children's
Hospital, Brisbane, Queensland, Australia

ROSAMUND L. HARRISON, DMD, MSc, MRCD(C)
Professor, Division of Pediatric Dentistry, University of British Columbia; Clinical
Investigator, Child and Family Research Institute, Vancouver, British Columbia,
Canada

MALCOLM KING, PhD
University of Alberta Pulmonary Research Group, CIHR Institute of Aboriginal Peoples' Health, University of Alberta, Edmonton, Canada

AMANDA J. LEACH, PhD
Child Health Division, Menzies School of Health Research; Institute of Advanced Studies, Charles Darwin University, Darwin, Northern Territory, Australia

JAMES McCARTHY, MD, FRACP
Associate Professor, Queensland Institute of Medical Research; School of Medicine, University of Queensland, Brisbane, Queensland, Australia

ROBERT I. MENZIES, MPH
The National Centre for Immunisation Research and Surveillance of Vaccine Preventable Diseases (NCIRS), Sydney, New South Wales, Australia

MICHAEL E.K. MOFFATT, MD, MSc, FRCPC
Professor, University of Manitoba; Research Scientist, The Manitoba Institute of Child Health; Executive Director, Division of Research and Applied Learning, Winnipeg Regional Health Authority, Winnipeg, Manitoba, Canada

KELLY MOORE, MD, FAAP
Associate Professor, Centers for American Indian and Alaska Native Health, University of Colorado, Aurora, Colorado

PETER S. MORRIS, MBBS, FRACP, PhD
Deputy Leader, Child Health Division, Menzies School of Health Research; Institute of Advanced Studies, Charles Darwin University, Darwin; Northern Territory Clinical School, Flinders University, Darwin, Northern Territory, Australia

K. O'GRADY, PhD
Child Health Division, Menzies School of Health Research, Charles Darwin University, Darwin, Northern Territory, Australia

POLLY OLSEN, BA
(Yakama Tribe), Director of Community Relations and Development, Indigenous Wellness Research Institute, School of Social Work, University of Washington, Seattle, Washington

GREGORY J. REDDING, MD
Professor of Pediatrics, Department of Pediatrics, University of Washington School of Medicine; Chief, Pulmonary Division, Seattle Children's Hospital, Seattle, Washington

EVERETT RHOADES, MD, FACP
Professor Emeritus of Medicine, University of Oklahoma Health Sciences Center, College of Public Health, University of Oklahoma, Oklahoma City, Oklahoma

ALAN R. RUBEN, MBBS, M.Appl.Epid, FRACP, FAFPHM
Associate Professor, Northern Territory Clinical School, Flinders University, Darwin, Northern Territory, Australia

SUSAN M. SAYERS, MBBS, DCH, FAAP, FRACP, PhD
Associate Professor, Child Health Division, Menzies School of Health Research, Institute of Advanced Studies, Charles Darwin University, Darwin, Northern Territory, Australia

ROBERT J. SCHROTH, DMD, MSc
Assistant Professor, Department of Pediatrics and Child Health and Department of Oral Biology, University of Manitoba; Research Scientist, The Manitoba Institute of Child Health, Winnipeg, Manitoba, Canada

ELIZABETH A.C. SELLERS, MD, MSc, FRCPC
Associate Professor, Department of Pediatrics and Child Health, University of Manitoba, Winnipeg, Manitoba, Canada

GURMEET R. SINGH, MBBS, DCH, DGO, MD, DNB, MPH&TM, FRACP, PhD
Senior Research Fellow, Child Health Division, Menzies School of Health Research; Institute of Advanced Studies, Charles Darwin University, Darwin, Northern Territory; Senior Lecturer, Northern Territory Clinical School, Flinders University, Adelaide, South Australia; Senior Lecturer, James Cook University, Townville, Queensland, Australia

ROSALYN J. SINGLETON, MD, MPH
Director, Immunization Program, Alaska Native Tribal Health Consortium; Arctic Investigations Program, National Center for Preparedness, Detection, and Control of Infectious Diseases, Coordinating Center for Infectious Diseases, Centers for Disease Control and Prevention, Anchorage, Alaska

ANDREW C. STEER, MBBS, BMedSc, FRACP
Department of Paediatrics, Centre for International Child Health, University of Melbourne, Melbourne, New South Wales, Australia; Division of Infectious and Immunologic Diseases, Department of Pediatrics, University of British Columbia, Vancouver, British Columbia, Canada

MICHAEL STORCK, MD
Associate Professor, Division of Child and Adolescent Psychiatry, Department of Psychiatry and Behavioral Sciences, University of Washington School of Medicine, Seattle, Washington; Co-chairman, Native American Child Committee, American Academy of Child and Adolescent Psychiatry

JUDITH THIERRY, DO, MPH, FAAP
Office of Clinical and Preventive Services, Indian Health Service, Rockville, Maryland

P.J. TORZILLO, MBBS, FRACP
Nganampa Health Council, Alice Springs, Northern Territory, Australia; Royal Prince Alfred Hospital, University of Sydney, Camperdown, New South Wales, Australia

L.J. DAVID WALLACE, MSEH
Consultant, Injury Prevention; Senior Injury Prevention Specialist (retired), US Public Health Service; Steamboat Springs, Colorado

Contents

An Overall Approach to Health Care for Indigenous Peoples

Malcolm King

Indigenous peoples across all the continents of the globe live with major gaps in health status and health outcomes associated with well-described social determinants of health, such as poverty and poor education. Indigenous peoples face additional health determinant issues associated with urbanization, isolation from traditional territories, and loss of cultural continuity. Indigenous children are particularly vulnerable as they grow up in isolation from their cultural and social roots and yet are also separated from the mainstream environment of their society. Programs to address these difficult health issues should be viewed as complex clinical interventions with health researchers, social scientists, and clinicians working together with Indigenous peoples to identify the most pressing needs and most appropriate and workable solutions that will result in effective policies and practices.

Indigenous Newborn Care

Susan M. Sayers

Infant mortality and morbidity disparities occur between non-Indigenous and Indigenous populations of Australia, Canada, New Zealand, and the United States. Neonatal mortality is due to high-risk births, which vary according to prevalence of the maternal risk factors of smoking, alcohol consumption, infection, and disorders of nutritional status, whereas postneonatal mortality is predominantly influenced by environmental factors. Aside from changing socioeconomic conditions, a continuum of maternal and child health care is likely to be the most effective measure in reducing these health disparities.

Vaccine Preventable Diseases and Vaccination Policy for Indigenous Populations

Robert I. Menzies and Rosalyn J. Singleton

There are many similarities regarding the health status of Indigenous people in the 4 English-speaking developed countries of North America and the Pacific (United States, Canada, Australia, New Zealand), where they are all now minority populations. Although vaccines have contributed to the reduction or elimination of disease disparities for many infections, Indigenous people continue to have higher morbidity and mortality from many chronic and infectious diseases compared with the general populations in their countries. This review summarizes the available data on the

Socially disadvantaged Indigenous infants and children living in western industrialized countries experience high rates of infectious diarrhea, no more so than Aboriginal children from remote and rural regions of Northern Australia. Diarrheal disease, poor nutrition, and intestinal enteropathy reflect household crowding, inadequate water and poor sanitation and hygiene. Acute episodes of watery diarrhea are often best managed by oral glucose-electrolyte solutions with continuation of breastfeeding and early reintroduction of feeding. Selective use of lactose-free milk formula, short-term zinc supplementation and antibiotics may be necessary for ill children with poor nutrition, persistent symptoms, or dysentery. Education, high standards of environmental hygiene, breastfeeding, and immunization with newly licensed rotavirus vaccines are all needed to reduce the unacceptably high burden of diarrheal disease encountered in young children from Indigenous communities.

The rising global burden of chronic renal disease, the high cost of providing renal replacement therapies, and renal disease also being a risk factor for cardiovascular disease is increasing focus on renal disease prevention. This article focuses on the aspects of renal disease (specifically poststreptococcal glomerulonephritis [PSGN] and chronic kidney disease [CKD]) in Indigenous populations in Australia, New Zealand, Canada, and the United States that diverge from those typically seen in the general population of those countries. The spectrum of renal and many other diseases seen in Indigenous people in developed countries is similar to that seen in developing countries. Diseases like PSGN that have largely disappeared in developed countries still occur frequently in Indigenous people. CKD during the childhood years is due to congenital anomalies of the kidney and urinary tract in up to 70% of cases and occurs later in polycystic kidney disease and childhood-onset diabetes. Several risk factors for CKD in adulthood are already present in childhood.

Otitis media (OM) is a common illness in young children. OM has historically been associated with frequent and severe complications. Nowadays it is usually a mild condition that often resolves without treatment. For most children, progression to tympanic membrane perforation and chronic suppurative OM is unusual (low-risk populations); this has led to reevaluation of many interventions that were used routinely in the past. Evidence from a large number of randomized controlled trials can help when discussing treatment options with families. Indigenous children in the United States, Canada, Northern Europe, Australia, and New Zealand experience more OM than other children. In some places, Indigenous children continue to suffer from the most severe forms of the disease. Communities with more than 4% of the children affected by chronic tympanic membrane perforation have a major public health problem (high-risk populations). Higher rates of invasive pneumococcal disease, pneumonia, and chronic suppurative lung disease (including bronchiectasis) are also seen. These children will often benefit from effective treatment of persistent (or recurrent) bacterial infection.

disease burden, treatment, and challenges in achieving successful clinical management of this disorder in Indigenous youth. Screening criteria and the complications and comorbidities of type 2 diabetes are also reviewed.

After first discussing historical, community and epidemiologic perspectives pertaining to mental health problems of Indigenous youth and families, this article reviews available research data on behavioral and mental health interventions and the roles that Native and Indigenous research programs are serving. Given the legacy of transgenerational trauma experienced by Indigenous peoples, community-based research and treatment methods are essential for solving these problems. The primary care provider stands in a unique position within the community to offer a "coinvestigator spirit" to youth and families in the pursuit of improving behavioral health. Strategies are presented for using the research literature, and collaborating with communities and families to help solve behavioral and mental health problems.

Dental caries in Indigenous children is a child health issue that is multifactorial in origin and strongly influenced by the determinants of health. The evidence suggests that extensive dental caries has an effect on health and well-being of the young child. This article focuses on early childhood caries as an overall proxy for Indigenous childhood oral health because decay during early life sets the foundation for oral health throughout childhood and adolescence. Strategies should begin with community engagement and always include primary care providers and other community health workers.

Developmental delay is common and often responds to early intervention. As with other health outcomes, the prevalence of developmental delay may be socially determined. Children in many Indigenous communities experience increased risk for developmental delay. This article highlights special conditions in Indigenous communities related to child development. It addresses the challenges of screening and evaluation for developmental delay in the context of Indigenous cultures, and in settings where resources are often inadequate. It is clear that careful research on child development in Indigenous settings is urgently needed. Intervention strategies tied to cultural traditions could enhance interest, acceptability, and ultimately developmental outcomes in children at risk.

Throughout the world, injuries and violence are a leading cause of mortality and suffering among Indigenous communities. Among American Indian and Alaska Native children aged 1 to 19 years, 71% of deaths are from injuries. Motor-vehicle accidents, attempted suicide, and interpersonal violence are the most common causes of injuries in highly industrialized countries. For Indigenous populations in middle- and low-income countries, trauma caused by motor-vehicle accidents, agricultural injuries, interpersonal violence, child labor, and the ravages of war are priorities for intervention. To be effective, injury-prevention efforts should be based on scientific evidence, be developmentally and culturally appropriate, and draw on the inherent strengths of Indigenous communities.

Most American Indian and Alaska Native Children (AIAN) receive health care that is based on the unique historical legacy of tribal treaty obligations and a trust relationship of sovereign nation to sovereign nation. From colonial America to the early 21st century, the wellbeing of AIAN children has been impacted as federal laws were crafted for the health, education and wellbeing of its AIAN citizens. Important public laws are addressed in this article, highlighting the development of the Indian Health Service (IHS), a federal agency designed to provide comprehensive clinical and public health services to citizens of federally recognized tribes. The context during which various acts were made into law are described to note the times during which the policy making process took place. Policies internal and external to the IHS are summarized, widening the lens spanning the past 200 years and into the future of these first nations' youngest members.

This article identifies significant historical and contemporary issues, programs, and progress to better understand the current policy in Australia relating to Aboriginal child health and well-being. A legislative perspective gives context to contemporary issues based on legally sanctioned historical practices specifically designed to make Aboriginal peoples disappear, particularly through the control and assimilation of Indigenous children.

FORTHCOMING ISSUES

February 2010
Bone Marrow Transplantation
Max Coppes, MD, PhD, MBA,
Terry Fry, MD, and
Crystal Mackall, MD, *Guest Editors*

April 2010
Solid Organ Transplantation
Vicky Lee Ng, MD, FRCPC, and
Sandy Feng, MD, PhD,
Guest Editors

June 2010
Pediatric Sports Medicine
Dilip R. Patel, MD, and
Donald E. Greydanus, MD,
Guest Editors

RECENT ISSUES

October 2009
Nutritional Deficiencies
Praveen S. Goday, MBBS, CNSP, and
Timothy S. Sentongo, MD,
Guest Editors

August 2009
Pediatric Quality
Leonard G. Feld, MD, PhD, MMM, FAAP,
and Shabnam Jain, MD, FAAP,
Guest Editors

April 2009
**Child Abuse and Neglect: Advancements
and Challenges in the 21st Century**
Andrew Sirotnak, MD, *Guest Editor*

RELATED INTEREST

Pediatric Clinics of North America Volume 52, Issue 5 (October 2005)
International Adoption: Medical and Developmental Issues
Lisa Albers, MD, MPH, Elizabeth Barnett, MD, Jerri Ann Jenista, MD,
and Dana E. Johnson, MD, PhD, *Guest Editors*
www.pediatric.theclinics.com

THE CLINICS ARE NOW AVAILABLE ONLINE!

Access your subscription at:
www.theclinics.com

Preface

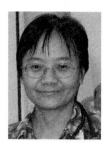

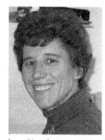

Anne B. Chang, MBBS, MPHTM, PhD, FRACP   Rosalyn Singleton, MD, MPH

Guest Editors

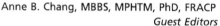

Why does the subject of health issues in Indigenous children deserve a special issue? Is the management of common disease in Indigenous children different from that for non-Indigenous children? Why adopt an evidence-based approach?

Globally, the disparity in health between Indigenous and non-Indigenous people is striking. It is most marked and well documented in affluent countries: Aboriginal and Torres Strait Islanders in Australia; Māori in New Zealand; First Nation, Inuit, and Metis People in Canada; and American Indians and Alaska Natives in the United States (here forth, all of these groups are referred to as Indigenous).[1] In these affluent countries, the disease patterns (frequency, age distribution, severity and/or contributors to disease) in Indigenous children are substantially different from those in non-Indigenous children. For example, trials of currently recommended antibiotic regimens for ear infections in Australian Indigenous children showed poorer resolution rates than trials published from studies in non-Indigenous children.[2] Also while the basic management of such illnesses as asthma in Indigenous children is identical to that in non–Indigenous children (eg, optimal treatment with use of appropriate asthma medications and devices, asthma action plan, etc.), the delivery of health care and asthma programs require modification. Thus, this issue is dedicated to health in Indigenous children.

Major advances in Indigenous child health will follow improvements in education and housing, and reductions in poverty; however, high-quality health care can also affect the outcome of many childhood conditions. High-quality care requires the application of the best evidence on prevention and management of common illnesses. In this issue, an evidence-based approach to common scenarios in Indigenous children is emphasized because significant advances in clinical care have occurred when long-held dogma were questioned and evidence applied.[3] William Silverman[3] eloquently articulated this in his book *Where's the Evidence?* He further challenges clinicians to reflect on where the line between "knowing" (the acquisition of new medical information) and "doing" (the application of that new knowledge) is drawn.

In this issue, authors from the United States, Canada, Australia, and New Zealand, with substantial clinical and research expertise in Indigenous child health, have shared

Pediatr Clin N Am 56 (2009) xvii–xix
doi:10.1016/j.pcl.2009.10.003
0031-3955/09/$ – see front matter © 2009 Elsevier Inc. All rights reserved.

pediatric.theclinics.com

their clinical experience and expertise. We thank the authors for their valuable contributions to this issue. The opening article is appropriately by Professor Malcolm King, an esteemed Canadian of First Nation heritage. He reminds us of the importance of issues outside the biomedical model. The closing articles are on health policies, which are empirically linked with politics and, subsequently, health outcomes, especially those aimed at reducing social inequalities.[4] The remaining articles take an evidence-based approach to guide the clinician in the care of Indigenous children with common conditions. The first few focus on generic preventative care (infant care, immunization, and nutrition) and the latter are disease-specific articles, with a focus on relatively common conditions affecting Indigenous children. Where relevant and possible, the updated GRADE[5] (Grading of Recommendations Assessment, Development and Evaluation) system for each recommended approach was undertaken. The steps are designed to answer the questions "What is the current evidence-based approach?" and "What is the strength of the recommendation and level of evidence?" In the updated GRADE system, a recommendation, if given, can be strong or weak.[5] The implications of a strong recommendation are:

- For patients: Most people in your situation would want the recommended course of action and only a small proportion would not; request discussion if the intervention is not offered.
- For clinicians: Most patients should receive the recommended course of action.
- For policy makers: The recommendation can be adopted as a policy in most situations.[5]

The implications of a weak recommendation are:

- For patients: Most people in your situation would want the recommended course of action, but many would not.
- For clinicians: You should recognize that different choices will be appropriate for different patients and that you must help each patient to arrive at a management decision consistent with her or his values and preferences.
- For policy makers: Policy making will require substantial debate and involvement of many stakeholders.[5]

A significant limiting factor in almost all articles is the lack of high-quality evidence for the suggested approaches taken. However, authors have provided the current evidence succinctly and have highlighted the evidence, or lack of, for managing conditions that health practitioners are likely to encounter in an Indigenous child. We hope readers will find these articles useful in their personal clinical practice and will do their best within their sphere to help reduce the health disparities between Indigenous and non-Indigenous children.

Anne B. Chang, MBBS, MPHTM, PhD, FRACP
Child Health Division, Menzies School of Health Research
Charles Darwin University, Darwin, Australia
Queensland Children's Respiratory Centre
and Qld Children's Medical Research Institute
Royal Children's Hospital, Brisbane, Queensland, Australia

Rosalyn Singleton, MD, MPH
Alaska Native Tribal Health Consortium and
Centers for Disease Control and Prevention
Anchorage, AK, USA

E-mail addresses:
annechang@ausdoctors.net (A.B. Chang)
ris2@cdc.gov (R. Singleton)

REFERENCES

1. Smylie J, Adomako P, editors. Indigenous children's health report. Available at: http://www.stmichaelshospital.com/crich/indigenous_childrens_health_report.php. 2009. Accessed April 22, 2009.
2. Morris PS, Leach AJ, Halpin S, et al. An overview of acute otitis media in Australian Aboriginal children living in remote communities. Vaccine 2007;25:2389–93.
3. Silverman WA. Where's the evidence? debates in modern medicine. Oxford: Oxford University Press; 1999.
4. Navarro V, Muntaner C, Borrell C, et al. Politics and health outcomes. Lancet 2006; 368:1033–7.
5. Guyatt GH, Oxman AD, Kunz R, et al. Going from evidence to recommendations. BMJ 2008;336:1049–51.

An Overall Approach to Health Care for Indigenous Peoples

Malcolm King, PhD

KEYWORDS

• Indigenous peoples • Sociocultural • Health care
• Health disparities

Indigenous peoples across all the continents of the globe live with major gaps in health status and health outcomes associated with well-described social determinants of health, such as poverty and poor education. Indigenous peoples face additional health determinant issues associated with urbanization, isolation from traditional territories, and loss of cultural continuity.[1] Indigenous children are particularly vulnerable as they grow up in isolation from their cultural and social roots and yet are also separated from the mainstream environment of their society.

Health practitioners need to be aware of the underlying causes of poor health among indigenous peoples. Addressing educational, economic, and cultural indicator deficits could potentially lead to greater health gains than solely focusing on conventional biomedical approaches. Initiatives targeting education, poverty, and other sociocultural inequities should be evaluated not only for themselves but for their potential to improve health. Health researchers need to be more involved in addressing these important health issues that could lead to improved health for indigenous peoples everywhere.[1,2]

There are many examples of health inequities to be found in indigenous children, as described in this volume. Poor living conditions, inadequate nutrition, and exposure to high rates of infection cause a heavy burden of disease in infants and children.[2] Childhood respiratory diseases, such as respiratory syncytial virus (RSV)-associated disease in northern indigenous populations in the United States and Canada, are much more common than in other populations.[3–5] Factors, such as inadequate housing (eg, overcrowding, poor ventilation),[4] remoteness, and lack of access to health services[5] lead to excess morbidity and risk of lifelong health deficits.

INDIGENOUS CONCEPTS OF HEALTH, ILLNESS, AND HEALING

Research on indigenous health has been largely focused on Western rather than indigenous concepts of health, disease, and treatment. By contrast, indigenous peoples

University of Alberta Pulmonary Research Group, CIHR Institute of Aboriginal Peoples' Health, University of Alberta, 173 HMRC University of Alberta, Edmonton, AB T6G 2S2, Canada
E-mail address: malcolm.king@ualberta.ca

Pediatr Clin N Am 56 (2009) 1239–1242
doi:10.1016/j.pcl.2009.09.005
0031-3955/09/$ – see front matter © 2009 Elsevier Inc. All rights reserved.

define wellbeing far more broadly than simply physical health or the absence of disease. For example, the Anishinabek (Ojibway) words *mno bmaadis*, which translate into "living the good life" or "being alive well", encapsulates beliefs in the importance of balance. The four elements of life, physical, emotional, mental and spiritual, are represented in the four directions of the medicine wheel. These four elements are intricately woven together and interact to support a strong and healthy person.[6] Balance extends beyond the individual realm such that good health and healing also require that an individual live in harmony with others, their community, and the spirit worlds. For indigenous peoples, land, food, and health are key components of being alive well.[7]

The root causes of poor health (ie, the social determinants of health) are generally to blame for the poor state of everyone's health,[8] but especially the health of indigenous peoples. Such determinants are universally thought to include the classic socioeconomic indicators, defined by the 1986 Ottawa Charter for Health Promotion: income, education, employment, living conditions, social support, and access to health services.[9] These factors certainly apply to the health of indigenous populations (see Anand and colleagues).[10] However, indigenous health is widely understood to also be impacted by a range of cultural factors including racism, along with various indigenous-specific factors, such as loss of language and connection to the land, environmental deprivation, and spiritual, emotional, and mental disconnectedness. The definition of indigeneity is, therefore, inherently social, and includes major elements of cultural identity. Being isolated from aspects of this identity is widely understood to impact negatively on indigenous health.[11]

Whole Health/Community Health

Holistic health is the vision most First Nations peoples articulate as they reflect upon their future. At the personal level this means each member enjoys health and wellness in body, mind, heart, and spirit. Within the family context, this means mutual support of each other. From a community perspective it means leadership committed to whole health, empowerment, sensitivity to interrelatedness of past, present, and future possibilities, and connected between cultures.[12]

The interactions among mental, emotional, and spiritual stress and physical health are relevant and important to indigenous health. For example, the increasing rates of diabetes in various indigenous populations have been associated with environmental factors related to the rapid sociocultural changes that occur with migration to the urban setting and acculturation.[13,14]

Interactions and comorbidities between mental and physical health are also important. Like illness, wellbeing is similarly multidimensional within the person, including a balance between the person and others (eg, their family/community) and the environment. The work of Chandler and Lalonde[15,16] delineated community factors related to empowerment and self-control that were protective of health in the particular case of youth suicide in British Columbia First Nations. The variation between communities was crucial to understanding the underlying factors. It was communities with programs and measures of self-determination that had the lowest suicide rates.

Social capital and resilience are also important relational concepts that impact on health. Social capital has been defined in various ways and refers to sociability, social networks and support, trust, reciprocity, and community and civic engagement.[17] Resilience, what keeps people strong in the face of adversity and stress, has many indigenous facets: spiritual connections, cultural and historical continuity, and the ties with family, community and the land.[18]

This is why factors like retention of Aboriginal languages, cultural practices, self-determination, and respect for elders are so important. And that is why we have so much to do to repair the damage done by so many disruptive assimilationist practices in the past, such as cutting off children from their families at residential schools or suppression of cultural practices that conflicted with European ideas.

THE POLITICS OF INDIGENOUS HEALTH

In most regions, indigenous peoples are geographically fragmented, living in urban environments, often ghettoized, and in scattered or isolated settlements. Services and supports for health and social programs are also typically fragmented in indigenous populations (see the Kirby Report in Canada[19] for an example). This fragmentation is true in the different levels of government that are all generally working without collaboration, which results in isolating symptomatic problems (eg, addiction, suicide, fetal alcohol, poor housing, lack of employment) and then designing stand-alone programs to try to manage each one separately. Many question the whole role of government in providing services, when indigenous peoples should be supported in the development of their own solutions rather than having solutions imposed on or provided for them. Such a change would foster the development of more culturally appropriate and effective services and supports.[15]

Although the need to improve overall socioeconomic conditions of vulnerable populations is self-evident, the actual health benefits that will result are less obvious. Intervention research in the social determinants of health is needed. The health benefits that will accrue from a social determinants intervention need to be delineated. Research is also needed to monitor the health benefits of interventions, such as programs to improve educational attainment in indigenous populations and programs to revitalize indigenous languages and support indigenous cultures. Such programs should be viewed as complex clinical interventions, and health researchers and clinicians should work with social scientists across a broad spectrum and with indigenous communities themselves to evaluate outcomes that will allow for knowledge translation to other communities.

We should be concerned about the over politicization of poor health and excessive blaming of external factors for the state of indigenous health.[20] As pointed out by Helin,[21] a Canadian First Nation author, indigenous peoples must reduce their culture of financial and psychological dependency on the external system and take more control over their own economic and social recovery, which would inevitably include striving for better health.

Programs to address these difficult health issues should be viewed as complex clinical interventions with health researchers, social scientists, and clinicians working together with indigenous peoples to identify the most pressing needs and most appropriate and workable solutions that will result in effective policies and practices.

REFERENCES

1. King M, Smith A, Gracey M. Indigenous perspectives on health: the underlying causes of the health gap. Lancet 2009;374:76–85.
2. Gracey M, King M. Indigenous health: determinants and disease patterns. Lancet 2009;374:65–75.
3. Singleton R, Morris A, Redding G, et al. Bronchiectasis in Alaska Native children: causes and clinical courses. Pediatr Pulmonol 2000;29:182–7.
4. Kovesi T, Gilbert NL, Stocco C. Indoor air quality and the risk of lower respiratory tract infections in young Canadian Inuit children. CMAJ 2007;177:155–60.

5. Banerji A, Greenberg D, White LF, et al. Risk factors and viruses associated with hospitalization due to lower respiratory tract infections in Canadian Inuit children. Pediatr Infect Dis J 2009;28:697–701.

6. Wilson K. Therapeutic landscapes and first nations peoples: an exploration of culture, health and place. Health Place 2003;9:83–93.

7. Settee P. *Pimatisiwin: indigenous knowledge systems, our time has come* [PhD thesis]. Saskatoon (SK): University of Saskatchewan;2007.

8. Marmot M. Achieving health equity: from root causes to fair outcomes. Lancet 2007;370:1153–63.

9. World Health Organization. Ottawa Charter for Health Promotion. Available at: http://www.who.int/hpr/NPH/docs/ottawa_charter_hp.pdf. Nov 1986. Accessed June 29, 2009.

10. Anand SS, Yusuf S, Jacobs R, et al. Risk factors, atherosclerosis, and cardiovascular disease among Aboriginal people in Canada: the study of health assessment and risk evaluation in Aboriginal peoples. Lancet 2001;358:1147–53.

11. World Health Organization. An overview of current knowledge of the social determinants of indigenous health. Compiled by Nettleton C, Napolitano DA, Stephens C. Symposium on the Social Determinants of Indigenous Health, Adelaide, April, 29–30, 2007.

12. Mussell WJ, Nichols WM, Adler MT. Making meaning of mental health challenges in first nations: a Freirean perspective. Chilliwack (BC): Sal'i'shan Institute Society; 1993. p. 26.

13. O'Dea K, Spargo RM, Akerman K. The effect of transition from traditional to urban life-style on the insulin secretory response in Australian Aborigines. Diabetes Care 1980;3:31–7.

14. Szathmary EJ, Ritenbaugh C, Goodby CS. Dietary change and plasma glucose levels in an Amerindian population undergoing cultural transition. Soc Sci Med 1987;24:791–804.

15. Chandler MJ, Lalonde CE. Cultural continuity as a hedge against suicide in Canada's First Nations. Transcult Psychiatry 1998;35:191–219.

16. Chandler MJ, Lalonde CE. Cultural continuity as a protective factor against suicide in First Nations youth. Horizons 2008;10:68–72.

17. Morrow V. Conceptualising social capital in relation to the well-being of children and young people: a critical review. Sociol Rev 1999;47:744–65.

18. Barlett JG, Robertson P. Thriving, not just surviving: developing Indigenous health workforce networks. Presentation to 3rd International Network for Indigenous Health Knowledge and Development. Rotorua (New Zealand): (INIHKD) 2007.

19. Kirby MJL, LeBreton M. The Health of Canadians – The federal role: final report of the standing senate committee on social affairs. Ottawa (Canada): Science and Technology; 2002.

20. Sutton P. The politicisation of disease and the disease of politicisation: causal theories and the indigenous health differential. Keynote address at 8th National Rural Health Conference, Alice Springs (Australia) 2005. Available at: http://nrha.ruralhealth.org.au/conferences/docs/8thNRHC/Papers/KN_sutton,%20peter.pdf.

21. Helin C. Dances with dependency: indigenous success through self-reliance. Accessed June 29, 2009. Vancouver (Canada): Orca Spirit Publishing; 2006.

Indigenous Newborn Care

Susan M. Sayers, MBBS, DCH, FAAP, FRACP, PhD

KEYWORDS

- Indigenous • Newborn • Preconception
- Prenatal • Neonatal care

In the economically developed counties of Australia, Canada, the United States, and New Zealand, indigenous people live as marginalized, socially disadvantaged, minority populations who have a determination to maintain traditional connections to their land, culture, and language. Compared with non-indigenous populations, they have lower incomes, poorer education outcomes, poorer food security, lower home ownership, and limited access to heath services. Overarching these social inequalities are long-standing issues relating to human rights, colonization, poverty, and self-determination.[1] These social circumstances are associated with specific health issues in indigenous populations, which have an adverse impact on infant health outcomes and infant mortality.

BACKGROUND AND BURDEN OF DISEASE

Similarities occur between the indigenous people of Australia,[2] Canada,[3] New Zealand,[4] and the United States[5] in that they all have higher infant mortality rates compared to the mainstream population (**Table 1**). The greatest disparity occurs in Australia, with infant mortality rates three times those of the non-Indigenous population, followed by Canada, with rates double those of the mainstream population. For indigenous populations in New Zealand and the United States, although infant mortality rates are higher than in the mainstream population, the gaps between the two are narrower. However if infant mortality is subcategorized into neonatal mortality (deaths per live births up to 28 completed days after birth) and post-neonatal mortality (deaths between 29 days and 364 days after birth), different patterns of mortality emerge for the different indigenous populations.

For Indigenous Australians and Canadians, infant mortality data is not disaggregated at a national level; however, based on studies from Western Australia and British Columbia, neonatal and postneonatal indigenous mortality rates are higher than in the non-indigenous populations with, again, the greatest differences occurring for Indigenous Australians. In contrast, for the indigenous people of New Zealand and the United States, the neonatal mortality rates are similar to the mainstream populations,

Child Health Division, Menzies School of Health Research, Institute of Advanced Studies, Charles Darwin University, PO Box 41096, Casuarina, NT 0811, Australia
E-mail address: sue.sayers@menzies.edu.au

Pediatr Clin N Am 56 (2009) 1243–1261
doi:10.1016/j.pcl.2009.09.009
0031-3955/09/$ – see front matter © 2009 Elsevier Inc. All rights reserved.

Table 1
Infant, neonatal, and postneonatal mortality for indigenous and nonindigenous populations of Australia, Canada, New Zealand, and United States

Indicator	Australia[2] Indige-nous	Australia[2] Non-Indige-nous	Canada[3] Indige-nous	Canada[3] Non-Indige-nous	New Zealand[4] Indige-nous	New Zealand[4] Non-Indige-nous	United States[5] Indige-nous	United States[5] Non-Indige-nous
Infant mortality	12.2	4.4	13.0	6.1	7.4	4.7	8.3	5.0
Neonatal mortality	9.7	3.9	5.6	3.8	2.8	3.3	3.9	3.1
Postneonatal mortality	11.2[6]	2.2[6]	8.2	2.3	4.6	1.4	4.4	1.9

with marked disparities between indigenous and non-indigenous populations occurring only in the postneonatal mortality rates (see **Table 1**). In Australia, Canada, and New Zealand, indigenous postneonatal mortality is higher than neonatal mortality, which is a pattern consistent with disadvantaged populations, with the reverse of that pattern seen in the non-indigenous populations in each country (see **Table 1**).

Deaths in the neonatal period are usually related to conditions associated with high-risk births and congenital abnormalities. Categories of high-risk births are low birth weight (LBW), which may be due to fetal growth-restricted (FGR) or preterm births, and large-for-gestational-age (LGA) or high-birth-weight births. **Table 2** shows the clinical conditions associated with the high-risk births that contribute to

Table 2
Clinical characteristics contributing to neonatal mortality in indigenous high-risk newborns

	Fetal Growth Restriction	Preterm	Large for Gestational Age or Macrosmia
Asphyxia, seizures	✔	✔	✔
Hypothermia	✔	✔	
Respiratory conditions	Meconium aspiration	Respiratory distress syndrome	
Cardiovascular conditions	Persistent pulmonary hypertension	Patent ductus arteriosus	
Hypoglycemia, hypocalcemia, hyperbilirubinemia	✔	✔	✔
Polycythemia, hyperviscosity	✔		✔
Birth injuries			Brachial plexus palsy fracture clavicle, humerus
Congenital abnormalities			Neural tube, cardiac, facial, extremities

neonatal morbidity and mortality. **Table 3** shows the percentages of the high-risk births in indigenous populations. The outstanding feature is the Australia Indigenous LBW rates, which are considerably higher than those of the other indigenous populations.

Low Birth Weight

LBW, defined as a birth weight less than 2500 g, is determined by the duration of gestation and fetal growth. Babies may be LBW because they are preterm (<37 weeks), FGR (birth weight <10th percentile of birth weight for gestational age), or both. Rates of LBW range from 7% in the developed countries to 16.5% in developing countries.[9] LBW is associated with increased mortality and morbidity.

The LBW rates of Indigenous Australians (12.7%) are double those of the indigenous populations of Canada and New Zealand and of non-Indigenous Australians and similar to those of the developing populations of Angola (12%), Guatemala (13%), and Uganda (12%).[9] In marked contrast, for the indigenous people of Canada, New Zealand, and the United States, the LBW rates are much lower, similar to their respective non-indigenous populations (see **Table 3**) and more consistent with the developed status of the countries in which they live.

The immediate and long-term consequences of LBW in a population depend on the relative proportions of FGR and preterm births within the heterogeneous LBW group. When LBW rates are more than 10% (as it is for Indigenous Australians), LBW is predominantly due to term-LBW babies (a proxy for FGR) but when the LBW rate is below 10%, it is predominantly due to preterm births.[10]

Reliable gestational age estimations are essential to avoid the common misclassification of small FGR babies as preterm births, but this information may not always be available. In a Northern Territory study of indigenous mothers, 6.5% were certain of their last menstrual period date and 8.2% had a fetal ultrasound at less than 14 weeks suitable for a gestational age estimation.[11] When gestation age estimates are unavailable, combining preterm birth and FGR into a single heterogeneous indicator of LBW is practical but likely to hinder health promotion efforts, as the causes and outcomes of the two conditions differ.[12]

Table 3
Birth characteristics for indigenous populations of Australia, Canada, New Zealand, and the United States

Characteristic	Australia[2]		Canada[3]		New Zealand[4]		United States[5]	
	Indige-nous	Non-Indige-nous	Indige-nous	Non-Indige-nous	Indige-nous	Non-Indige-nous	Indige-nous	Non-Indige-nous
LBW (%)	12.7	6	5.4	5.6	7.3	5.7	6.6	7.4
Preterm (%)	14	8	9.5	5.6	7.6	7.3	12.2	11.2
FGR (%)	25[7]	10[7]	7.5	10.2	—	—	—	—
LGA or macrosomia (%)	1.4	1.8[8]	15.5	9.6	—	—	12.6	10.2

Abbreviations: FGR, birth weight <10th percentile of birth weight for gestational age; LBW, birth weight <2500 g; LGA, birth weight >90th percentile for gestational age; macrosomia, birth weight >4500 g or birth weight >4000 g; Preterm, gestational age <37 weeks gestation.

Fetal Growth Restriction

The high LBW in the Australian Indigenous population suggests the majority of the LBW births are FGR, but difficulties with reliable gestational aging means confirming evidence is limited. High rates of LBW FGR births are unlikely in indigenous populations of Canada, New Zealand, and the United States, because the LBW rates are below 10% and higher birth weights are more frequent (see **Table 3**).

One Northern Territory study with careful attention to gestational aging, using postnatal clinical estimations, showed 25% of indigenous newborns were FGR instead of the expected 10%.[7] Furthermore, in the neonatal period, Australian Indigenous babies are consistently shown to have better survival rates than non-Indigenous babies of the same birthweight.[13] The most likely explanation is that these surviving babies are FGR, with increased maturity relative to their birthweights.

Morbidity of FGR extends beyond the neonatal period. FGR children have higher rates of neurodevelopmental impairments[14] and there is a body of literature describing relationships of FGR to adult coronary heart disease, hypertension, type 2 diabetes mellitus, insulin resistance, and kidney disease.[15] The main risk factors for FGR births in the Northern Territory study were maternal smoking, maternal undernutrition, and maternal age of less than 19 years.[16]

Preterm

Preterm (gestation <37 weeks) birth rates are higher for the indigenous populations of Australia, Canada, and the United States compared to the non-indigenous populations, with Australian Indigenous people having the highest rates of all (see **Table 3**). The disparity between preterm rates in indigenous and non-indigenous people is also greatest in Australians (see **Table 3**), although this may in part be due to preterm misclassification because of gestational aging errors

The consequences of preterm births extend from childhood to adult life. Neurodevelopmental disabilities occur in approximately 25% of preterm births; the major disabilities are cerebral palsy, mental retardation, and epilepsy but other abnormalities, such as visual and auditory deficits and long term respiratory consequences of respiratory distress syndrome, occur more commonly.[17]

The causes of indigenous preterm births are unknown but factors, including smoking, infection, and stress associated with socioeconomic conditions, are likely.

Large for Gestational Age and Macrosomia

In contrast to Indigenous Australians, LGA (birthweight >90th percentile of birthweight for gestational age) and macrosomic births (birthweight >4.5 kg or >4 kg) occur more commonly in the indigenous populations of Canada and United States compared to the non-indigenous population. The percentage of First Nation babies with birthweights greater than 4 kg was 21% compared to 13% for the general Canadian population and for the American Indian and Alaska Native (AIAN) population in 1997, 12.6% of births were greater than 4 kg compared to the United States all-birth rate of 10.2%.[5] For Indigenous Australians, the high-birth-weight cutoff is greater than 4.5 kg and, therefore, cannot be compared directly to the other indigenous populations, but rates of 1.4% for Indigenous Australians[2] compare variably with the 1.8% reported for the non-Indigenous Australian population.[8]

High birthweight is associated with operative deliveries, shoulder dystocia, and asphyxia.[18] Morbidity extends beyond the neonatal period, with long-term consequences of neurologic injury to the brachial plexus and higher risks of adolescent obesity, diabetes, and metabolic syndrome.[19] The causes for the higher birthweights in the indigenous populations of Canada and the United States are not completely understood. In part they are due to the higher prevalence of maternal obesity and diabetic risk in these groups but in addition there may be ethnic differences in the effects of maternal diabetes on birthweight.[20]

RISK FACTORS FOR ADVERSE PREGNANCY OUTCOMES IN INDIGENOUS POPULATIONS

The risk factors for adverse pregnancy outcomes are important for all indigenous populations but are more important for the indigenous populations of Australia and Canada, which have marked neonatal mortality disparities from the mainstream populations. The importance of these risk factors varies according to the pattern of high-risk births. Factors relating to LBW, preterm and FGR, are important for Indigenous Australians, whereas those relating to preterm births and LGA births are important for Canada and the United States.

Smoking

Smoking during pregnancy is known to have harmful effects on mothers and babies. The smoking rates of indigenous women of childbearing age and during pregnancy are considerably higher than for non-indigenous women. In New Zealand, 47% of Maori women aged 15 to 64 years were smokers, more than twice the smoking prevalence reported for European women.[21] In the United States, 20.2% of AIAN smoked during pregnancy compared to 13.2% of mothers nationwide.[5] The highest smoking rates of all and the greatest disparities between Indigenous and non-Indigenous occur in Australia, with 54% of Indigenous mothers recorded as smoking in pregnancy compared to 17% of non-Indigenous mothers.[8]

Fetal effects of exposure to maternal smoking are LBW, FGR, and preterm birth.[22,23] Infants born to mothers who smoke are on average 200 g lighter, with the risk of a lower birthweight being dose dependent.[22,23] Studies suggest there is a more direct and stronger association between maternal smoking and fetal growth than gestational age. In a recent Australian study of Indigenous mothers, smoking multiplied the risk of having a full-term LBW baby more than threefold (ie, >200% increase) in comparison to the risk of preterm birth, which was approximately 1.3 times higher (ie, 30% increase).[24]

Evidence for effective intervention is present in a Cochrane meta-analysis of 64 trials, which demonstrated that women receiving a smoking cessation intervention during pregnancy were more likely to stop smoking and had a 15% to 20% reduction in preterm and LBW rates and a 33-g increase in mean birthweight. Cognitive–behavioral interventions, including incentives and social supports, were shown to be the most effective.[25] Currently, there is a lack of information about the most effective and culturally appropriate smoking interventions for indigenous populations prior to and during pregnancy. There are strong recommendations for cessation of smoking during pregnancy based on high-quality evidence, but cessation of smoking before conception should be the aim.

Alcohol Consumption

There is a spectrum of abnormalities associated with exposure of the developing fetus to alcohol. These range from fetal alcohol syndrome, with a triad of prenatal or postnatal growth retardation, distinctive abnormal facial features, and neurodevelopmental abnormalities, to alcohol-related neurodevelopmental disorder and alcohol-related birth defects, which are associated with lesser degrees of alcohol exposure.[26]

In surveys of fetal alcohol syndrome, indigenous populations are over-represented. In an Australian study, Indigenous population rates were 14 times higher than those of the non-Indigenous population.[27] In Canada, the prevalence of fetal alcohol syndrome/fetal alcohol effects may be as high as 20% in First Nations and Inuit communities compared to 0.2% for the general population.[28] There are concerns, however, about these high rates because of lack of standardized and culturally appropriate testing instruments and because the typical facial features were originally established in populations of Caucasion children.

There is still uncertainty about level of alcohol consumption, but as there is no guarantee about the safe lower limits, complete abstinence is recommended based on moderate evidence. A Cochrane evaluation of supportive counseling and educational sessions to reduce alcohol consumption in pregnancy was inconclusive.[29]

Obesity, Gestational Diabetes, and Maternal Diabetes

Obesity, gestational diabetes mellitus (GDM), and types 1 and 2 diabetes mellitus are independently associated with an increased risk of LGA births, preterm births, birth injury, and macrosomia.[19,30–32] There is a threefold to fourfold increase in major congenital anomalies occurring in women with these conditions and even higher absolute and relative risks for particular malformations, such as neural tube defects. The most common defects involve the cardiovascular system, central nervous system, face, and extremities.[32] Exposure to a hyperglycemic intrauterine environment is associated with later increased risk of childhood obesity, metabolic syndrome, and type 2 diabetes mellitus.[32]

Globally, indigenous populations are undergoing a nutritional transition, which is associated with sedentary lifestyles and diet changes linked to overweight and obesity. As a result, in each country, the prevalence of overweight and obesity is higher in the indigenous population than in the non-indigenous population. In Canada, 64% of indigenous women (off-reserve) are overweight or obese compared to 47% of non-indigenous women, and in New Zealand, 43% of Maori women were obese compared to 23% for Europeans.[21] A similar pattern is present for Indigenous Australians and Native Americans.[33] Prevalence data for pregnant indigenous women are not available but it is likely the disparities are repeated.

Accompanying rising obesity rates in indigenous populations are increasing rates of type 2 diabetes mellitus in childbearing years and GDM.[21,34] Between 1990 and 1998, for AIAN attending United States Indian health services, the prevalence of type 2 diabetes mellitus increased by 68% for adolescents and by 50% for adults 25 to 34 years old.[35] In New Zealand and the United States, the indigenous population has an almost threefold higher diabetes prevalence than the majority populations. The highest rates of type 2 diabetes mellitus are recorded for Native Americans in the southern United States (38%–40%) and Torres Strait Islanders in Australia (33%).[36] This epidemic of type 2 diabetes mellitus in indigenous populations, which is increasing in younger age groups, has resulted in increasing diabetes in pregnancy.

Because of strong associations between glycemic control as measured by glycosylated hemoglobin levels and congenital abnormalities and LGA, glycemic targets are central to management. Folic acid supplementation recommended for all women planning a pregnancy or capable of conception is especially pertinent for those women of diabetogenic risk because of higher rates of neural tube defects. In a Cochrane review of four trials with 6425 women, periconception folate significantly reduced neural tube defects.[37]

Management strategies to reduce macosomia and LGA births associated with obesity and diabetes can best be delivered in the preconception period with recommendations for all women with diabetes and obesity to be counseled about the importance of diabetes control before considering pregnancy. Contraceptive consultation is suggested with pregnancy delay until as near normal glycosylated hemoglobin levels as possible can be achieved. A Cochrane meta-analysis evaluating energy restriction and exercise for overweight pregnant women found that fetal growth may be impaired,[38] emphasizing the optimum time for weight reduction is before pregnancy, with folic acid supplementation for those at risk of conception.

Controversies exist about GDM, defined as glucose intolerance with onset or first recognition during pregnancy, and there is generally a paucity of high-quality evidence and lack of consensus about screening and management of GDM and pre-existing diabetes of pregnancy.[39] Recognized management includes close glucose monitoring and dietary and physical activity advice.[40] A Cochrane analysis found no difference in the prevalence of macrosomic babies between women with dietary and no specific treatment programs.[41] However, as there is a twofold to fourfold increase of LGA in untreated GDM compared to treated GDM, there are recommendations for active management of GDM based on weak evidence.

Undernutrition

Maternal undernutrition is associated with an increased risk preterm and FGR with the maternal undernutrition occurring, as low prepregnant weight before conception and/or low gestational weight gain due to inadequate diet during pregnancy.[12]

Despite the high rates of obesity reported for indigenous populations, maternal undernutrition is still described in some Australian Indigenous populations. This may be due to the high rates of teenage pregnancies in these populations[2]; the changes from low body mass index (BMI) to high BMI are strongly age related in Aboriginal women.[42] In the Northern Territory, 15% of postpartum women had a BMI less than 18.5 kg/m^2, with 28% of LBW and 15% of FGR attributable to maternal undernutrition. In a Kimberley (Western Australia) survey, 16% of women of childbearing age were underweight,[42] and in three Northern Territory communities, women aged 19 to 24 years had a prepregnant BMI of 19.9 kg/m^2 compared to the all-Australian average of 23.6 kg/m^2.[43]

Interventions to decrease the risk of FGR by improving maternal weight can be delivered in preconception and prenatal primary health care. Evidence for effective intervention in pregnancy is present in a Cochrane meta-analysis of 13 trials of 4665 pregnant women. Those receiving a balanced energy/protein supplementation during pregnancy showed modest improvements in maternal weight and mean birthweights.[38] Hence, there are strong recommendations for balanced energy/protein supplementation during pregnancy based on high-quality evidence; however, maternal weight gain before conception is likely to achieve better birth outcomes. In contrast, high protein supplementation during pregnancy is not recommended.[38]

Infection

Preterm births are associated with asymptomatic genital and urinary tract infections. Bacterial vaginosis, an overgrowth of anaerobic bacteria and reduction of normal vaginal lactobacillus, is the most common lower genital tract condition in women of reproductive age. In a large US cohort study, 6% of preterm births were attributable to bacterial vaginosis.[44] Bacterial vaginosis can be eradicated by antimicrobial therapy but meta-analyses and reviews have shown this treatment does not reduce the occurrence of preterm birth.[45]

Asymptomatic infection of the urine may occur in 2% to 10% of pregnancies associated with increased risk of maternal pyelonephritis and preterm births. Fourteen studies of 2302 women showed antibiotics were effective in clearing the urine of infection and reducing the incidence of LBW.[46] Urine culture is the most accurate method for detecting asymptomatic bacteriuria and the most effective time for screening and treating is in early pregnancy.

Other genital infections—chlamydia, gonorrhea, and group B streptococcus (GBS)—acquired from the colonized birth canal can infect neonates at the time of delivery, causing opthalmia neonatorium, pneumonia, and serious systemic infection. One of the leading causes of neonatal sepsis is early-onset GBS infection. Approximately 10% to 30% of pregnant women are colonized with GBS in the vagina or rectum. For those women with vaginal carriage of GBS, 1% to 2% of babies become infected and 6% die if they have early onset of disease. Infants usually present with sepsis or pneumonia and, less often, meningitis, osteomyelitis, or septic arthritis. LBW babies are the most vulnerable.[47]

Population-based comparisons of strategies to prevent early-onset GBS show a better protective effect of a universal screening strategy relative to a risk-based strategy.[48] Therefore, strong recommendations are made for all pregnant women to be screened at 35 to 37 weeks' gestation for vaginal and rectal GBS colonization. A Cochrane review of five trials shows intrapartum antibiotics significantly reduce the rate of neonatal infection.[49] Screening should be performed in each pregnancy.

Indigenous women have high rates of genital tract infections compared to non-indigenous women. In Australia, young Indigenous women have infections of chlamydia 5 to 7 times and gonorrhea 50 to 140 times higher than non-indigenous women of the same age.[50] In Australian Indigenous women at first prenatal visit, the prevalence of urinary tract infections was reported as 15.7%.[51]

Stress

Mothers experiencing high levels of stress and clinical depression are at increased risk of preterm birth (approximately double), even after adjusting for confounding factors.[52] Data on the prevalence of stress in pregnancy in indigenous populations is limited but, in general, indigenous populations have higher exposures to life stressor events and report higher rates of stress and related disorders. It is seems likely the experiences of pregnant indigenous women are similar or even higher as pregnancy may be associated with increased stresses.

In a Native American study, there was a 21% prevalence of posttraumatic stress disorder (a rate similar to survivors of mass shootings and major burns) compared to 1% to 9% for the non-indigenous population.[53] For Indigenous Canadians, up to 18% had a major depression during the previous year; 15% had attempted suicide at some time in their lives, and approximately 30% report having been physically abused in some way.

Compared with non-Indigenous Australians, Indigenous Australians were twice as likely to report high levels of psychologic distress (27%–13%)[54] and 3.5 times as likely to have been affected by alcohol/drug-related problems or abuse/violent crime.[54] For Indigenous women, hospitalizations for injury due to assault are 33 times higher than for non-Indigenous women.[55]

The mechanisms underlying the associations between stress and preterm delivery are unknown, but relationships between stress and corticotrophin-releasing hormone and inflammatory pathways initiating labor have been implicated.[56] Screening during preconception and prenatal care may help indigenous women reduce their exposure to stress and violence through access to specialist care, including police and legal support services. However, programs offering extra emotional support, practical assistance, and advice to disadvantaged women during pregnancy, have not been shown to decrease LBW or preterm births.[57]

Teenage Pregnancies

Teenage pregnancy (maternal age <19 years) is a risk factor for preterm delivery, LBW, and FGR.[58] In Australia, 23% of Indigenous pregnancies were teenage pregnancies compared with 4% for non-Indigenous pregnancies.[2] In New Zealand, the teenage birth rate for Maori is reported at nearly five times that of European teenagers,[59] and in the United States, the proportion of pregnancies for young mothers is significantly higher for AIAN than in the general population.

Teenage pregnancies are associated with the risky behaviors of tobacco smoking, alcohol use, and poor prenatal attendance. After adjusting for these confounders, however, teenage pregnancy still is shown independently associated with increased risks of preterm delivery, LBW, and FGR.[60]

Evidence about effective interventions to decrease teenage pregnancies, which are specific to indigenous populations, is currently lacking. Research directions regarding indigenous sexuality education, availability of contraception, and attitudes toward sex, parenthood, and sole parenthood need to be investigated to achieve delayed childbearing in indigenous people.[59]

POST-NEONATAL MORTALITY

Although the factors associated with postneonatal mortality are important for each indigenous population, for the indigenous populations of New Zealand and the United States, they are more important. In these populations, neonatal mortality rates are similar to the corresponding non-indigenous populations, so mortality in the postneonatal period is the main contributor to the excess indigenous infant mortalities reported. Nevertheless, based on the Western Australian population, the highest indigenous postneonatal mortality rates are reported for Indigenous Australians.[6]

For the indigenous populations of Australia, Canada, New Zealand, and the United States, postneonatal mortality relates to the potentially preventable causes of sudden infant death syndrome (SIDS), infections, and unintentional injuries, with SIDS the leading cause of postneonatal death in all the indigenous populations.[3-6] For the Indigenous population in Western Australian (1980–2001), infections ranked second to SIDS, with rates highest in remote regions, followed by congenital abnormalities.[6] For the AIAN population (1998–2000), injuries ranked second to SIDS followed by congenital abnormalities and respiratory infections,[61] whereas for indigenous Canadians in British Columbia (1981–2000), infection ranked second to SIDS followed by external causes.[3] Apart from the perinatal associations with congenital abnormalities and SIDS, these findings suggest that for indigenous infants, after completion of the neonatal period, it is the postneonatal environment that is strongly influential on survival in the first year of life.

In each country, compared with the non-indigenous populations, indigenous people are disadvantaged regarding the key socioeconomic factors of employment, income, and education. In Australia in 2004–2005, the unemployment rate for the Indigenous population was three times higher than for non-Indigenous people, and in a similar period, the Indigenous weekly household income was almost half that of non-Indigenous households. Results from the 2006 Aboriginal Peoples Survey in Canada show unemployment rates were four to five times higher for indigenous people and that 41% of young First Nation children were from low-income families compared to 18% of non-indigenous children. In New Zealand, 27% of Maori children live in poverty compared with 16% of New Zealand European children population.[62] Similarly, educational outcomes are lower for Indigenous populations. Year 12 retention rates are 36% for Indigenous Australians compared with 73% for the total population,[63] and in New Zealand, 49% of Maori leave school without a National Certificate of Educational Achievement Qualification compared with 22% of non-Maori students.[62]

The United Nations Development Programme's Human Development Index (HDI) is a composite index with equal ratings for life expectancy, educational attainment, and median income. Using this index, Australia, Canada, New Zealand, and the United States are consistently placed near the top of the rankings with a high human development classification. According to the HDI, however, the indigenous people within these countries are rated at only medium human development level. Based on the HDI, recent improvements have occurred for indigenous people in Canada, New Zealand, and the United States, but for Indigenous Australians, the HDI decreased slightly and relative to improvements in the HDI for non-Indigenous Australians, the overall result has been a increasing gap between the two.[64]

It is these broad socioeconomic factors that influence the social and physical environment of indigenous infants during their first years of life. Downstream factors, such as poor housing, overcrowding, cosleeping, cigarette smoke exposure, food insecurity, inability to access health services, and poor appreciation of infant illness and safety needs, all contribute to the SIDS, injuries, and infection rates associated with high postneonatal mortality rates.

Sudden Infant Death Syndrome

SIDS refers to the sudden death of an infant younger than 1 year that remains unexplained after a thorough case investigation, including the performance of a complete autopsy, an examination of the death scene, and a review of an infant's clinical history. International comparisons are difficult due to inconsistencies of identification, coding, and terminology. However considerable disparities between the indigenous and nonindigenous populations, are consistently reported. In New Zealand, 72.5% of all SIDS cases are Maori.[4] In Western Australia, Aboriginal SIDS rates are seven times those of non-Aboriginal.[6] In the United States, the SIDS rate for AIAN was 2.1 times the US all-races rate in 1997,[5] and in Quebec (1985–1997), with ethnicity based on language groups, the First Nations had rates 6 times greater than those based on English language.

SIDS may be an endpoint of a variety of causes, with delayed maturation of arousal pathways the current hypothesis. Young maternal age, inadequate prenatal care, preterm and LBW births, environmental smoke exposure, and cosleeping have all been implicated, but the risk factors that have the greatest potential for modification are prone sleeping position, sleeping on a soft surface, overheating, and maternal smoking.[65] In the United States, recommendations to place babies supine in 1992 augmented by a Back to Sleep national program changed the frequency of prone sleeping over the course of a decade from 70% to approximately 20%, with a concurrent SIDS reduction greater than 40%. Hence, there are strong recommendations for the supine sleeping position of babies based on moderate evidence.[65]

Others

The injuries and infections contributing to the high postneonatal mortality rates of indigenous infants are discussed in articles by Chang and colleagues, Grimwood and Forbes, Andrews and colleagues, and Berger and colleagues elsewhere in this issue.

RECOMMENDED STRATEGIES TO REDUCE INFANT MORBIDITY AND MORTALITY IN INDIGENOUS POPULATIONS

Apart from alleviating the underlying socioeconomic conditions, improvement in infant mortality rates involves the delivery of primary health care in concert with focused community programs supported by government policy and legislation. The continuum of primary health care begins before conception and continues through the prenatal (preconception and prenatal), newborn, and postnatal periods. Most of these are generic to all people. Those with evidence specific to indigenous populations are highlighted when available (**Tables 4–6**).

Preconception Care

Some of the most powerful influences on pregnancy and subsequent infant health are related to the health and the well-being of the mother long before the beginning of pregnancy. Many maternal risk factors associated with adverse birth outcomes are characterized by a need to start and sometimes finish interventions before conception occurs.[77] The time available in the prenatal period may be insufficient to achieve effective interventions, particularly as indigenous women are more likely to have inadequate prenatal care.[5] In addition, many pregnancies are unplanned and early teratogen exposure to the fetus may occur before pregnancy is recognized.[77]

Recommendations relating to preconception health care are published by the US Centers for Disease Control[77] but adaptations tailored to indigenous care settings are not available. Opportunistic incorporation of preconception care into appropriate clinical encounters before pregnancy are likely to be the easier to implement in the first instance.[78] Adaptations of the five A's strategy recommended by the US Preventive Services Task Force may be used to initiate clinical counseling[79] with the strategy repeated at each contact to accommodate changed motivation and relapses (**Box 1**).

Currently, there is no evidence assessing preconception care delivered as a complete program but evaluations of interventions focusing on single risk factors are reported[80]; some are based on preconception care but others are extrapolated from pregnancy and basic primary interventions (see **Table 4**).

Prenatal Care

Current guidelines and protocols for prenatal care focus on providing information about birth and parenthood, screening and managing problems likely to have adverse impacts on mothers and the babies, and monitoring progress of pregnancy.

There are no randomized controlled trials on the impact of traditional prenatal care programs on perinatal and neonatal outcomes, but studies linking birth/death data based on up to 22 million women show relationships between neonatal mortality and inadequate prenatal care.[81]

There is debate on the number of prenatal visits and the components of prenatal care. Systematic analyses of the most effective components of care show tetanus toxoid immunization, iron-folate supplementation, detection and management of preeclampsia, screening and treatment for bacteriuria, and, where appropriate, screening and treatment for syphilis and malaria are priority activities.[70]

Table 4
Strength of recommendations and quality of evidence for selected preconception care interventions to improve newborn outcomes in indigenous populations

Preconception Intervention	Grade	Quality	Recommendation
Smoking	Strong	High	All women of childbearing age should be screened for smoking, with benefits discussed of not smoking before, during, and after pregnancy. Discussion of medication and referral.[66]
Alcohol	Strong	Moderate	All women of childbearing age should be screened for alcohol consumption. Information about the consequences of alcohol during the early first trimester and warnings that, as no safe level is established, abstinence required. Identify alcohol dependence and assist with cessation and long-term abstinence. Contraceptive consultation with suggested pregnancy delay until alcohol-free pregnancy can be achieved.[67]
Weight status	Weak	Moderate	All women should have BMI assessed. Women with BMI ≥ 26 kg/m^2 should be counseled about risks to own health and future pregnancies, including infertility. Offer strategies to decrease caloric intake and increase physical activity, encourage enrollment in structured weight loss program. Commence folic acid supplementation. Testing for diabetes of asymptomatic women who are overweight and have one or more risk factors, including history of gestational diabetes should be undertaken.[68] Women with BMI ≤ 19.8 kg/m^2 should be counseled about risk to future pregnancy.
Diabetes	Strong	Moderate	All women with diabetes should be counseled about the importance of diabetes control before considering pregnancy. Contraceptive consultation with suggested pregnancy delay until as near normal as possible glycosylated hemoglobin should be achieved to decrease congenital defects.[69] Folic acid supplementation should be commenced.
Folic acid	Strong	High	All women planning pregnancy or capable of conception take folic acid supplementation.[37]

An evaluation of only four prenatal visits compared with more frequent visits in a large multicenter trial by the World Health Organization showed no impact on FGR or preterm birth outcomes.[82]

Similar to preconception care approaches, screening and behavior counseling interventions using the five A's strategy are recommended, but evidence about effective prenatal interventions specific to indigenous populations is currently lacking. Cochrane evaluations have been undertaken on single interventions in general populations (see **Table 5**).

Neonatal Care

The newborn care of indigenous babies includes all the elements of routine care recommended for every newborn.[83] High-risk births are more likely to require active

Table 5
Strength of recommendations and quality of evidence for selected prenatal care interventions to improve newborn outcomes in indigenous populations

Prenatal Intervention	Grade	Quality	Recommendation
Smoking	Strong	High	All pregnant women should be screened for smoking. Cognitive-behavioral intervention effective.[25]
Alcohol	Strong	Moderate	All pregnant women should be screened for alcohol consumption. Psychologic and education intervention inconclusive.[29]
Overweight	Strong	Moderate	BMI assessed. Energy restriction and physical exercise may increase FGR—not recommended[38]
Underweight	Strong Strong	Low Moderate	Balanced energy/protein supplementation improved mean birthweight—recommended[38]
Underweight	Strong	Moderate	High protein supplementation may increase FGR—not recommended.[38]
Folic acid	Strong	High	Folic acid supplementation decreases congenital defects—recommended.[37]
Asymptomatic bacteriuria	Strong	High	Screening at 12–16 weeks with antibiotic if positive decreases LBW delivery—recommended.[46]
Group B streptococcus	Strong	High	Universal screening better than risk based only—recommended.[48]
Group B streptococcus	Strong	High	All pregnant women screened 35–37 weeks with intrapartum antibiotic if positive decreases neonatal infection.[49]
Bacterial vaginosis	Strong	High	Antibiotics eradicate infection but do not reduce preterm delivery—not recommended.[45]

resuscitation at delivery and specific management of their associated clinical complications (see **Table 6**).

A recent extensive review confirms the outstanding benefits of breastfeeding in regard to infant morbidity and mortality, intellectual and motor development, and later chronic disease risk.[84] In case-controlled studies and cohort studies, rates of diarrhea, respiratory tract infections, otitis media, and deaths due to these diseases are all lower in breastfed babies compared with nonbreastfed babies. Dose-response relationships are demonstrated with rates lower in the first 6 months for those exclusively breastfed compared with those partially breastfed.

The World Health Organization and the United Nations Children's Fund have developed a comprehensive and successful program to promote institutional support for breastfeeding through the Baby Friendly Hospital Initiative, entitled, "Ten Steps to Successful Breastfeeding." Attitudes are changed within hospitals by banning free gifts and formula from formula companies, removing all advertisements of formula, training all staff who have any contact with mothers from cleaners through to medical staff about breastfeeding, promoting skin-to-skin contact of mother and baby at delivery, feeding on demand with no other food and drink, no pacifier use, and support groups in the postnatal time.

Table 6
Strength of recommendations and quality of evidence for selected early neonatal care interventions to improve newborn outcomes in indigenous populations

Neonatal Intervention	Grade	Quality	Recommendation
Resuscitation training programs	Strong	Moderate	Neonatal mortality improved—recommended.[70]
Room air instead of 100% oxygen	Strong	Moderate	Mortality less in room air resuscitated—recommended but supplementary oxygen should be available.[71]
Laryngeal mask versus endotracheal intubation	Weak	Weak	Mask quicker, less skill, no difference outcome—insufficient evidence to recommend.[72]
Delayed clamping of cord	Weak	Moderate	Less transfusion, better iron stores, more hyperbilirubinemia—not recommended.[73]
Plastic wrap, skin to skin, warmed mattress	Strong	Moderate	Heat loss reduced—recommended.[74]
Stockinet cap, double walled incubator	Weak	Moderate	No significant differences—not recommended.[74]
Vitamin K	Strong	Strong	Single dose of intramuscular vitamin K prevents hemorrhagic disease of the newborn—recommended.[75]
Breastfeeding initiation	Strong	Strong	Education and peer support increase breastfeeding rates—recommended.[76]
Duration of exclusive breastfeeding	Strong	Strong	Six months' less morbidity and no growth deficit—recommended.[73]
Supine sleeping	Strong	Strong	Decrease SIDS rates—recommended.[65]

Postnatal Care

Current postnatal care interventions are based on home visiting programs aimed primarily at the prevention of child maltreatment and neglect. In the United States, the Nurse-Family Partnership program, targeting first-time disadvantaged mothers, resulted not only in fewer injury- and ingestion-related hospitalizations but also fewer deaths occurring from birth to 9 years from preventable causes.[85] In New Zealand,

Box 1
Five A's strategy: ask, assess, advise, assist, arrange

Ask about risk factor

Assess level of risk by brief screening

Advise about risk to maternal health and subsequent newborn

Assist with motivation, self-help skills, and support

Arrange follow-up support, repeat counseling, and referral if needed a randomized controlled trial comparing outcomes between control families and those enrolled in an Early Start program with home visits from soon after birth showed program families had greater contact with family physicians and dentists and were less likely to have hospital visits due to ingestions and accidents.[86]

Home visiting programs adapted for indigenous mother and child care need initial focus on immunization status, the sleeping environment of the baby, maternal smoking reduction, breastfeeding support, and maternal interconception care. Recently, Health@Home Plus, a nurse-led home visiting program for Indigenous mothers and babies, was commenced in Australia with aims to improve children's health during the first weeks of life and reduce maternal smoking, childhood injuries, and child abuse and neglect. Research programs evaluating culturally appropriate applications of postnatal programs to remote and rural Indigenous communities, Indigenous attitudes to home visiting, available resources, and potential work force are needed for the development of effective postnatal Indigenous programs.

Health promotion activities supporting primary health care include community-based interventions of mass media campaigns, youth programs, sporting sponsorships, and pamphlets, posters, and booklets directed toward the reduction of high-risk behaviors and promotion of healthy lifestyles. The most powerful behavior-modifying effects, however, at a population level have been achieved through government legislation. This has been demonstrated in Australia by government restrictions and taxation of tobacco products. There have been no evaluations of these measures on Indigenous people in Australia, but increased taxation of tobacco products, restrictions of sales to minors, and restricted smoking in public places are all likely to be as effective for Indigenous people as non-Indigenous people.

Future directions in closing the gaps in indigenous infant mortality include improving the translation of research into policy, increasing the indigenous work force capacity, and developing sustainable working partnerships with indigenous communities.

REFERENCES

1. Who. Social determinants and indigenous health: the international experience and its policy implications. Available at: http://www.who.int/social_determinants/resources/indigenous_health_adelaide_report_07.pdf. Accessed July, 2009.
2. Leeds KL, Gourley M, Laws PJ, et al. Indigenous mothers and their babies, Australia 2001–2004. Canberra: AIHW; 2007. AIHW Cat no PER 38. Perinatal statistics series no. 19.
3. Luo ZC, Kierans WJ, Wilkins R, et al. Infant mortality among First Nations versus non-First Nations in British Columbia: temporal trends in rural versus urban areas 1981–2000. Int J Epidemiol 2004;33:1252–9.
4. New Zealand Health Information Service. Fetal and infant deaths 2003 & 2004. Wellington: Ministry of Health; 2007.
5. Alexander GR, Wingate MS, Boulet S. Pregnancy outcomes of American Indians: contrasts among regions and other ethnic groups. Matern Child Health J 2008; 12:S5–11.
6. Freemantle C, Read AW, de Klerk NH, et al. Patterns, trends and increasing disparities in mortality for Aboriginal and non-Aboriginal infants born in Western Australia, 1980–2001: population database study. Lancet 2006;367:1758–66.
7. Sayers SM, Powers JR. Birth size of Australian aboriginal babies. Med J Aust 1993;159(9):586–91.
8. Laws PJ, Sullivan EA. Australia's mothers and babies 2002 [report]. AIHW Cat no PER 28. Sydney.

9. United Nations Children's Fund and World Health Organization, low birthweight: country, regional and global estimates [report]. UNICEF, New York, 2004.

10. Villar JM, Belizan JM. The relative contribution of prematurity and fetal growth retardation to low birth weight in developing and developed societies. Am J Obstet Gynecol 1982;143:793–8.

11. Sayers SM, Powers. An evaluation of three methods to access gestational age in Aboriginal neonates. J Paediatr Child Health 1995;31(3):261.

12. Kramer MS. Determinants of low birth weight: methodological assessment and meta-analysis. Bull World Health Organ 1987;65(5):663–737.

13. Gogna N, Smiley M, Walker AC, et al. Low birthweight and mortality in Australian Aboriginal babies at the Royal Darwin Hospital: a 15 year study. Aust Paediatr J 1986;22:281–4.

14. Yanney M, Marlow N. Paediatric consequences of fetal growth restriction. Semin Fetal Neonatal Med 2004;9(5):411–8.

15. Victora CG, Adair L, Fall C, et al. Maternal and child undernutrition: consequences for adult health and human capital. Lancet 2008;371(9609):340–57.

16. Sayers SM, Powers J. Risk factors for Aboriginal low birth weight, intra-uterine growth retardation and preterm births in the Darwin health region. Aust N Z J Public Health 1997;21:524–30.

17. Saigal S, Doyle LW. An overview of mortality and sequelae of preterm births from infancy to adulthood. Lancet 2008;371:261–9.

18. Baxley EG, Gobbo RW. Shoulder dystocia. Am Fam Physician 2004;67:1707–14.

19. Gillman MW, Rifas-Shiman S, Berkey CS, et al. Maternal gestational diabetes, birth weight and adolescent obesity. Pediatrics 2003;111(3):e221–5.

20. Rodrigues S, Robinson EJ, Kramer MS, et al. High rates of infant macrosmia: a comparison of Canadian native and non-native population. J Nutr 2000;130:802–12.

21. Ministry of Social Development. The social report 2006. Auckland: New Zealand; 2006. Available at: http://www.socialreport.msd.govt.nz/health/obesity.html. Accessed July, 2009.

22. Ward C, Lewis S, Coleman T. Prevalence of maternal smoking and environmental tobacco smoke exposure during pregnancy and impact on birth weight: retrospective study using Millennium Cohort. BMC Public Health 2007;7:81.

23. Ananth CV, Platt RW. Reexaming the effects of gestational age, fetal growth and maternal smoking on neonatal mortality. BMC Pregnancy Childbirth 2004;4:22.

24. Wills R-A, Coory MD. Effect of smoking among Indigenous and non-Indigenous mothers on preterm birth and full-term low birthweight. Med J Aust 2008;189(9):490–4.

25. Lumley J, Oliver SS, Chamberlain C, et al. Interventions for promoting smoking cessation in pregnancy. Cochrane Database Syst Rev 2008;(4):CD001055. DOI:10.1002/14651858.

26. Hoyme HE, May PA, Kalberg WO, et al. A clinical approach to diagnosis of fetal alcohol spectrum disorders: clarification of the 1996 Institute of Medicine criteria. Pediatrics 2005;115(1):39–47.

27. Elliott EJ, Payne J, Morris A, et al. Fetal alcohol syndrome: a prospective national surveillance study. Arch Dis Child 2008;93:732–7.

28. Canada Health. Fetal alcohol syndrome/fetal alcohol effects First Nations, Inuit and Aboriginal health. Health Canada Available at: http://www.hc-sc.gc.ca/fniah-spnia/famil/preg-g. Accessed July, 2009.

29. Stade BC, Bailey C, Dzendoletas D, et al. Psychological and/or educational interventions for reducing alcohol consumption in pregnant women and women planning pregnancy. Cochrane Database Syst Rev 2009;(2):CD004228. DOI:10.1002/14651858.

30. Callaway LK, Prins J, Chang AM, et al. The prevalence and impact of overweight and obesity in an Australian population. Med J Aust 2006;184(2):56–9.

31. Feig DS, Palda VA. Type 2 diabetes in pregnancy: a growing concern. Lancet 2002;359(9318):1690–2.

32. Reece EA, Leguizmanon G, Wiznitzer A. Gestational diabetes: the need for common ground. Lancet 2009;373:1735–51.

33. Story M, Evans M, Fabsitz RR, et al. The epidemic of obesity in American Indian communities and the need for childhood obesity prevention programs. Am J Clin Nutr 1999;69(4):747S–54S.

34. Opogonowski J, Miazgowski T, Kuczyriska M, et al. Pregravid body mass index as predictor of gestational diabetes mellitus. Diabet Med 2009;26(4):334–8.

35. Acton KJ, Burrows NR, Moore K, et al. Trends in diabetes prevalence among American Indian and Alaskan native children, adolescents, and young adults. Am J Public Health 2002;92(9):1485–90.

36. Yu C, Zinman B. Type 2 diabetes and impaired glucose tolerance in aboriginal populations: a global perspective. Diabetes Res Clin Pract 2007;72(2):159–70.

37. Lumley J, Watson L, Watson M, et al. Periconceptional supplementation with folate and/or multivitamins for preventing neural tube defects. Cochrane Database Syst Rev 2001;(2):CD001056. DOI:10.1002/14651858.

38. Kramer MS, Kakuma R. Energy and protein intake in pregnancy. Cochrane Database Syst Rev 2006;(4):CD000032. DOI:10.1002/14651858.

39. Chappell LC, Germain SJ. Commentary: controversies in management of diabetes from preconception to postnatal period. BMJ 2008;336:717–8.

40. The Guideline Development Group. Management of diabetes from preconception to the postnatal period: summary of nice guidance [report].

41. Tuffnell DJ, West J, Walkinshaw SA. Treatments for gestational diabetes and impaired glucose tolerance in pregnancy. Cochrane Database Syst Rev 2008;(4):CD003395. DOI:10.1002/14651858.

42. Gracey M, Spargo RM, Bottrell C, et al. Maternal and childhood nutrition among Aborigines of the Kimberley region. Med J Aust 1996;141:506–8.

43. Mackerras D. Birthweight changes in pilot phase of the Strong Women Strong Babies Strong Culture Program in the Northern Territory. Aust N Z J Public Health 2001;25:34–41.

44. Hillier SL, Nugent RP, Eschenbach DA, et al. Association between bacterial vaginosis and preterm delivery of a low-birth-weight infant. N Engl J Med 1995;333: 1737–42.

45. McDonald HM, Brocklehurst P, Gordon A. Antibiotics for treating bacterial vaginosis in pregnancy. Cochrane Database Syst Rev 2006;(3):CD000262. DOI:10. 1002/14651858.

46. Smaill F, Vazquez JC. Antibiotics for asymptomatic bacteriuria in pregnancy. Cochrane Database Syst Rev 2007;(1):CD000490. DOI:10.1002/14651858.

47. Early onset group B streptococcus in Aboriginal and non-Aboriginal infants Australasian Study Group for Neonatal Infections. Med J Aust 1995;163(6):302–6.

48. Schrag SJ, Zell ER, Lynfield R. A population based comparison of strategies to prevent early onset group B streptococcal disease in neonates. N Engl J Med 2002;347:233–9.

49. Smaill FM. Intrapartum antibiotics for group B streptococcal colonization. Cochrane Database Syst Rev 1996;(2):CD000115. DOI:10.1002/14651858.

50. Australian Institute of Health and Welfare. Aboriginal and Torres Strait Islander health performance framework 2008 [report]. Detailed analyses. Canberra: AIHW; 2008. Cat no IHW 22.

51. Bookallil M, Chalmers E, Bell A. Challenges in preventing pyelonephritis in pregnant women in Indigenous communities. Rural Remote Health 2005;5:395. Available at: http://www.rrh.org.au/publishedarticles/article_print_395.pdf. Accessed October, 2009.
52. Goldenberg R, Culhane JF, Iams J. Epidemiology and causes of preterm birth. Lancet 2007;371:73–82.
53. Robin RW, Chester B, Rasmussen JK, et al. Prevalence and characteristics of trauma and posttraumatic stress disorder in a southwestern American Indian community. Am J Psychiatry 1997;154:1582–8.
54. Australian Institute of Health and Welfare. Measuring the social and emotional wellbeing of Aboriginal and Torres Strait Islander peoples. Canberra: AIHW; 2009. Cat no IHW 24.
55. Pink B, Allbon P. The Health and Welfare of Australia's Aboriginal and Torres Strait Islander Peoples 2008. Commonwealth of Australia, 2008.
56. Austin NP, Leader L. Maternal stress and obstetric and infant outcomes: epidemiological findings and neuroendocrine mechanisms. Aust N Z J Obstet Gynaecol 2000;40:331–7.
57. Hodnett ED, Fredericks S. Support during pregnancy for women at increased risk of low birthweight babies. Cochrane Database Syst Rev 2009;(1):CD000198. DOI:10.1002/14651858.
58. Paranjothy S, Broughton H, Adappa R, et al. Teenage pregnancy: who suffers? Arch Dis Child 2009;94:239–45.
59. Dickson N, Sporle A, Rimene C, et al. Pregnancies among New Zealand teenagers: trends, current status and international comparisons. N Z Med J 2000;113:241–5.
60. Chen XK, Wen SW, Fleming N, et al. Teenage pregnancy and adverse birth outcomes: a large population based retrospective cohort study. Int J Epidemiol 2007;36:368–73.
61. Tomashek KM, Qin C, Hsia J, et al. Infant mortality trends and differences between America Indians/Alaskan Native infants and White infants in the United States 1989–1991 and 1998–2000. Am J Public Health 2006;96(12):2222–7.
62. Smylie J, Adomako P, Crengle S. Health of Maori Children in Aotearoa/New Zealand. In: Smylie J, Adomako P, editors. Indigenous Children's Health Report: health assessment in action. Toronto: The Centre for Research on Inner City Health; 2009. p. 97.
63. Ring IT, Brown N. Indigenous health: chronically inadequate responses to damning statistics. Med J Aust 2002;177(11):629–31.
64. Cooke M, Mitrou F, Lawrence D, et al. Indigenous well-being in four countries. An application of the UNDP'S human development index to indigenous peoples in Australia, Canada, New Zealand and the United States. BMC Int Health Hum Rights 2007;7:9.
65. American Academy of Pediatrics Policy Statement Task Force on Sudden Infant Death Syndrome. The changing concept of sudden infant death syndrome: diagnostic coding shifts, controversies regarding sleeping environment and new variables to consider in reducing risk. Pediatrics 2005;116:1245–55.
66. Fiore M, Jain CR, Baker TB, et al. A clinical practice guideline for treating tobacco use and dependence: 2008 update. A U.S. Public Health Service report. Am J Prev Med 2008;35:158–76.
67. Floyd LR, Sobell M, Velasquez MM, et al. Preventing alcohol-exposed pregnancies. A randomized controlled trial. Am J Prev Med 2007;32:1–10.
68. Dunlop A, Jack BW, Bottalico JN, et al. The clinical content of preconception care: women with chronic medical conditions. Am J Obstet Gynecol 2008; 199(6 Suppl 2):S310–27.

69. Ray JG, O'Brien TE, Chan WS. Preconception care and the risk of congenital anomalies in the offspring of women with diabetes mellitus: a meta-analysis. QJM 2001;94:435–44.

70. Bhutta ZA, Darmstadt GL, Hasan BS, et al. Community-based interventions for improving perinatal and neonatal health outcomes in developing countries: a review of the evidence. Pediatrics 2005;115:519–617.

71. Rabi Y, Rabi D, Yee W. Room air resuscitation of the depressed newborn: a systematic review and meta-analysis. Resuscitation 2007;72:353–63.

72. Grein AJ, Weiner GM. Laryngeal mask airway versus bag-mask ventilation or endotracheal intubation for neonatal resuscitation. Cochrane Database Syst Rev 2005;(2):CD003314. DOI:10.1002/14651858.

73. McDonald SJ, Middleton P. Effect of timing of umbilical cord clamping of term infants on maternal and neonatal outcomes. Cochrane Database Syst Rev 2008;(2):CD004074. DOI:10.1002/14651858.

74. McCall EM, Alderdice F, Halliday HL, et al. Interventions to prevent hypothermia at birth in preterm and/or low birthweight infants. Cochrane Database Syst Rev 2007;(3):CD004210. DOI:10.1002/14651858.

75. Puckett RM, Offringa M. Prophylactic vitamin K for vitamin K deficiency bleeding in neonates. Cochrane Database Syst Rev 2000;(4):CD002776. DOI:10.1002/14651858.

76. Dyson L, McCormick FM, Renfrew MJ. Interventions for promoting the initiation of breastfeeding. Cochrane Database Syst Rev 2007;(3):CD001688. DOI:10.1002/14651858.

77. CDC. Recommendations to improve preconception health and health care—United States. A report of the CDC/ATSDR Preconception Care Work Group and the Select Panel on Preconception Care. MMWR Recomm Rep 2006; 55(No. RR-6):1–23.

78. Moos MK, Dunlop AL, Jack BW, et al. Healthier women, healthier reproductive outcomes: recommendations for routine care of all women of reproductive age. Am J Obstet Gynecol 2008;199(6 Suppl 2):S280–9.

79. U.S. Preventive Services Task Force. Screening and behavioral counseling interventions in primary care to reduce alcohol misuse: recommendation statement. Ann Intern Med 2004;140:554–6.

80. Jack BW, Atrash H, Coonrod DV, et al. The clinical content of preconception care: an overview and preparation of this supplement. Am J Obstet Gynecol 2008; 199(6 Suppl 2):S266–79.

81. Chen WK, Wen SW, Yang Q, et al. Adequacy of prenatal care and neonatal mortality in infants born to mothers with and without antenatal high risk conditions. Aust N Z J Obstet Gynaecol 2007;47(2):122–7.

82. Villar J, Carroli G, Khan-Neelofur D, et al. Patterns of routine antenatal care for low-risk pregnancy. Cochrane Database Syst Rev 2001;(3):CD000934. DOI:10.1002/14651858.

83. WHO. Integrated management of pregnancy and childbirth. Pregnancy, childbirth, postpartum and newborn care: a guide for essential practice. Geneva: WHO; 2006.

84. Leon-Cava N, Lutter C, Ross J, et al. Quantifying the benefits of breast feeding. A summary of the evidence. Washington, DC: PAHO; 2002.

85. Olds DL, Kitzman H, Hanks C, et al. Effects of nurse home visiting on maternal and child functioning: age-9 follow-up of a randomized trial. Pediatrics 2007; 120:e832–45.

86. Fergusson DM, Grant H, Horwood LJ, et al. Randomized trial of the early start program of home visitation: parent and family outcomes. Pediatrics 2007;72:353–63.

Vaccine Preventable Diseases and Vaccination Policy for Indigenous Populations

Robert I. Menzies, MPH[a], Rosalyn J. Singleton, MD, MPH[b,c],*

KEYWORDS

- Vaccine-preventable disease • Indigenous population
- Vaccination strategy • Health policy

There are many similarities between the historical experiences, current social situations, and health status of indigenous people in the 4 English-speaking developed countries of North America and the Pacific, where they are all now minority populations. In the United States, American Indians and Alaska Native (AI/AN) people make up 1.5% of the population overall[1] while Alaska Native (AN) people make up 19.0% of the Alaska population[2]; in Canada the First Nations and Inuit people constitute 3.2%[3]; and in Australia, Aboriginal and Torres Strait Islander people are 2.4% of the population.[4] Finally, in New Zealand, Maori make up 14% of the population.[5] Indigenous populations have experienced European colonization, loss of traditional lands, devastation from introduced infections,[6,7] cultural marginalization, and reduced access to health services. Although vaccines have contributed to the reduction or elimination of disease disparities for many infections, indigenous people continue to have higher morbidity and mortality from many chronic and infectious diseases compared with the general populations in their countries.[8–11]

This review summarizes the available data on the epidemiology of vaccine-preventable diseases in indigenous populations in these 4 countries in the context of the vaccination strategies used and their impact, with the aim of identifying successful strategies with the potential for wider implementation.

[a] The National Centre for Immunisation Research and Surveillance of Vaccine Preventable Diseases (NCIRS), Sydney, Australia
[b] Arctic Investigation Program–CDC, 4055 Tudor Center Drive, Anchorage, AK 99508, USA
[c] Alaska Native Tribal Health Consortium, D-CHS Clinical and Research Services, 4315 Diplomacy Drive, Anchorage, AK 99508
* Corresponding author. Alaska Native Tribal Health Consortium, D-CHS Clinical and Research Services, 4315 Diplomacy Drive, Anchorage, AK 99508.
E-mail address: ris2@cdc.gov (R.J. Singleton).

Pediatr Clin N Am 56 (2009) 1263–1283
doi:10.1016/j.pcl.2009.09.006
0031-3955/09/$ – see front matter. Published by Elsevier Inc.

pediatric.theclinics.com

METHODS

Information for this review was collected systematically through searches of Medline and government websites from the United States, Canada, Australia, and New Zealand.

A major focus of this report is nationally recommended and funded vaccination schedules. Nationally recommended vaccines are funded in New Zealand[12]; and in the United States, all nationally recommended childhood vaccines are funded for all indigenous children, through the Vaccines for Children Program.[13] In Australia, most nationally recommended childhood vaccines have been funded,[14] whereas in Canada recommendations are made at a national level, but funding and delivery of vaccines is the responsibility of provinces.[15] The term "indigenous" in this report refers to the range of peoples who inhabited these countries before European colonization, that is, AI/AN, First Nations and Metis people of Canada, Canadian Inuit, Australian Aboriginal people, Torres Strait Islanders, and New Zealand Maori.

HAEMOPHILUS INFLUENZAE TYPE B DISEASE (INVASIVE)
Epidemiology

The highest rates of invasive *Haemophilus influenzae* type b (Hib) disease reported in the prevaccine era were in indigenous populations (**Table 1**), characterized by a younger age of onset[32,33] and rarity of epiglottitis.[32]

Vaccination Schedules

The available Hib vaccines have differences relevant to the specific epidemiology in indigenous populations. The polyribosylribitol phosphate *Neisseria meningitidis* outer membrane protein vaccine (PRP-OMP) gives significant immune response following the first dose at 2 months of age, whereas the other conjugated vaccines require at least 2 doses to reach similar levels.[34,35] PRP-OMP is therefore frequently recommended for indigenous populations because of their earlier average age of Hib disease.[31] PRP-OMP does not achieve as high a peak antibody concentration after a full course,[36] suggesting that it may have less impact on nasopharyngeal carriage of Hib compared with other vaccines. However, although high carriage rates have been shown in highly vaccinated populations in Alaska,[37] they have not been found in highly vaccinated White Mountain Apache or Navajo populations.[38] The reemergence of Hib disease in Alaska in 1996, following replacement of PRP-OMP by a Diphtheria-Tetanus-whole cell Pertussis (DTPw)-HbOC vaccine, highlighted the importance of early immunity to Hib in indigenous children.[34] Control of Hib disease improved after reintroduction of PRP-OMP into Alaska in 2001.

The vaccination schedules used in the 4 countries are shown in **Table 1**. All countries with the exception of Canada have had a specific role for PRP-OMP vaccine. However, this changed in 2008 due to the shortage of PRP-OMP vaccine, with PRP-OMP being prioritized for use in AI/AN children in the United States,[24] and in indigenous children in the Northern Territory in Australia, and non-OMP recommended for all New Zealand children.[18]

Disease Impact

Universal conjugate Hib vaccine programs for infants have resulted in spectacular decreases in the reported incidence of invasive Hib disease for all children younger than 5 years in all 4 countries, by 98% by 1995 in the United States,[38] more than 99% in Canada by 2000,[15] 95% by 2000 in Australia,[16] and 92% in New Zealand by 1995 to 2000.[27] Although the declines in indigenous populations were also considerable (eg, 95% decrease in Alaska Native children), the relative burden in indigenous

Table 1
Haemophilus influenzae type b vaccines currently used for indigenous infants, and disease incidence in indigenous children younger than 5 years, before and after widespread infant vaccination

Country	Hib Vaccine	Cases Per 100,000 Per Year, Age <5 Years	
		Prevaccine	Postvaccine
Australia	PRP-OMP/Other[a]	278–529,[d] 6 times higher than nonindigenous[16]	4.3[f] (3–5 times higher than nonindigenous)
Canada	PRP-T[b,17]	N/A	8.3,[g] 17.0[h] (8–15 times higher than nonindigenous)
New Zealand	PRP-T[b,18]	28[e] (38 for all children <5)	4.1[i]
United States	PRP-OMP/Other[c]	250–500,[19–21] 5–10 times higher than nonindigenous	5.4,[j] 6.0,[k] 9[l] (>5 times higher than nonindigenous)

Abbreviation: N/A Not available.

[a] Polyribosylribitol phosphate *Neisseria meningitidis* outer membrane protein conjugate vaccine (PRP-OMP) was funded for all indigenous infants from 1993 to 2005[22]; from November 2005, it was funded only for indigenous infants in Queensland, the Northern Territory, South Australia, and Western Australia, and from October 2009 OMP vaccines were no longer available due to an international vaccine shortage. Non-OMP vaccines were used in other jurisdictions.

[b] Polyribosylribitol phosphate tetanus toxoid conjugate vaccine (PRP-T). In New Zealand, changed from PRP-OMP in March 2008.

[c] National universal recommendations are for either PRP-OMP or other vaccines[23]; PRP-OMP is recommended for AI/AN populations.[24]

[d] Northern Territory 1985 to 1988[25] and 1989 to 1993.[26]

[e] Based on hospitalizations for *Haemophilus influenzae* meningitis and epiglottitis, notification data not available.[27]

[f] 2003 to 2006.[28]

[g] 2000 to 2004.[17]

[h] 2001 to 2007 Northern Canada (Arctic Investigations Program—CDC, International Circumpolar Surveillance, unpublished, 2009).

[i] 2006 to 2007.[29,30]

[j] Alaska 2001 to 2004.[31]

[k] Alaska 2001 to 2007 (Arctic Investigations Program—CDC, International Circumpolar Surveillance, unpublished, 2009).

[l] 9 (95% confidence interval: 3, 18) Navajo and White Mountain Apache, 2006 to 2008. (Katherine O'Brien, personal communication, 2009).

children has remained several orders of magnitude higher than the general population in United States AI[38] and AN children,[31] Australia[39] and New Zealand,[27] and Canada.[40] Possible explanations for the continuing higher rates include persistent nasopharyngeal colonization[34] (possibly due to environmental factors such as crowding and lack of running water), poorer immunologic responses due to environmental factors,[41] and delayed vaccination.[37]

Recent data suggest that in the New Zealand,[29,30] the United States,[31,38] Australia,[39] and Canada,[9,40] indigenous Hib disease incidence remains higher than that of comparator populations, although the absolute numbers of cases are small (see **Table 1**).

HEPATITIS A
Epidemiology

In the absence of funded vaccination programs, indigenous populations experienced higher rates of hepatitis A in all 4 countries,[42–44] with the possible exception of

New Zealand (**Table 2**). The epidemic patterns ranged from being hyperendemic in young children,[49] to regular community-wide epidemics in older children and adults, including deaths.[44,46,50–52]

Vaccination Schedules

Nationally funded hepatitis A vaccination programs are in place only in the United States and Australia. In the United States a recommendation for high-rate populations, including AI/AN children, was implemented in 1996[53] followed by a universal childhood recommendation in 2006.[23] In Australia, hepatitis A was recommended in 2005 for indigenous children in high prevalence areas (see **Table 2**).[54] Local or regional programs targeting children in regions with large indigenous populations have previously been implemented in Canada[9] and Australia,[50] and the Province of Quebec currently funds universal hepatitis A (with hepatitis B as Twinrix) immunization in primary schools.[55]

Disease Impact

Nationally and regionally funded vaccination programs, whether targeted solely at indigenous populations or the broader population, have proved very effective in reducing hepatitis A in indigenous populations. In the United States, since 2001 rates among AI/ANs have been lower than or similar to those for other races.[56] Programs targeting Indigenous people in specific geographic regions have been very successful in reducing disease incidence in Canada[9] and Australia[50] (see **Table 2**), including reductions in nontarget populations (ie, nonindigenous children).[50]

HEPATITIS B
Epidemiology

In nonindigenous populations the predominant modes of hepatitis B virus transmission were in adulthood, via sexual or parenteral means. In contrast, in indigenous

Table 2
Funded hepatitis A vaccination for indigenous children, and disease incidence in indigenous populations before and after widespread infant vaccination

Country	Hepatitis A Vaccination Program	Yearly All-Age Incidence	
		Prevaccine	Postvaccine
Australia	High prevalence areas[a]	110/100,000[d] 4 times nonindigenous rate[45]	4/100,000[e,45]
Canada	None[b]	12 times higher than nonindigenous[9]	N/A
New Zealand	None[18]	0.8/100,000 (2.0 for all races/ethnicities combined)[29,30]	N/A
United States	Universal, 1 year of age[c]	3–10 times higher than non-AI/AN[46]	0.5/100,000, no different to rates in non-AI/AN[47]

[a] 1999 to 2005, indigenous children in north Queensland only[45]; from November 2005, indigenous children age 1 to 5 years in Queensland, the Northern Territory, South Australia, and Western Australia.[22]
[b] Funded vaccination in Quebec Province only, primary school children in fourth grade.[48]
[c] From 2006. Previously all children in states, counties or areas with notification rates ≥20/100,000 population, from 1999.[47]
[d] North Queensland, 1996 to 1999.[45]
[e] North Queensland, 2000 to 2003.[45]

populations infection usually occurred in early childhood, and though largely asymptomatic, led to high rates of chronic carriage and hepatic cancer.[57] High rates of infection, chronic carriage, and hepatocellular carcinoma have been reported from indigenous populations in all 4 countries, especially among AN people in whom 5% to 29% were hepatitis B surface antibody positive,[58,59] before routine vaccination programs (**Table 3**). There seem to be some exceptions in Canada, where rates in First Nations populations were similar to nonindigenous rates, and a less virulent hepatitis B strain among Inuit was postulated.[67]

Vaccination Schedules

In Alaska a vaccine trial was conducted in 1981 to assess adequate response to the vaccine in AN,[68] which was followed by a comprehensive vaccination program of AN in 1984.[69] This trial included screening of pregnant women, routine infant vaccination at birth, and an extensive catch-up program. Elsewhere in the United States and in Canada, Australia, and New Zealand, vaccination strategies initially targeted infants of carrier mothers or those from racial or risk groups from the mid-1980s.[70–73] Following the limited success of these targeted approaches, universal infant or adolescent vaccination was adopted, first in New Zealand[71] and the United States (see **Table 3**).[63]

Disease Impact

The comprehensive vaccination program in AN people was highly successful in preventing disease in all age groups.[68,74] However, other targeted programs, which were often conducted in a less intensive manner or in regions where high-risk populations were more difficult to target, had limited impact.[75,76] Universal infant or adolescent vaccination programs have been very successful in preventing disease

Table 3
Funded hepatitis B vaccination, disease incidence, and prevalence in indigenous populations, before and after widespread infant vaccination

Country	Vaccination Program	Indigenous Incidence/Prevalence	
		Prevaccine	Postvaccine
Australia	Universal infant and adolescent catch-up[22]	5%–30% carriers,[60] HCC[b] (10 times higher than nonindigenous)	Indigenous <5 y 0.6/ 100,000, nonindigenous 0.3/ 100,000[c]
Canada	Universal preadolescent and infant[a]	Inuit 5% carriers (20 times higher than nonindigenous First Nations 0.3%–3%, same as nonindigenous)[15,61]	0 cases[d]
New Zealand	Universal infant and <16 y catch-up[18]	7% carriers, HCC 10 times higher than nonindigenous[62]	Maori all age 1.6/ 100,000, European 1.5/100,000[e]
United States	Universal infant and ≤18 y catch-up[63]	5%–29% carriers[57–59]	84% decline, 0–18 y[63]

[a] Preadolescent programs in all provinces, infant programs in 6 of 13 provinces.[64]
[b] Hepatocellular carcinoma (HCC), Northern Territory Aboriginals.[65]
[c] 2003 to 2006.[28]
[d] British Columbia, 2001.[66]
[e] 2007.[30]

in vaccinated indigenous age groups, while higher incidence continues in young adults.[28,68] A significant decline in national indigenous notification rates has been reported in the United States[77] and one Canadian province, and low hepatitis B incidence rates were reported post vaccination in Australia and New Zealand (see **Table 3**).

HUMAN PAPILLOMAVIRUS
Epidemiology

Mortality from cervical cancer is at least 5 times higher in indigenous than in nonindigenous women in Australia and New Zealand, and the United States Northern Plains (**Table 4**) In Australia there is also a strong gradient toward higher mortality in remote compared with metropolitan indigenous women. Although the disparity in cancer incidence is lower than that for mortality (approximately twofold higher in indigenous women), diagnoses in indigenous women are more often at a later stage of tumor development. There is no clear difference in rates of human papilloma virus (HPV) infection[83] or cervical intraepithelial neoplasia[79] in indigenous compared with nonindigenous Australian women, suggesting the major contributing factor to higher mortality is access to the highly successful cervical screening programs.[79] In the United States, cervical cancer incidence is also up to 3 times higher in indigenous AI/AN women than in non-Hispanic white women, but rates vary dramatically by region.[84]

Vaccination Schedules

Two vaccines have recently been licensed in most developed countries, both of which contain the 2 HPV types responsible for at least 70% of cervical cancer (16 and 18), while one also includes types 6 and 11, which cause 90% of genital warts. Funded

Table 4
Currently funded human papillomavirus vaccination programs for adolescents, and disease incidence before and after widespread vaccination

Country	Funded HPV Vaccination Program	Cervical Cancer Mortality Rate, Indigenous Women	
		Prevaccine	Postvaccine
Australia	Yes[a]	9.9/100,000, >4 times higher than in nonindigenous women[c]	N/A
Canada	Yes[48]		N/A
New Zealand	Yes[b]	10.9/100,000, >4 times higher than in non-Maori women[d]	N/A
United States	Yes[78]	15.6/100,000, 5 times higher than in nonindigenous women[e] 1.8/100,000, similar to nonindigenous[f]	N/A

[a] Females age 10 to 13 years with catch-up to 27 years, from 2007. Vaccine also licensed but not funded for adolescent males.[22]
[b] Females age 12 years, with catch-up to 18 years, from 2008.[18]
[c] Age 20 to 69 years, 2001 to 2004.[79]
[d] 1996 to 2000.[80]
[e] 1989 to 1993, Northern Plains.[81]
[f] 1994 to 1998, Alaska.[82]

universal vaccination programs for adolescent girls commenced in the United States in 2006, in Australia in 2007,[22] and in New Zealand in 2008.[18]

Disease Impact

No data on disease impact are yet available.

INFLUENZA
Epidemiology

Influenza hospitalization rates have been reported as severalfold higher in indigenous than in nonindigenous children in Australia.[28,85] In the United States, numerous reports have noted high attack rates and high burden of morbidity and mortality associated with influenza outbreaks in AI/AN, and a greater burden of pneumonia and influenza mortality compared with the United States population.[86] The role of influenza as a major cause of morbidity in children,[87] the high frequency of secondary pneumonia,[87] and high rates of morbidity and mortality due to pneumonia in indigenous populations, are well documented and indicate the importance of influenza as a cause of vaccine-preventable disease.[8,11]

Vaccination Schedules

The United States recently expanded universal influenza recommendations to include children 6 months to 18 years,[88] while influenza remains recommended in Canada for children age 6 to 23 months.[89] (**Table 5**). In New Zealand influenza vaccine is funded for children with high-risk medical conditions, while in Australia this is recommended but not funded. All 4 countries have funded vaccination for the elderly, with varying age

Table 5
Currently funded influenza vaccination programs, and hospitalization or death rates due to influenza or pneumonia in indigenous people, before and after widespread vaccination

Country	Funded Influenza Program	Hospitalization or Death Rates Due to Influenza and/or Pneumonia	
		Prevaccine	Postvaccine
Australia	Indigenous ≥50 y Indigenous 15–49 y with risk factors All ≥65 y[22]	N/A	Hospitalizations: 46/100,000 (3.0 times higher than nonindigenous)[d]
Canada	All ≥65 y, <65 y with risk factors[a] All 6–23 mo[89]	N/A	Cause of 6% of deaths aged ≥65 y[e]
New Zealand	All ≥65 y, <65 y with risk factors[18]	Hospitalizations: Maori 9.5/100,000, nonindigenous 7.3/100,000[b]	N/A
United States	All ≥50 y All 6 mo to 18 y[88]	Deaths: 22/100,000 (1.5 times United States all races rate)[c]	N/A

[a] Eligibility expanded to ≥55 years in Nunavut province.
[b] 1990 to 1999 all ages, influenza only, pneumonia not included.[12]
[c] 1987 to 1996.[11]
[d] 2003 to 2006, age ≥50 years.[28]
[e] 1999.[9]

cutoffs, and including young adults with medical risk factors in Canada and New Zealand. Programs specific to indigenous adults are in place in Australia (age 50–64 years and 15–49 years with risk factors), and one Canadian Territory with a large indigenous population has extended age eligibility (Nunavut, 55–64 years).

Disease Impact

Data are generally not available comparing influenza and pneumonia rates in indigenous populations before and after immunization programs. However, where data are available, influenza and pneumonia remain significant causes of morbidity and mortality, particularly in indigenous adults (see **Table 5**).

PNEUMOCOCCAL DISEASE (INVASIVE)
Epidemiology

Invasive pneumococcal disease (IPD) rates are highest in young children and the elderly. The rates in indigenous populations in central Australia and certain indigenous groups in the United States (AN, White Mountain Apache, and Navajo people) were among the highest ever reported for both children and adults[90–92] (**Table 6**), but case-fatality rates were about the same as in the nonindigenous population.[99]

Vaccination Schedules

The 23-valent polysaccharide pneumococcal vaccine (23 vs PPV) includes the serotypes of an estimated 90% of IPD cases internationally[106]; however, as with other

Table 6
Currently funded pneumococcal vaccination programs for indigenous children, and disease incidence before and after widespread vaccination

Country	Funded Childhood Pneumococcal Vaccination Program	Cases Per 100,000 Per Year, Indigenous Children	
		Prevaccine	Postvaccine
Australia	Yes[a]	180–2053 (up to 15 times higher than nonindigenous)[d]	73[i]
Canada	Yes[b]	225 (0 nonindigenous cases)[e]	39[f]
New Zealand	Yes[18]	127 (107 for all races/ethnicities <2)[g]	N/A
United States	Yes[c]	300–1820 (18–52 times higher than United States non-natives)[h]	6,[j] 244,[k] 120[l]

[a] Indigenous infants from 2001, all infants from 2005.[22]
[b] Recommended from 2002,[15] funded in all provinces by 2005.[64]
[c] From 2000, with catch-up for AI/AN and other high-risk children <5 years.[93]
[d] Indigenous children <2 years of age, central Australia 1985 to 1990,[92] Northern Territory 1994 to 1998,[94] Western Australia 1993.[95]
[e] 2001, North Canadian indigenous children.[96]
[f] Alberta indigenous children 0 to 6 years, 2006.[97]
[g] 1984 to 1992.[98]
[h] <2 years old, White mountain Apache 1983 to 1990,[99] Alaskan natives 1980 to 1986,[100] Navajo 1996.[101]
[i] Australian indigenous children <2 years, 2006.[102]
[j] AI/AN children <5 years, 2003.[103]
[k] AN children <2 years, 2004 to 2006.[104]
[l] White Mountain Apache children <5 years, 2001 to 2006.[105]

polysaccharide vaccines, 23vPPV is poorly immunogenic in children younger than 2 years and has no impact on mucosal carriage.[106] The currently licensed 7-valent pneumococcal conjugate vaccine (7vPCV) is highly efficacious against IPD in infants, and also has some effectiveness against pneumonia and acute otitis media.[107,108] However, the proportion of IPD that was caused by vaccine serotypes in the prevaccine era, and was therefore vaccine preventable, was generally lower in indigenous (67%–77%) than in nonindigenous children (84%–86%).[91,92,109,110] New expanded valency 10-valent and 13-valent pneumococcal conjugate vaccines are on the verge of licensure in several countries.

Funded universal infant conjugate vaccination programs are in place in all 4 countries. Such a program was first introduced in the United States with a 4-dose series in 2000, followed by Canada from 2002 (used in a 4-dose series in most provinces and in the indigenous population) and Australia (a 3-dose primary series followed by 23vPPV at 18 months in Aboriginal children from 2001, and a 3-dose primary series for other Australian children from 2005), and a 4-dose schedule was introduced in New Zealand in mid 2008 (see **Table 6**).

Disease Impact

The impact of infant conjugate vaccination programs on vaccine serotype IPD in indigenous children has been impressive; however, increases in nonvaccine serotypes have limited the impact of 7vPCV vaccination in some populations. Before use of 7vPCV vaccine the incidence of IPD in the United States among AI/AN children in the southwest and Alaska was 5 to 24 times higher than the incidence among other United States children.[91,99,105] Since the routine use of PCV there has been a virtual elimination of vaccine serotype IPD among previously high-risk AI/AN children from the Southwest United States and Alaska.[90,104,111] Despite the tremendous effectiveness of 7vPCV, Southwest and Alaska AI/AN children have continued to have disproportionate rates of IPD due to nonvaccine serotypes. Whereas the rate of nonvaccine serotypes has been stable in most populations including Southwest AI children, in AN children an increase in the annual rate of nonvaccine serotype disease led to a doubling of the rate of IPD between the periods 2001 to 2003 and 2004 to 2006.[111] In Australia, 5 to 7 years after commencement of the targeted program 7vPCV vaccine serotype, IPD had decreased by more than 80% in indigenous children younger than 2 years and rates of nonvaccine serotype IPD were unchanged.[95,102,112]

Otitis media has been identified as a significant cause of morbidity among indigenous children from the United States and Australia, and approximately one-third of otitis media is mediated by *Streptococcus pneumoniae*. Despite the low efficacy in clinical trials, greater serotype diversity, greater potential for serotype switching, and early colonization,[113] a significant decrease in otitis media visits has been identified in the general child populations in the United States[114] and Australia,[115] and in AI populations in the United States, but decreases have not been observed in AN[116] or remote Australian Aboriginal children.[117] Available regional data on IPD in Canadian indigenous children continues to show disparity in IPD (at least fourfold higher than the general population in Alberta).[118]

ROTAVIRUS
Epidemiology

Diarrhea is a leading cause of morbidity and mortality in developing countries, and even in the United States results in 50,000 to 70,000 hospitalizations per year.[119] In the period 1980 to 1982, the rate of diarrhea-associated hospitalizations in AI/AN children younger than 5 years was nearly twice as high as the United States rate.[120] By 2000 to 2004, this disparity had disappeared in the under-5 age group, whereas in infants the rate remained nearly twice as high in AI/AN compared with all United States infants.[121] In Australia it is estimated that 1 in 27 children are hospitalized with rotavirus by the age of 5 years, and in indigenous children the rates are 3 to 5 times higher, occur at a younger age, and have a longer duration of stay compared with nonindigenous children (**Table 7**).[22]

Vaccination Schedules

A live pentavalent rotavirus vaccine was tested in a large multicenter trial that included AI/AN children from the Navajo and Apache reservations in the United States. Among Navajo and Apache infants, the vaccine had 98% efficacy (95% confidence interval: 88.3%, 100%) against severe rotavirus disease.[122] Rotavirus vaccine was licensed in the United States in 2006 and is recommended for all United States children. In Australia vaccination was funded for all children in the Northern Territory in 2006 and nationally from 2007.[123,124] The vaccine is licensed in Canada for infants 6 to 32 weeks old; however, it is not funded by any Provincial/Territorial programs.[125] The vaccine is not part of the New Zealand Immunization Schedule.[18]

Disease Impact

At this stage data on the impact of vaccination are limited. During the second season of vaccine use, rotavirus activity in the United States was substantially delayed in onset and diminished in magnitude compared with the 15 previous years.[126]

OTHER VACCINE-PREVENTABLE DISEASES

Indigenous children historically experienced higher measles and pertussis morbidity than the general child populations of their respective countries. For measles, pertussis, and meningococcal disease, vaccination strategies have not been specifically targeted to indigenous populations. Universal 2-dose childhood vaccination for measles has been implemented in all 4 countries,[14,127–129] and incidence has been reduced to local outbreaks related to imported cases.[15,130] For pertussis, universal childhood and, in some cases, adolescent programs are in place.[14,127–129] Pertussis epidemics continue to occur due to waning vaccine-induced immunity, and there

Table 7
Currently funded rotavirus vaccination programs for indigenous children, and disease incidence before and after widespread vaccination

Country	Funded Rotavirus Vaccination Program	Hospitalizations Per Year, Indigenous Children	
		Prevaccine	Postvaccine
Australia	Yes[22]	1–3/1000 (4–8 times higher than nonindigenous)[a]	N/A
Canada	No[48]		N/A
New Zealand	No[18]	N/A	N/A
United States	Yes[78]	26.2/1000 (2 times higher than nonindigenous)[b]	

[a] Age <1 year, 1993 to 2002, rotavirus gastroenteritis (ICD9 008.61, ICD10 A08.0) as principal or contributing cause of hospitalization.
[b] Age <1 year, 2000 to 2004, diarrhea hospitalizations.[119]

have been reports of higher mortality,[131] hospitalization,[132] and disease notification rates[9] in indigenous infants, possibly related to delayed vaccination.[132] Universal childhood vaccination for meningococcal disease has been introduced in Canada[129] and Australia,[14] and for adolescents in the United States.[133] In New Zealand, a national 15-year epidemic of a serotype B clone was particularly focused in Maori and Pacific Island children, and led to the development of a clone-specific vaccine and national vaccination program for all children younger than 18 years.[134] A national vaccination program for all younger than 20 years commenced in 2004 and ended in 2008, following a substantial decline in reported cases to slightly higher than preepidemic levels.[135]

VACCINATION COVERAGE

In the United States, analysis of the National Immunization Survey (NIS) data from 2000 to 2005 showed that AI/AN children overall had lower immunization rates than white children at 24 months; however, in 2007 the NIS reported comparable coverage rates in AI/AN (83% AI/AN vs 78% white children fully vaccinated for DTaP, IPV, Hib, Hep B).[136] Although national data on immunization coverage is unavailable for Canada, in the Alberta region coverage for First Nations children is 30% lower than rates for the general Alberta population.[118]

In Australia, vaccination coverage in indigenous children was in the past substantially lower than in nonindigenous children.[28] In more recent years, however, the disparities are less pronounced. In 2007 coverage was 7% lower in indigenous than in nonindigenous children at 12 months of age (83% vs 90% fully vaccinated for DTP, IPV, Hib, Hep B), due to less timely vaccination of indigenous children, which has been frequently reported.[137,138] At 24 months of age vaccine coverage in indigenous children was no different to that in nonindigenous children (91% vs 92% fully vaccinated for doses of DTP, IPV, Hib, Hep B, and MMR, 2007).[28] Coverage for vaccines recommended only for indigenous children is consistently lower than for that universally recommended. For example, in Australia only 45% of indigenous children received PPV23 and less than 30% received 2 doses of hepatitis A vaccine within 6 months of the due date, in contrast to 83% vaccinated with DTP, IPV, Hib, and Hep B at 12 months.[28] Coverage in Maori children was reported as lower than other racial or ethnic groups in 2005 (69% Maori vs 77% all children fully vaccinated with DTaP, polio, Hib, Hep B, MMR at 2 years of age), and timeliness was also poorer, with 29% of Maori compared with 39% of all children age 2 to 3 years receiving all doses on time.[139]

SUMMARY

Important lessons and points of continuity emerge from this review that are of relevance to immunization programs for indigenous people in developed countries. There is a higher incidence and earlier age of onset for almost all diseases in all countries, consistent with adverse environmental factors, including household crowding,[2,140] low income,[11] lack of running water,[141] high rates of chronic lung disease, and other medical risk factors.[142] Some differences in immunologic responses to vaccines have been demonstrated in indigenous people in some instances, including hepatitis B[143] and Hib.[41,144] However, the causes of these different responses are not entirely clear, as in at least one study the difference was present at 1 year of age but not at birth, suggesting a role for the environmental conditions in immunologic responses.[41] In addition, several vaccine trials have demonstrated high efficacy in indigenous children, no different to that in other populations.[145–148] Given the lack of racial links but similarities in cultural and economic situations between indigenous people in North America, Australia, and New Zealand, the cause of the greater burden of vaccine-preventable diseases is much more likely to be related to adverse living conditions (poverty, overcrowding, lack of running water, poor indoor air quality) than genetic factors. Therefore, the evidence strongly supports the conclusion that, even in the presence of higher prevaccination rates of morbidity in indigenous children, vaccines have been highly effective and immunization programs have contributed to correcting health inequity for indigenous people. Although the causes of disease disparity are most likely to be socioeconomic, vaccines have contributed to the reduction or elimination of disease disparities while socioeconomic inequities have remained.

There do seem, however, to be some policy options that are more effective than others in achieving high population coverage and disease control (**Table 8**). Nationally

Table 8
Grading of immunization recommendations

Intervention	Recommendation	Grading of Recommendation	Quality of Supporting Evidence
Nationally funded universal vaccination (eg, pertussis, measles, Hib, S pneumoniae, hepatitis B)	1. Highly effective in vaccinated individuals	Strong	High[a]
	2. Highly effective in achieving high population coverage and disease control	Strong	Moderate[b]
Nationally funded targeted universal vaccination in geographic regions of high incidence (eg, hepatitis A)	1. Highly effective in vaccinated individuals	Strong	High[a]
	2. Highly effective in achieving high population coverage and disease control	Strong	Moderate[b]
Funded targeted vaccination of indigenous people in specific geographic areas	Highly effective in vaccinated individuals	Strong	High[a]
	Variable effectiveness in achieving high population coverage and disease control	Moderate[b]	Moderate[b]
Nationally funded targeted vaccination of indigenous people	Highly effective in vaccinated individuals	Strong	High[a]
	Low effectiveness in achieving high population coverage and disease control	Moderate[b]	Moderate[b]

[a] Pre-licensure placebo-controlled efficacy trials and post-licensure surveillance.
[b] Post-licensure surveillance.

funded universal vaccination programs are clearly the most effective way of reducing disease in indigenous populations, as well as reducing racial disparities. The most successful of these have been for viral diseases in which strain variations are not important and herd immunity is high, such as measles and hepatitis B. For the bacterial infections, significant decreases in disease burden have also occurred. However, strain variations (pneumococcal disease), heavy nasopharyngeal colonization of young infants (pneumococcal and Hib disease), low vaccine effectiveness in adults with high risk factor prevalence (polysaccharide pneumococcal vaccine), and waning immunity (pertussis), have been associated with continuing or widening of disparities between indigenous and nonindigenous populations. Where the conditions are not ideal, environmental factors as well as lower coverage or delayed vaccination have limited program effectiveness. In these situations it seems likely that new, more effective vaccines and vaccine delivery will be needed to achieve further progress.

Universal vaccination programs are not always possible. The cost-effectiveness of universal vaccination programs can be limited by low disease rates in nonindigenous populations, especially for expensive vaccines. On the other hand, the high disease burden has sometimes led to vaccines being tested, or programs implemented, in indigenous populations first. However, successful wider implementation has not been limited to fully national universal programs. Geographic targeting, whereby all individuals within certain regions with high disease rates are targeted, has reduced incidence and disparities between high and low incidence populations for hepatitis A in the United States,[46] and also influenza in some North American regions.[149] Targeting indigenous populations in regions where they are larger proportions of the population have also been pursued successfully.[150] The evidence from this review would suggest that national programs targeting only indigenous people are the least effective approach, particularly in urban areas where identifying indigenous people to achieve high vaccine coverage is more difficult.[132] Innovative program approaches are particularly needed in these situations.

ACKNOWLEDGMENTS

The authors thank Michael Young (Pediatrics, Northwest Territories, Canada), Katherine O'Brien (Johns Hopkins University), and Amy Groom (Indian Health Service) for their critical review and data contributions. This article includes material from, and updates and expands on, a previous publication: Menzies R, McIntyre P. Vaccine preventable disease and vaccination policy in indigenous populations. Epidemiol Rev 2006;28:71–80.

REFERENCES

1. US Census Bureau. The American Indian and Alaska native population. Report num. C2KBR/01–15. Washington, DC: US Census Bureau; 2002.
2. Bulkow LR, Singleton RJ, Karron RA, et al. Alaska RSV Study Group. Risk factors for severe respiratory syncytial virus infection among Alaska native children. Pediatrics 2002;109:210–6.
3. Statistics Canada. Canada e-book. Available at: http://142.206.72.67/r000_e. htm. Accessed April 20, 2006.
4. Australian Bureau of Statistics (ABS). Australian demographic statistics. Report num. 3101.0. Canberra, Australian Capital Territory: ABS; 2003.
5. Statistics New Zealand. Census snapshot: Maori. Available at: http://www. stats.govt.nz/products-and-services/Articles/census-snpsht-maori-Apr02.htm. Accessed April 20, 2006.

6. Boughton CR. Smallpox and Australia. Intern Med J 2002;32:59–61.
7. Newman MT. Aboriginal new world epidemiology and medical care, and the impact of old world disease imports. Am J Phys Anthropol 1976;45:667–72.
8. Australian Bureau of Statistics (ABS). Australian Institute of Health and Welfare (AIHW). The health and welfare of Australia's Aboriginal and Torres Strait Islander peoples: 2003. Cat. No. 4704.0. Report num. 4704.0. Canberra: ABS; 2003.
9. First Nations and Inuit Health Branch. A statistical profile on the health of First Nations in Canada. Ottawa (ON): Health Canada; 2003.
10. New Zealand Ministry of Health. Our health, our future. Hauora pakari, koiora roa. The health of New Zealanders 1999. Wellington NZ: New Zealand Ministry of Health; 1999.
11. Palagiano C, Shalala DE, Trujillo MH, et al. Trends in Indian Health, 1998–99 [report]. Indian Health Service, US Department of Health and Human Services, 1999.
12. Ministry of Health. Immunisation handbook 2006. Wellington: Ministry of Health; 2006.
13. Hutchins SS, Jiles R, Bernier R. Elimination of measles and of disparities in measles childhood vaccination coverage among racial and ethnic minority populations in the United States. J Infect Dis 2004;189 (Suppl 1):S146–52.
14. National Health and Medical Research Council. The Australian immunisation handbook. 8th edition. Canberra, Australian Capital Territory: Australian Government Department of Health and Ageing; 2003.
15. National Advisory Committee on Immunization. Canadian immunization guide. 6th edition. Ottawa (ON): Health Canada; 2002.
16. Horby P, Gilmour R, Wang H, et al. Progress towards eliminating Hib in Australia: an evaluation of *Haemophilus influenzae* type b prevention in Australia, 1 July 1993 to 30 June 2000. Commun Dis Intell 2003;27:324–41.
17. Scheifele DW, Law BJ, Gold R, et al. Recent trends in pediatric *Haemophilus influenzae* type b infections in Canada. Can Med Assoc J 1996;154:1041–7.
18. Ministry of Health. 2008 National immunisation schedule health provider booklet. Wellington: Ministry of Health; 2008.
19. Coulehan JL, Michaelis RH, Hallowell C, et al. Epidemiology of *Haemophilus influenzae* type b disease among Navajo Indians. Public Health Rep 1984;99:404–9.
20. Losonsky GA, Santosham M, Sehgal VM, et al. *Haemophilus influenzae* disease in the white mountain apaches: molecular epidemiology of a high risk population. Pediatr Infect Dis J 1984;3:539–47.
21. Ward JI, Margolis HS, Lum MK, et al. *Haemophilus influenzae* disease in Alaskan Eskimos: characteristics of a population with an unusual incidence of invasive disease. Lancet 1981;1:1281–5.
22. National Health and Medical Research Council. The Australian immunisation handbook. 9th edition. Canberra: Australian Government Department of Health and Ageing; 2008.
23. Centers for Disease Control and Prevention (CDC). Recommended childhood and adolescent immunization schedule—United States, 2006. MMWR Morb Mortal Wkly Rep 2006;54:Q1–4.
24. Centers for Disease Control and Prevention (CDC). Interim recommendations for the use of *Haemophilus influenzae* type b (Hib) conjugate vaccines related to the recall of certain lots of Hib-containing vaccines (PedvaxHIB and Comvax). MMWR Morb Mortal Wkly Rep 2007;56:1318–20.
25. Hanna JN. The epidemiology of invasive *Haemophilus influenzae* infections in children under five years of age in the Northern Territory: a three year study. Med J Aust 1990;152:234–40.

26. Markey P, Krause V, Boslego JW, et al. The effectiveness of *Haemophilus influenzae* type b conjugate vaccines in a high risk population measured using immunization register data. Epidemiol Infect 2001;126:31–6.
27. Wilson N, Wenger J, Mansoor O, et al. The beneficial impact of Hib vaccine on disease rates in New Zealand children. N Z Med J 2002;115:U122–8.
28. Menzies R, Turnour C, Chiu C, et al. Vaccine preventable diseases and vaccination coverage in Aboriginal and Torres Strait Islander people, Australia, 2003 to 2006. Commun Dis Intell 2008;32(Suppl):S2–67.
29. Population and Environmental Health Group Institute of Environmental Science and Research Limited. Notifiable and other diseases in New Zealand 2007 [report]. 2009.
30. Population and Environmental Health Group Institute of Environmental Science and Research Limited. Notifiable and other diseases in New Zealand Annual Report 2006 [report]. 2009.
31. Singleton R, Hammit L, Hennessey T, et al. The Alaska *Haemophilus influenzae* type b experience: lessons in controlling a vaccine-preventable disease. Pediatrics 2006;118:e421–9.
32. Hanna J. The epidemiology and prevention of *Haemophilus influenzae* infections in Australian aboriginal children. J Paediatr Child Health 1992;28:354–61.
33. Hansman D, Hanna J, Morey F. High prevalence of invasive *Haemophilus influenzae* disease in central Australia, 1986 (letter). Lancet 1986;2:927.
34. Galil K, Singleton R, Levine OS, et al. Reemergence of invasive *Haemophilus influenzae* type b disease in a well-vaccinated population in remote Alaska. J Infect Dis 1999;179:101–6.
35. Santosham M, Wolff M, Reid R. The efficacy in Navajo infants of a conjugate vaccine consisting of *Haemophilus influenzae* type b polysaccharide and *Neisseria meningitidis* outer-membrane protein complex. N Engl J Med 1991;324:1767–72.
36. Decker MD, Edwards KM, Bradley R, et al. Comparative trial in infants of four conjugate *Haemophilus influenzae* type b vaccines. J Pediatr 1992;120:184–9.
37. Singleton R, Bulkow LR, Levine OS, et al. Experience with the prevention of invasive *Haemophilus influenzae* type b disease by vaccination in Alaska: the impact of persistent oropharyngeal carriage. J Pediatr 2000;137:313–20.
38. Millar EV, O'Brien KL, Levine OS, et al. Toward elimination of *Haemophilus influenzae* type B carriage and disease among high-risk American Indian children. Am J Public Health 2000;90:1550–4.
39. Wang H, Deeks S, Glasswell A, et al. Trends in invasive *Haemophilus influenzae* type b disease in Australia, 1995–2005. Commun Dis Intell 2009;32:316–25.
40. Scheifele D, Halperin S, Law B, et al. Invasive *Haemophilus influenzae* type b infections in vaccinated and unvaccinated children in Canada, 2001–2003. CMAJ 2005;172:53–6.
41. Guthridge S, McIntyre P, Isaacs D, et al. Differing serologic responses to an *Haemophilus influenzae* type b polysaccharide-*Neisseria meningitidis* outer membrane protein conjugate (PRP-OMPC) vaccine in Australian Aboriginal and Caucasian infants—implications for disease epidemiology. Vaccine 2000; 18:2584–91.
42. Centers for Disease Control and Prevention (CDC). Hepatitis A vaccination programs in communities with high rates of hepatitis A. MMWR Morb Mortal Wkly Rep 1997;46:600–3.
43. Peach D, McMahon BJ, Bulkow L, et al. Impact of recurrent epidemics of hepatitis A virus infection on population immunity levels: Bristol Bay, Alaska. J Infect Dis 2002;186:1081–5.

44. Adams L, Johnson G. Hepatitis A virus infection, immunisation and the Kimberley Public Health Bulletin [letter]. Kimberley P.H. Bull 2003;13.9

45. Hanna JN, Hills SL, Humphreys JL. Impact of hepatitis A vaccination of Indigenous children on notifications of hepatitis A in north Queensland. Med J Aust 2004;181:482–5.

46. Bialek SR, Thoroughman DA, Hu D, et al. Hepatitis A incidence and hepatitis A vaccination among American Indians and Alaska Natives, 1990–2001. Am J Public Health 2004;94:996–1001.

47. Advisory Committee on Immunization Practices (ACIP), Fiore AE, Wasley A, Bell BP. Prevention of hepatitis A through active or passive immunization: Recommendations of the Advisory Committee on Immunization Practices (ACIP). MMWR Recomm Rep 2006;55(RR-7):1–23 Centers for Disease Control and Prevention (CDC).

48. National Advisory Committee on Immunization. Canadian immunization guide. 7th edition. Ottawa (ON): Public Health Agency of Canada; 2006.

49. Bowden FJ, Currie BJ, Miller NC, et al. Should aboriginals in the "top end" of the Northern Territory be vaccinated against hepatitis A? Med J Aust 1994;161: 372–3.

50. Hanna JN, Hills SL, Humphreys JL. The impact of hepatitis A vaccination of Indigenous children on the incidence of hepatitis A in North Queensland. Med J Aust 2004;181(9):482–5.

51. Bulkow LR, Wainwright RB, McMahon BJ, et al. Secular trends in hepatitis A virus infection among Alaska Natives. J Infect Dis 1993;168:1017–20.

52. Welty TK, Darling K, Dye S, et al. Guidelines for prevention and control of hepatitis A in American Indian and Alaska Native communities. [erratum appears in S D J Med 1997 May;50(5):179]. S D J Med 1996;49:317–22.

53. Centers for Disease Control and Prevention (CDC). Prevention of hepatitis A through active or passive immunization: Recommendations of the Advisory Committee on Immunization Practices. MMWR Recomm Rep 1996;45(RR-15): 15–20.

54. Australian Government Department of Health and Ageing. Indigenous immunisation program. Available at: http://www.immunise.health.gov.au/internet/immunise/publishing.nsf/Content/atsi2. Accessed January 24, 2006.

55. Sante et services sociaux. Regular vaccination schedule. Available at: http://www.msss.gouv.qc.ca/sujets/santepub/vaccination/index.php?calendrier_de_vaccination_en. Accessed June 12, 2009.

56. Centers for Disease Control and Prevention (CDC). Surveillance for acute viral hepatitis, 2007. MMWR Surveill Summ 2009;58(SS-3):1–27.

57. Centers for Disease Control and Prevention (CDC). Protection against viral hepatitis: recommendations of the Immunization Practices Advisory Committee. MMWR Recomm Rep 1990;39(RR-2):2–3.

58. McMahon BJ, Schoenberg S, Bulkow L, et al. Seroprevalence of hepatitis B viral markers in 52,000 Alaska Natives. Am J Epidemiol 1993;138:544–9.

59. Schreeder MT, Bender TR, McMahon BJ, et al. Prevalence of hepatitis B in selected Alaskan Eskimo villages. Am J Epidemiol 1983;118:543–9.

60. Kaldor JM, Plant AJ, Thompson SC, et al. The incidence of hepatitis B infection in Australia: an epidemiologic review. Med J Aust 1996;165:322–6.

61. Minuk GY, Uhanova J. Viral hepatitis in the Canadian Inuit and First Nations populations. Can J Gastroenterol 2003;17:707–12.

62. Blakely T, Salmond C, Tobias M. Hepatitis B virus carrier prevalence in New Zealand: population estimates using the 1987 police and customs personnel survey. N Z Med J 1998;111:142–4.

63. Centers for Disease Control and Prevention (CDC). Acute hepatitis B among children and adolescents—United States, 1990–2002. MMWR Morb Mortal Wkly Rep 2004;53:1015–8.
64. Canadian Nursing Coalition on Immunization. Provincial and territorial immunization programs. Available at: http://www.phac-aspc.gc.ca/im/ptimprog-progimpt/table-1_e.html. Accessed April 20, 2006.
65. Wan X, Mathews JD. Primary hepatocellular carcinoma in Aboriginal Australians. Aust N Z J Public Health 1994;18:286–90.
66. Patrick DM, Bigham M, Ng H, et al. Elimination of acute hepatitis B among adolescents after one decade of an immunization program targeting Grade 6 students. Pediatr Infect Dis J 2003;22:874–7.
67. Minuk GY, Zhang M, Wong SG, et al. Viral hepatitis in a Canadian First Nations community. Can J Gastroenterol 2003;17:593–6.
68. McMahon BJ, Rhoades ER, Heyward WL, et al. A comprehensive programme to reduce the incidence of hepatitis B virus infection and its sequelae in Alaskan natives. Lancet 1987;2:1134–6.
69. Heyward WL, Bender TR, McMahon BJ, et al. The control of hepatitis B virus infection with vaccine in Yupik Eskimos. Demonstration of safety, immunogenicity, and efficacy under field conditions. Am J Epidemiol 1985;121:914–23.
70. National Health and Medical Research Council. The Australian immunisation procedures handbook. 5th edition. Canberra, Australian Capital Territory: Australian Government Publishing Service; 1994.
71. New Zealand Ministry of Health. Immunisation handbook. Wellington, New Zealand: New Zealand Ministry of Health; 2002.
72. Carlson J, Stratton F, Delage G, et al. Report of the hepatitis B working group. Can Commun Dis Rep 1994;20:105–12.
73. Centers for Disease Control and Prevention (CDC). Hepatitis B virus: a comprehensive strategy for eliminating transmission in the US through universal childhood vaccination: Recommendations of the Immunization Advisory Committee. MMWR Recomm Rep 1991;40(RR-13):1–25.
74. Harpaz R, McMahon BJ, Margolis HS, et al. Elimination of new chronic hepatitis B virus infections: results of the Alaska immunization program. J Infect Dis 2000; 181:413–8.
75. Oman KM, Carnie J, Ruff TA. Hepatitis B immunisation rates among infants in ethnic groups with high prevalences of hepatitis B surface antigen carriers. Aust N Z J Public Health 1997;21:293–6.
76. Alter MJ, Hadler SC, Margolis HS, et al. The changing epidemiology of hepatitis B in the United States. JAMA 1990;263:1218–22.
77. Centers for Disease Control and Prevention (CDC). Surveillance for acute viral hepatitis—United States, 2006. MMWR Surveill Summ 2008;57(SS-2):1–24.
78. Centers for Disease Control and Prevention (CDC). Recommended immunization schedules for persons aged 0 through 18 years—United States, 2009. MMWR Morb Mortal Wkly Rep 2009;57:Q1–4.
79. O'Brien ED, Bailie RS, Jelfs PL. Cervical cancer mortality in Australia: contrasting risk by Aboriginality, age and rurality. Int J Epidemiol 2009;29:813–6.
80. Dachs GU, Currie MJ, McKenzie F, et al. Cancer disparities in indigenous Polynesian populations: Maori, Native Hawaiians, and Pacific people. Lancet 2009;9:473–84.
81. Leman RF, Espey DK, Cobb N. Invasive cervical cancer among American Indian women in the Northern Plains, 1994–1998. Public Health Rep 2005;120:283–7.
82. Ehrsam G, Lanier A, Sandidge J. Cancer mortality among Alaska Natives, 1994–1998. Ala Med 2001;43:50–60.

83. Bowden FJ, Tabrizi SN, Paterson BA, et al. Determination of genital human papillomavirus genotypes in women in Northern Australia using a novel, self-administered tampon technique. Int J Gynecol Cancer 2009;8:471–5.

84. Becker TM, Espey DK, Lawson HW, et al. Regional differences in cervical cancer incidence among American Indians and Alaska Natives, 1999–2004. Cancer 2008;113:1234–43.

85. D'Onise K, Raupach CAJ. The burden of influenza in healthy children in South Australia. Med J Aust 2009;188:510–3.

86. Groom AV, Jim C, Laroque M, et al. Pandemic influenza preparedness and vulnerable populations in tribal communities. Am J Publ Health 2009;99(Suppl 2):S271–8 [Epub 2009 May 21].

87. Centers for Disease Control and Prevention (CDC)Prevention and control of influenza. Recommendations of the Advisory Committee on Immunization Practices. MMWR Recomm Rep 2004;53(RR-6):1–40.

88. Centers for Disease Control and Prevention (CDC). Prevention and control of influenza: recommendations of the Advisory Committee on Immunization Practices (ACIP), 2008. MMWR Morb Mortal Wkly Rep 2008;57(RR-7):1–60.

89. National Advisory Committee on Immunization (NACI). Statement on influenza vaccination for the 2008-2009 season. An Advisory Committee Statement (ACS). Can Commun Dis Rep 2008;34(ACS-3):1–46.

90. Lacapa R, Bliss SJ, Larzelere-Hinton F, et al. Changing epidemiology of invasive pneumococcal disease among White Mountain Apache persons in the era of the pneumococcal conjugate vaccine. Clin Infect Dis 2008;47:476–84.

91. Rudolph KM, Parkinson AJ, Reasonover AL, et al. Serotype distribution and antimicrobial resistance patterns of invasive isolates of Streptococcus pneumoniae: Alaska, 1991–1998. J Infect Dis 2000;182:490–6.

92. Torzillo PJ, Hanna J, Morey F, et al. Invasive pneumococcal disease in central Australia. Med J Aust 1995;162:182–6.

93. Hanna JN, McCall B, Murphy D. Invasive meningococcal disease in north Queensland, 1990–1994. Commun Dis Intell 1996;20:320–4.

94. Krause VL, Reid SJ, Merianos A. Invasive pneumococcal disease in the Northern Territory of Australia, 1994–1998. Med J Aust 2000;173(Suppl):S27–31.

95. Giele C, Moore H, Bayley K, et al. Has the seven-valent pneumococcal conjugate vaccine had an impact on invasive pneumococcal disease in Western Australia? Vaccine 2009;25:2379–84.

96. Bruce M, Cottle T, Parkinson A. International Circumpolar Surveillance (ICS) summary report. Arctic investigations program, Centers for Disease Control, 2005.

97. Nicolaeva MA, Huntly P, Dumaresq G. Immunization coverage and incidence rates in Canadian First Nations children on-reserve. 2009. (GENERIC) Ref Type: Conference Proceeding.

98. Voss L, Lennon D, Okesene-Gafa K, et al. Invasive pneumococcal disease in a pediatric population, Auckland, New Zealand. Pediatr Infect Dis J 1994;13:873–8.

99. Cortese MM, Wolff M, Almeido-Hill J, et al. High incidence rates of invasive pneumococcal disease in the White Mountain Apache population. Arch Intern Med 1992;152:2277–82.

100. Davidson M, Parkinson AJ, Bulkow LR, et al. The epidemiology of invasive pneumococcal disease in Alaska, 1986 to 1990—ethnic differences and opportunities for prevention. J Infect Dis 1994;170:368–76.

101. O'Brien KL, Shaw J, Weatherholtz R, et al. Epidemiology of invasive Streptococcus pneumoniae among Navajo children in the era before use of conjugate pneumococcal vaccines, 1989–1996. Am J Epidemiol 2004;160:270–8.

102. Roche P, Krause V, Cook H. Invasive pneumococcal disease in Australia, 2006. Commun Dis Intell 2008;32:18–30.
103. Centers for Disease Control and Prevention (CDC). Summary of notifiable diseases—United States, 2003 [report]. MMWR Surveill Summ 2005;52(54):1–85.
104. Hennessy TW, Singleton RJ, Bulkow LR, et al. Impact of heptavalent pneumococcal conjugate vaccine on invasive disease, antimicrobial resistance and colonization in Alaska natives: progress towards elimination of a health disparity. Vaccine 2005;23:5464–73.
105. Zangwill KM, Vadheim CM, Vannier AM, et al. Epidemiology of invasive pneumococcal disease in southern California: implications for the design and conduct of a pneumococcal conjugate vaccine efficacy trial. J Infect Dis 1996;174:752–9.
106. Plotkin SA, Orenstein WA, editors. Vaccines. 4th edition. Philadelphia: WB Saunders; 2004.
107. Lucero MG, Dulalia VE, Parreno RN, et al. Pneumococcal conjugate vaccines for preventing vaccine-type invasive pneumococcal disease and pneumonia with consolidation on X-ray in children under two years of age. Review. Cochrane Database Syst Rev 2004;(4):CD004977.
108. Straetemans M, Sanders EAM, Veenhoven RH, et al. Pneumococcal vaccines for preventing otitis media. Review. Cochrane Database Syst Rev 2005;(1): CD001480.
109. McIntyre PB, Nolan TM. Conjugate pneumococcal vaccines for non-Indigenous children in Australia. Med J Aust 2000;173:S54–7.
110. Scheifele D, Law B, Vaudry W, et al. Invasive pneumococcal infections among Canadian aboriginal children. Can Commun Dis Rep 2003;29:37–42.
111. Singleton RJ, Hennessey T, Bulkow L, et al. Invasive pneumococcal disease caused by nonvaccine serotypes among Alaska Native children with high levels of 7-valent pneumococcal conjugate vaccine coverage. JAMA 2007;297:1784–92.
112. Hanna JN, Humphreys JL, Murphy DM. Invasive pneumococcal disease in Indigenous people in north Queensland: an update, 2005–2007. Med J Aust 2009;189:43–6.
113. Morris PS. A systematic review of clinical research addressing the prevalence, aetiology, diagnosis, prognosis and therapy of otitis media in Australian Aboriginal children. J Paediatr Child Health 1998;34:487–97.
114. Grijalva CG, Poehling KA, Nuorti JP, et al. National impact of universal childhood immunization with pneumococcal conjugate vaccine on outpatient medical care visits in the United States. Pediatrics 2006;118:865–73.
115. Jardine A, Menzies R, Deeks S, et al. The impact of pneumococcal conjugate vaccine on rates of myringotomy with ventilation tube insertion in Australia. Pediatr Infect Dis J 2009;28(9):761–5.
116. Singleton RJ, Holman RC, Plant R, et al. Trends in otitis media and myringotomy with tube placement among American Indian/Alaska native children and the US general population of children. Pediatr Infect Dis J 2009;28:102–7.
117. Leach AJ, Morris PS. The burden and outcome of respiratory tract infection in Australian and Aboriginal children. Pediatr Infect Dis J 2009;26:S4–7.
118. Health Canada. First nations health status report, Alberta region, 2007–2008. Ottawa (ON): Health Canada; 2009.
119. Glass RI, Lew JF, Gangarosa RE, et al. Estimates of morbidity and mortality rates for diarrheal diseases in American children. J Pediatr 1991;118(4[Pt 2]):S27–33.
120. Holman RC, Parashar UD, Clarke MJ, et al. Trends in diarrhea-associated hospitalizations among American Indian and Alaska native children, 1980–1995. Pediatrics 1999;103:E11.

121. Singleton RJ, Holman RC, Yorita KL, et al. Diarrhea-associated hospitalizations and outpatient visits among American Indian and Alaska Native children younger than five years of age, 2000–2004. Pediatr Infect Dis J 2007;26:1006–13.

122. Vesikari T, Matson DO, Dennehy P, et al. Safety and efficacy of a pentavalent human-bovine (WC3) reassortant rotavirus vaccine. N Engl J Med 2006;354: 23–33.

123. Northern Territory Government. Territory to fund rotavirus vaccine. Available at: http://newsroom.nt.gov.au/index.cfm?fuseaction=printRelease&ID=287. Accessed June 12, 2009.

124. Commonwealth Department of Health and Ageing. Fact sheets: Australian government funding of rotavirus vaccine. Available at: http://www.health.gov.au/internet/main/publishing.nsf/Content/rotavirus_vaccine.htm. Accessed June 12, 2009.

125. National Advisory Committee on Immunization (NACI). Statement on the recommended use of pentavalent human-bovine reassortant rotavirus vaccine. An Advisory Committee Statement (ACS). Can Commun Dis Rep 2008; 34(ACS-1):1–33.

126. Centers for Disease Control and Prevention (CDC). Delayed onset and diminished magnitude of rotavirus activity—United States, November 2007–May 2008. MMWR Morb Mortal Wkly Rep 2008;57:697–700.

127. Centers for Disease Control and Prevention (CDC). Recommended childhood and adolescent immunization schedule—United States, January-June 2004. MMWR Morb Mortal Wkly Rep 2004;53:Q1–4.

128. New Zealand Ministry of Health. Immunisation schedule. Available at: http://www.moh.govt.nz/mohnsf/indexmh/immunisation-schedule. Accessed April 20, 2006.

129. Public Health Agency of Canada. Immunization schedule. Available at: http://www.phac-aspc.gc.ca/im/is-cv/index.html. Accessed April 20, 2006.

130. Miller M, Roche P, Yphannes K, et al. Australia's notifiable disease status, 2003: annual report of the National Notifiable Diseases Surveillance System. Commun Dis Intell 2005;29:1–61.

131. Vitek CR, Pascual FB, Baughman AL, et al. Increase in deaths from pertussis among young infants in the United States in the 1990s. Pediatr Infect Dis J 2003;22:628–34.

132. Menzies R, McIntyre P, Beard F. Vaccine preventable diseases and vaccination coverage in Aboriginal and Torres Strait Islander people, Australia, 1999 to 2002. Commun Dis Intell 2004;28(Suppl 1):S1–S45.

133. Centers for Disease Control and Prevention (CDC) Prevention and control of meningococcal disease. [report]. MMWR Recomm Rep 2005;54:RR07, 1–21.

134. O'Hallahan J, Lennon D, Oster P. The strategy to control New Zealand's epidemic of group B meningococcal disease. Pediatr Infect Dis J 2004;23: S293–8.

135. Martin D, Lopez L. The epidemiology of meningococcal disease in New Zealand in 2007. Report num. FW 0841. Environmental Science and Research Ltd, 2008.

136. Centers for Disease Control and Prevention (CDC). Estimated vaccination coverage with individual vaccines and vaccination series among children 19-35 months of age by race/ethnicity. US, National Immunization Survey, Q1/2007-Q4/2007. Available at: http://www.cdc.gov/vaccines/stats-surv/nis/tables/07/tab30_race_nat.xls. Accessed June 12, 2009.

137. Hull BP, McIntyre PB. Timeliness of childhood vaccination in Australia. Vaccine 2006;24:4403–8.

138. Vlack SA, Foster R, Menzies R, et al. Immunisation coverage of Queensland Indigenous 2 year old children by cluster sampling and by register. Aust N Z J Public Health 2007;31:67–72.
139. Ministry of Health. The National childhood immunisation coverage survey 2005. Wellington: Ministry of Health; 2009.
140. National American Indian Housing Council (NAIHC). Too few rooms: residential crowding in Native American communities and Alaska Native villages [report]. Washington, DC: NAIHC; 2001.
141. Hennessy TW, Ritter T, Holman RC, et al. The relationship between in-home water service and the risk of respiratory tract, skin, and gastrointestinal tract infections among rural Alaska natives. Am J Public Health 2008;98:2072–8.
142. Australian Bureau of Statistics (ABS), Australian Institute of Health and Welfare (AIHW). The health and welfare of Australia's Aboriginal and Torres Strait Islander peoples, 2005. Cat. No. 4704.0. Report num. Report Num 4704.0. Canberra: ABS; 2005.
143. Hanna JN, Faoagali JL, Buda PJ, et al. Further observations on the immune response to recombinant hepatitis B vaccine after administration to aboriginal and Torres Strait Island children. J Paediatr Child Health 1997;33:67–70.
144. Siber G, Santosham M, Reid R. Impaired antibody response to *Haemophilus influenzae* type b polysaccharide and low IgG2 and IgG4 concentrations in Apache children. N Engl J Med 1990;323:1387–92.
145. Miernyk KM, Parkinson AJ, Rudolph KM, et al. Immunogenicity of a heptavalent pneumococcal conjugate vaccine in Apache and Navajo Indian, Alaska native, and non-native American children aged <2 years. Clin Infect Dis 2000;31:34–41.
146. O'Brien KL, Moulton LH, Reid R, et al. Efficacy and safety of seven-valent conjugate pneumococcal vaccine in American Indian children: group randomised trial. Lancet 2003;362:355–61.
147. Watt JP, O'Brien KL, Benin AL, et al. Invasive pneumococcal disease among Navajo adults, 1989–1998. Clin Infect Dis 2004;38:496–501.
148. Bulkow L, Wainwright R, Letson GW, et al. Comparative immunogenicity of 4 *Haemophilus influenzae* type b conjugate vaccines in Alaskan Native infants. Pediatr Infect Dis J 1993;12:484–92.
149. Squires SG, Pelletier L. Publicly-funded influenza and pneumococcal immunization programs in Canada: a progress report. Can Commun Dis Rep 2000;26:141–8.
150. Hanna JN, Young DM, Brookes DL, et al. The initial coverage and impact of the pneumococcal and influenza vaccination program for at-risk indigenous adults in Far North Queensland. Aust N Z J Public Health 2001;25:543–6.

Undernutrition and Obesity in Indigenous Children: Epidemiology, Prevention, and Treatment

Alan R. Ruben, MBBS, M.Appl.Epid, FRACP, FAFPHM

KEYWORDS

- Indigenous • Child • Obesity • Malnutrition
- Prevention • Intervention

NORMAL GROWTH AND GROWTH STANDARDS

The categorization of normal growth and desirable body habitus in children (and adults) is problematic. First, what the general population considers normal for growth patterns and body size are strongly influenced by cultural values.[1,2] Second, population growth and weight distribution may be influenced by child-rearing practices, which vary between ethnic groups; these may influence the rate of growth and even final adult size compounded because growth patterns may vary within ethnic groups depending on variations in diet.[3,4] Third, abnormal growth or size can be defined statistically but depends on the growth patterns and size of the reference (standard) population.[4,5] Finally, a disease basis for normality may be used whereby certain patterns of growth or size are constituted as conferring a risk on a child or even as a disease.[6]

Therefore there are difficulties in the definitions of normal growth and body size. For example, within the same sociocultural groupings, healthy breastfed babies have different growth patterns in early infancy from healthy bottle-fed babies[3]; using standards from one group may cause healthy babies in the other group to be statistically defined as failing to thrive or as overweight[a] (depending on source, body mass index [BMI] more than 1 or 2 SD scores above the median of the reference population or weight above the 85th or 95th percentile of the reference population) and using combined data may lower the positive and negative predictive values of nutritional status for both groups.[7] Similarly, it is generally recognized that in developed countries over the past 30 years, the average weight for height and BMI in children have

---

Northern Territory Clinical School, P.O. Box 41326, Casuarina, NT 0811, Australia
E-mail address: alan.ruben@flinders.edu.au

[a] In this article, the terms, *overweight* and *obesity*, are as they appeared in the referenced studies or reviews.

Pediatr Clin N Am 56 (2009) 1285–1302
doi:10.1016/j.pcl.2009.09.008
0031-3955/09/$ – see front matter © 2009 Published by Elsevier Inc.

significantly increased.[8] By what standards should children be measured in this new millennium to distinguish those children whose growth patterns are normal from those whose are not?[9,10]

Attempts to address these problems are compounded by changing growth standards; over the past decade, three different standards have been accepted internationally. From 1977 to 2006, the World Health Organization (WHO) endorsed the use of the National Center for Health Statistics (NCHS) standards but over time recognized there were problems with their use in breastfed babies and with definitions of obesity (depending on source, BMI > 2 or 3 SD scores above the median of the reference population or weight above the 95th or 99th percentile of the reference population).[11] In 2000, the US Centers for Disease Control (CDC) and the NCHS introduced a new set of standards, which were endorsed by several international bodies, including the American Academy of Pediatrics and the Australian National Health and Medical Research Council; however, the issues, in particular for breastfed babies and obese children, remained.[12,13] In addition, the International Obesity Taskforce produced its own standards. Field workers, including the author, found that the new CDC standards categorized children at either end of the weight range in a manner that did not fit with clinical findings; compared with clinical findings, the CDC standards had poor positive predictive values for underweight (weight < 2 SD scores below the median of the reference population) and poor negative predictive values for overweight in children aged over 6 months. This had the effect of labeling children as underweight and requiring intervention when they were clinically well nourished and labeling children as not requiring intervention when they were clinically overweight or obese. The problems of differing standards has been well described, including by Guillaume, who showed that, depending on age group, there was up to a 15% difference in children classified as obese depending on which standards were used.[6] For undernutrition, a study from Canada showed that of 548 children aged under 2 years referred for assessment of failure to thrive, the NCHC/WHO 1977 standards classified 15.9% of them as underweight compared with 22.5% for CDC/NHCS 2000 standards.[4]

In the interim, the WHO has been working on a new set of standards from international populations of healthy children.[14] These standards were accepted by the WHO in 2006 and have been endorsed by several organizations. It is anticipated that these will become the new international standards.

To illustrate these difficulties, **Figs. 1** and **2** show comparative classifications for a theoretic child whose weight and weight for height were at the cutoff for underweight and wasting (weight for height < 2 SD scores below the median of the reference

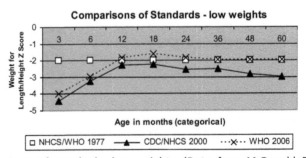

Fig. 1. Comparisons of standards—low weights. (*Data from* McDonald EL, Baillie RS, Rumbold AR, et al. Preventing growth faltering among Australian Indigenous children: implications for policy and practice. Med J Aust 2008;188(8 Suppl):S84–6.)

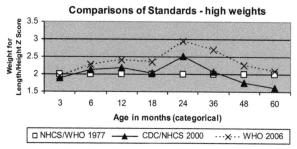

Fig. 2. Comparisons of standards—high weights. (*From* McDonald EL, Baillie RS, Rumbold AR, et al. Preventing growth faltering among Australian Indigenous children: implications for policy and practice. Med J Aust 2008;188(8 Suppl):S84–6; with permission.)

population; 2 z scores) on the NCHS/WHO 1977 standards at ages 3, 6, 12, 24, 36, 48, and 60 months and then compared these to the CDC/NCHS 2000 and the new WHO 2006 standards.

Compared with the new WHO 2006 standards, the NCHS/WHO 1977 standards underestimate underweight in infants aged under 6 months and CDC/NHCS 2000 data increasingly overestimate underweight through 5 years old. For high-weight children, the NCHC/WHO 1977 and CDC/NHCS 2000 underestimate overweight in children aged over 3 years, the latter more so as age increases.[7] For older children and adolescents, there are several publications that describe the difficulties presented by the different reference standards in the definition and management of obesity at individual and population levels.[9,10,15]

The introduction of three standards within a short space of time creates significant difficulties not only for field workers but also for those monitoring population child health. Many countries have population data sets on obesity and underweight and have published data using the earlier two standards. With the introduction of a third standard, careful consideration is needed in the compiling and comparisons of longitudinal data, including the need to convert data from the old to the new standards.[16]

DOES UNDERNUTRITION OR OBESITY IN CHILDHOOD MATTER?

Since Barker first suggested that poor nutrition in early life increases susceptibility to the effects of an affluent life,[17–21] there has been considerable interest in this area. Although the initial studies were ecologic and thus hypothesis generating, in recent years the results of several large cohort studies have become available: there is an increasing body of evidence that health in the prenatal period and early life may have lifelong and even intergenerational consequences. There is evidence that intrauterine growth retardation, poor growth in infancy, and obesity in childhood are associated with the development in later life of obesity, cardiovascular disease, hypertension, renal disease, adult-onset diabetes, and cerebrovascular disease and that the risks for some of these conditions may be increased if small for gestational age infants (< the 10th percentile of the reference population) undergo rapid postnatal and early childhood growth.[22–26] Although currently available evidence is moderate for association, the evidence for a causal relationship remains low.

The evidence for childhood growth having an impact on adult health from indigenous populations in developed countries is increasing but remains low. For example, examining the results of a cross-sectional population screening program and retrospective retrieval of birth weights, Singh and colleagues concluded that low birth weight (under 2.5 kg) is significantly associated with higher blood pressure in adult life; the effect is amplified by higher current weight. The investigators concluded that special attention should be paid to children with low birth weight to prevent their becoming overweight in adult life.[27] Wang and Hoy found that being overweight was protective for mortality in adults compared with being normal, obese, or underweight.[28]

Sayers has been leading a team that has followed a birth cohort of Australian Aboriginal children from the Northern Territory for almost 20 years. In 2004, the research team reported that at ages 8 to 14 years, small for gestational age children were significantly lighter than normal birth weight children. After adjustment for childhood size, there was no relationship between any birth measures and fasting glucose or insulin concentrations; current child size, not postnatal growth, was related to glucose and insulin metabolism[29] and the metabolic syndrome was common despite low rates of overweight or obesity.[30] In 2006, Bucens and colleagues[31] reported that for Northern Territory Aboriginal children, factors related to childhood environment are more important than perinatal factors in determining childhood lung function. Sayers' team has concluded that as some markers of health differ between peripubertal Indigenous children living in urban areas and those in remote areas, results of surveys in remote areas cannot be generalized to urban Indigenous populations.[32] Regarding overweight or obesity in childhood, the effects may have an impact on a child's health or may confer risk factors for diseases in adult life, and children who are currently obese, in particular those less than 8 years old, are at the greatest risk of becoming obese adults.[33] The consequences in childhood and beyond may include cardiovascular disease and metabolic, gastrointestinal, pulmonary, orthopedic, neurologic, psychologic, and social disorders.[34] Others have suggested these concerns are exaggerated and that medical care may ameliorate long-term impacts.[35] The epidemic of obesity and diabetes in Indigenous adults and, increasingly, children is well described.[29,36-39]

As the studies from Indigenous populations are limited, are the results from the general population applicable? Wang and Hoy have concluded that the Framingham function substantially underestimates the actual risk of coronary heart disease observed in Indigenous people in a remote community, especially for women and younger adults. The investigators concluded that traditional risk factors have different degrees of impact or that other factors are contributing to risk; a population-specific risk function is needed.[40]

Outcomes from a population-based cohort in Pelotas, in Southern Brazil, showed that for small for gestational age babies, rapid weight gain in infancy is associated with fewer hospitalizations but no differences in mortality from normal birth weight babies.[41] In a commentary on this study Victora and Barrow discussed the catch-up dilemma for small for gestational age babies—that later weight gain may be associated with risks of chronic diseases in adult life, the timing and detail of which are poorly understood. They conclude that in developing countries it is reasonable to promote growth in young children but that it is a priority to assess the full impact for the short and long term.[42]

A systematic review of data from five longstanding prospective cohort studies from Brazil, Guatemala, India, the Philippines, and South Africa suggests that lower birth weight and undernutrition in childhood are risk factors for high glucose concentrations, high blood pressure, and harmful lipid profiles once adult BMI and height are adjusted for, suggesting that rapid postnatal weight gain—especially after infancy—is linked to these conditions. Birthweight was positively associated with lung function and with the incidence of some cancers, and undernutrition could be associated with mental illness. The investigators note that low height for age at 2 years was associated with lower human capital and conclude that damage suffered in early life leads to permanent impairment and might also affect future generations. They conclude that prevention will probably bring about important health, educational, and economic benefits and that chronic diseases are especially common in undernourished children who experience rapid weight gain after infancy[43]; the same group found that rapid early growth is associated with prevalence of obesity in later life.[44]

CURRENT SITUATION

The International Group for Indigenous Health Measurement has been established in recognition that in the USA, Australia, Canada and New Zealand there are problems with the availability of high-quality data and that there are differences in the availability of indigenous health data between these countries. The group most recently met in Canberra, Australia, in 2006. The purpose of the meeting was to further international collaboration to tackle health measurement issues for indigenous populations, building on the work that began at the inaugural meeting in Vancouver, Canada, in 2005. The Group concluded that indigenous sample sizes in national surveys are generally too small to enable accurate indigenous rates to be estimated, and because of differences in methodology, there should be a cautious approach to international comparisons.

Although the Group considered that high-quality data are necessary to measure the health of indigenous people and to prioritize health needs, they also reported that indigenous people in all four countries are concerned with being over-researched— being research subjects; indigenous people in all four countries want strategies put in place to build capacity within their communities so that they can collect, manage, and "own" data.[45] Fremantle and colleagues[46] recently called for improved data to underpin better health outcomes in Indigenous children in Australia.

Health in general and growth in particular are reflections of prenatal health influences, history, and socioeconomic status, including modern diet these factors may account for the health disparities between indigenous people and the wider population.[47,48] With the exception of small numbers of Aboriginal children in the remote northern parts of Australia, there has been a marked transition in the nutritional status of indigenous children over the past 50 years, from a high prevalence of undernutrition to one of obesity. For this manuscript, all available reports since 1960 through PubMed and the Cochrane Central Register of Controlled Trials were reviewed, and, where available, respective government, university, and indigenous health organization Web sites. Although the data are incomplete, they do provide an overview of the recent history and current status of growth in indigenous children in developed countries.

United States

Changes in indigenous growth and nutritional status have been reasonably well documented in the United States. For example, in 1976, Van Duzen and colleagues[49] reported a substantial fall in undernutrition rates in hospitalized Navajo children from 1963–1967 to 1969–1973. In 1998, Story and colleagues[50] reported, based on data from 1969 to 1972, that the prevalence of being underweight (less than the third percentile) was between 18% and 33% in selected indigenous communities; in the same report, the 1994 underweight rate at 2.1% was lower than for all other ethnic groups. In 1999, Story and colleagues[51] reported that obesity had become a major health problem in American Indians, with the prevalence of overweight/obesity ranging from 9% to 17% in preschool children and 27% to 40% in school-aged children. In 2000, Eisenmann and colleagues[52] reported on the increasing weight and BMI in

Navajo children from 1955 to 1997. A review by Crawford and colleagues[53] in 2001 reported similar overweight rates from studies that included approximately 50,000 indigenous preschool children and obesity rates as high as 77% from small populations of school-aged children but approximately 40% for the majority of schools. In 2003, Story and colleagues[54] reported that obesity in American Indian communities was widespread, although there is considerable variation across tribes. They cited a CDC survey of 30,630 children aged 24 to 59 months: 29.3% had a BMI greater than the 85th percentile and 13.7% greater than the 97th percentile.

Canada

In Canada there are few published early reviews; in 1969, Partington and Roberts reported on the growth of schoolchildren in James Bay and Hudson Bay. They found that compared with nonindigenous Canadians, Mohawk children were slightly heavier and taller, Cree children were comparable, and Inuit children were slightly smaller.[55] In 1978, Coondin and colleagues wrote there was no evidence to support an assertion made in the *Canadian Medical Association Journal* that marasmus and kwashiorkor still occurred in Indian and Inuit children. Gunn replied that 24 of 25 children she had seen with chronic diarrhea were underweight and mircocephalic.[56] A comprehensive review of overweight in indigenous Canadian children was undertaken by Willows in 2005. She reported that knowledge of the rate of overweight and obese children in indigenous Canadian children is restricted to a few intensely studied communities and that in schoolchildren the rates for overweight vary between 24% and 38% and for obesity between 10% and 35%. Willows also writes that there are limited quality data on preschool-aged children and little information on potential associations or antecedents for these obesity data.[57] In 2007, Willows and colleagues[58] reported overweight and obesity rates of 32% and 21%, respectively, for 5-year-old Cree children; 14.7% of children categorized as normal weight at age 2 years were obese at age 5 years, using International Obesity Taskforce definitions.

New Zealand

Although Bryder reports that undernutrition was common in Maori children immediately after World War II,[59] there are no available reports describing malnutrition in Maoris in New Zealand after 1960. In 2007, Utter and colleagues[60] reported obesity rates of 41% in Maori children aged 5 to 14 years in data from 2002; using the same data set, Goulding and colleagues[61] reported obesity rates (>95th percentile for BMI) of 21%, 19%, and 17% for Maori children aged 5 to 6 years, 7 to 10 years, and 11 to 14 years, respectively; the extreme obesity rates (>99th percentile for BMI) in the same age groups were 8.3%, 4.5%, and 4%, respectively. The 2006/2007 New Zealand Health Survey indicated an obesity rate in Maori children aged 2 to 14 years of 11.8%, lower than the 23.3% for Pacific Islander children but higher than the 5.5% for European/Other. Overall, the obesity rates for Maori children were approximately 8% for children up to 9 years old, rising to 14% for children aged 10 to 14 years. Obesity rates were highest in neighborhoods classified as "most deprived," almost three times that of "least deprived" neighborhoods.[62]

Australia

Australia is the only developed country with high rates of undernutrition in its Indigenous population, with wasting rates of more than 10% reported in some rural and remote areas.[63–65] There is a dichotomy in Indigenous children, however, who are overrepresented in underweight and overweight categories. In 1994, Cunningham and Mackerras reported underweight rates of 15% and 11% for boys and girls, respectively, ages 7 to 15 years, and overweight rates of 13% and 19%, respectively, using definitions of less than the 5th percentile for underweight and greater than the 95th percentile for overweight for BMI.[66] In 2008, O'Dea reported from a 2006 survey of 47 schools nationwide that 8.6% of Indigenous children aged 6 to 11 years were obese and 16.0% overweight.[67] In Western Australian hospitals, failure to thrive has been noted as an admission diagnosis in 11% of Aboriginal children (0–4 years) compared with 5% of non-Aboriginal children.[68] In 2007–2008, a survey of 7733 Indigenous children, aged 2 to 16 and living in remote areas of Australia, found a wasting rate of 11.8% that was uniform across all age groups; the obesity rate was 4.8% overall but strongly associated with age: 3.7% in children ages 2 to 5 years, rising to 8% in children ages 12 to years.[65] The CDC 2000 reference standards were used and, as discussed previously, may have overestimated wasting and underestimated obesity. Detailed findings on childhood obesity from the 2007 Australian National Children's Nutrition and Physical Activity Survey have yet to be released but the National Aboriginal and Torres Strait Islander Health Survey, 2004–2005, used self-reported weights and heights to estimate adult overweight and obesity rates at 56%, up from 48% in 1995.

INTERVENTIONS

In 1999, Morris reported that there was a profound lack of well-designed studies assessing medical interventions specifically addressing the health needs of Aboriginal Australians[69] and this situation, for nutritional issues, has not changed in Australia or the other developed countries with large indigenous populations. Furthermore, the evidence of effective interventions in the prevention or treatment of undernutrition and obesity is limited to the general or developing country populations and almost absent from indigenous communities. Where limited evidence does exist, issues around generalizability arise, as the underlying causes of these conditions are more sociocultural than biomedical (**Table 1**).[32,70,79,86,87]

Obesity

The evidence for effectiveness of interventions in obesity prevention in children is weak and the outcomes of systematic reviews on obesity prevention in children may be contradictory and open to bias, depending on the methodology of the reviewers. For example, in 2005, Summerbell and colleagues[8] concluded from a systematic review that studies that focused on combining dietary and physical activity approaches did not significantly improve BMI, but some studies that focused on dietary or physical activity approaches showed a small but positive impact on BMI status; in 2006, Doak and colleagues[76] concluded from a review of school-based interventions that the majority of overweight/obesity prevention programs included in their review were effective. The two principal investigators then combined the results of their reviews but could not agree on the inclusion or exclusion criteria, in particular whether or not studies with aims not specific to preventing weight gain should be included and the manner of assessment of anthropometric measures.[77]

In 2008, Kamath and colleagues[78] summarized evidence on the efficacy of interventions aimed at changing lifestyle behaviors (increased physical activity, decreased sedentary activity, increased healthy dietary habits, and decreased unhealthy dietary habits) to prevent obesity and concluded that although obesity prevention programs caused small changes in behavior, there was no evidence of significant effect on BMI. Reilly discussed that one of the reasons for the failure of many preventive interventions is that by targeting behavior modification at the microlevel (individual

Table 1
Key recommendations for prevention and treatment of undernutrition and obesity in indigenous children living in affluent countries

Intervention	Recommendation[a]	Recommendation Grade	Quality of Supporting Evidence
Undernutrition			
Preventing children from becoming malnourished	Antenatal care and breastfeeding (including weaning)	Covered in article elsewhere in this issue by Sayers	Covered in article elsewhere in this issue by Sayers
	Environmental improvements, such as better housing and sanitation	Strong for	Low[47–49,63,70,71]
	Community-based nutrition/counseling interventions that focus on nutrition behavior change and interventions that are well integrated into primary health care systems	Strong for	Moderate[47,48,63,70,71]
	Not to change current practices for supplementary/complementary feeding programs for children or pregnant/lactating women	Strong for	Moderate[47,48,70,72]
	Growth-monitoring programs, micronutrient supplementation and de-worming unless population known to be affected	Weak against	Moderate[47,48,70,72]
Treatment of children who are malnourished	Ready-to-use therapeutic and ambulatory foods,	Strong for	Moderate[73,74]
	High volume intravenous fluid for undernourished children in shock	Strong against	Moderate[73,75]
	Broad spectrum antibiotics in severe undernutrition	Strong for	Moderate[73,75]
	Micronutrient supplementation in populations known to be affected	Strong for	Moderate[47,73–75]
Obesity			
Preventing children from becoming obese	Antenatal care and breastfeeding (including weaning)	Covered in article elsewhere in this issue by Sayers	Covered in article elsewhere in this issue by Sayers
	Physical exercise and dietary modification, alone or combined, as part of school-based programs or otherwise	Strong for	Low[8,76–78,b]
Treatment of children who are obese	Combined behavioral lifestyle interventions	Strong for	Moderate[79,80]
	Orlistat, sibutramine, or metformin selected children in conjunction with lifestyle changes	Weak for	Moderate[79–81]
	Surgery for morbid obesity in carefully selected cases	Weak for	Low[33,79,82–84]

[a] See text for further explanation.
[b] Includes information from a randomized trial in indigenous children in affluent countries, remainder of randomized trials from nonindigenous children.

children, their families, or schools), they were unable to have an impact on the many other influences on weight status that determine the environment at the macrolevel, such as those suggested by Nestle, which include education, food labeling, food assistance programs, transport, and taxes.[86-88]

Similarly the evidence on any protective effects of breastfeeding on the later development of obesity is unclear. The longitudinal studies from Pelotas in Brazil do not support the hypothesis that breastfed babies are less likely to become obese in later life[89,90] whereas, in contrast, Gillman and colleagues[91] study suggested that infants who were fed breast milk more than infant formula, or who were breastfed for longer periods, had a lower risk of being overweight during older childhood and adolescence. A systematic review concluded that BMI may be lower in breastfed subjects but the effect was small and likely influenced by publication bias.[92] In summary, although there may be other benefits from interventions to prevent obesity, any effect on BMI and obesity is at best small.

In indigenous communities, there have been no systematic reviews on interventions for obesity prevention because there have been few randomized controlled trials. In 2003, Story suggested that intervention measures include access to healthier food choices and safe, affordable, physical activity opportunities.[54] In the same year, the Pathways study reported on a 9-year trial which had the objective of evaluating the effectiveness of a school-based, multicomponent intervention for reducing percentage of body fat in American Indian schoolchildren. The study concentrated on school curriculum, physical activity, food service, and family. The intervention and control groups in the study showed significant differences in self-reported dietary and physical activity behaviors but fewer or no differences in these outcomes when measured objectively; there were no differences in the main outcome of reduction in measures of adiposity.[93] The study faced many difficulties, with important lessons learned for the design and implementation of future studies.[94]

Regarding treatment of obesity, systematic reviews have suggested some interventions may be effective. A systematic review published in 2008, which included trials of pharmacologic treatments and dietary and physical activity intervention, alone or combined, concluded that limited evidence supports the short-term efficacy of medications (sibutramine and orlistat) and lifestyle interventions but concluded that the long-term efficacy and safety of pediatric obesity treatments remain unclear.[80] They noted the conclusions were not different from those drawn from a Cochrane review in 2003,[95] that most studies were too small to detect treatment effects and that outcomes measured were inconsistent across studies. The investigators commented that perhaps measures of fat distribution are more sensitive to change than BMI.

The 2003, the Cochrane review concluded that most of the 18 studies included were small and drawn from homogenous, motivated groups in hospital settings, so generalizable evidence from them is limited and there is a limited amount of quality data on the components of programs to treat childhood obesity that favor one program over another.[95] The Cochrane review was updated in 2009 with new investigators and concluded that although there are limited quality data to recommend one treatment program over another, that combined behavioral lifestyle interventions compared with standard care or self-help can produce a significant and clinically meaningful reduction in overweight in children and adolescents, and that in obese adolescents consideration should be given to the use of orlistat or sibutramine (but not metformin) as an adjunct to lifestyle interventions, although this approach needs to be carefully weighed against the potential for adverse effects.[79] These two medications have also been found to be modestly effective in weight loss for adults in another Cochrane review,[96] but a randomized, double-blind, placebo-controlled trial showed that metformin may be a useful agent to promote short-term weight loss in girls making modest lifestyle changes[81]; the results are supported by other systematic reviews.[80] The limited evidence, mostly from adults, suggests surgery is more effective than conventional management for weight loss in morbid obesity.[33,82–85]

The author considered if the issue of differing study inclusion criteria may have influenced the outcomes of the two Cochrane reviews.[79,95] The 2003 Cochrane review included 18 studies published between 1985 and 2001; the 2009 review included 64 studies published between 1985 and 2008; the 2009 review also considered for inclusion into the review studies of drug and surgical interventions but found no studies met their inclusion criteria. All studies from the 2003 review were included in the 2009 review; no studies were used in the 2009 review that had been available to the 2003 investigators. It is, therefore, reasonable to conclude that study inclusion bias does not account for stronger recommendations in the latter review and that these arise from new studies.

The investigators of the 2009 review noted that it is unlikely that the implications for practice can be directly extrapolated from one group to another. The practicalities of delivering effective advice on lifestyle changes to obese children and adolescents vary with the wide span of social, ethnic, and economic circumstances and with the many variations in available resources for local health service delivery. These aforementioned issues are discussed by Maziak and colleagues,[97] who note that recent systematic reviews of childhood obesity prevention and intervention programs indicate limited success at best and that as a lifestyle risk, obesity requires a lifestyle approach.

Several other studies of indigenous communities have been published; these have not been randomized trials and although they have shown effects on behavior and knowledge, they have not shown significant benefit in terms of reduced obesity levels.[98–112] For indigenous children, there have been no systematic reviews because there have been no randomized trials.

Undernutrition

In 1976, van Duzen and colleagues[49] discussed whether or not the improvements in rates of undernutrition in Navajo children might be ascribed to the lower rates of infectious diseases, such as diarrhea and pneumonia, seen in the well-baby clinics, which may have been the result of environmental improvements, such as better housing and sanitation. Hood and Elliott found the health of elite Maori and Caucasian New Zealander children to be the same.[113] This is in accordance with the improvement in Maori rates of undernutrition coincident with efforts to improve socioeconomic status[59] and the findings from Australia that undernutrition in Aborigines is more prevalent in the most socioeconomically deprived communities located in remote areas.[63] This association between poverty and growth has been long recognized.[71]

There have been few systematic reviews and no meta-analysis on the prevention or treatment of undernutrition in developed countries, again because there have been so few randomized controlled trials, including in indigenous communities. Except in cases of chronic disease, the antecedents of childhood undernutrition in developed countries are socioeconomic in their indigenous and nonindigenous communities; solutions must, therefore, come from outside of the health sector.[86] As discussed previously, undernutrition is now confined to Indigenous communities in rural and remote Australia; as a consequence, this discussion is largely confined to Australia.

In 2006, in a systematic review, McDonald and colleagues[48] examined which preventive or health promotion program models and approaches are most likely to improve patterns of growth faltering in children 5 years old or younger in the Australian remote Indigenous community context and if the models or the nature of the evidence vary depending on the age of the child. They examined evidence for supplementary and complementary feeding programs for children, supplementary feeding programs for pregnant or lactating women, growth monitoring, nutrition education and counseling, deworming, and vitamin and mineral supplementation (zinc, iron, iron and zinc, multiple micronutrient supplementation, vitamin A, multifaceted interventions, and other measures of relevance). The results were summarized in 2008.[72]

The investigators indicated that "there was a clear need for high-quality evidence to support specific preventive interventions, in addition to better evidence on approaches to implementing interventions." They continued that this is especially relevant to remote Indigenous communities, where the primary cause of disadvantage is largely related to social exclusion and poverty. They concluded that international experience indicated that coordinating interventions between the health sector and other sectors do more to improve children's health in the context of poverty than a series of single interventions or than one sector trying to address a problem alone and that strengthening resources and capacity at the community level for preventive programs that are culturally appropriate, participatory, and focus on the family seem to be the key to success and sustainability of interventions (**Box 1**).[72]

Brewster[73] has published a series of four critical appraisals on undernutrition. Concordant with MacDonald and colleagues, Brewster concluded that in the treatment of malnourished Australian Aboriginal children in northern Australia, the emphasis needs to change from hospital case management to improved community management with a focus on environmental health (eg, housing, hygiene, and overcrowding) and child care issues. Regarding treatment of undernutrition, he concluded that not only is the evidence base deficient but also the external generalizability of even good-quality studies was seriously compromised by the great variability in

---

Box 1
Review findings from MacDonald and colleagues

Although the evidence is not strong and the effects are modest, the interventions for which there is some evidence of benefit in general populations include community-based nutrition and counseling interventions that focus on nutrition, behavior change, and interventions that are well integrated into primary health care systems.

Interventions for which there is some evidence of benefit in specific populations include vitamin A supplementation in populations with moderate to severe vitamin A deficiency and deworming treatment in populations with high infestation rates.

Interventions for which the research evidence clearly supports neither implementation of new programs nor withdrawal of existing programs[a] include supplementary and complementary feeding programs for children or pregnant or lactating women and multiple micronutrient supplementations.

Interventions where the research shows no clear evidence of benefit include growth-monitoring programs, population iron supplementation for children, and iron and zinc supplementation in general. There is clear evidence that zinc supplementation was of no benefit in preventing growth faltering. Supplementation, however, was associated with increases in height.

[a] Interventions for which there is no evidence of benefit or harm (in some studies, there were methodologic concerns)

From McDonald, EL, et al. Preventing growth faltering among Australian Indigenous children: implications for policy and practice. Med J Aust 2008;188(8 Suppl):S84–6.

clinical practice between regions and types of health facilities in the developing world, which is much greater than between developed countries.[70] He made recommendations based on formulas used in developing countries for malnourished children and the beneficial use of micronutrients, namely zinc and vitamin A.[73] A randomized controlled trial by Chang and colleagues, however, found that Australian Aboriginal children given zinc had increased risk of readmission with acute lower respiratory infection. These investigators concluded that vitamin A and zinc therapy may not be useful and the effect of supplementation may depend on the prevalence of deficiency of these micronutrients in the population.[114] Brewster also found good evidence that severely malnourished children do not tolerate excessive fluid administration and that wide-spectrum antibiotics need to be given empirically for severe undernutrition to prevent otherwise unavoidable early mortality.[75] Severe undernutrition is becoming less frequent in Australia but still occurs.

Brewster and colleagues[47] have published a comprehensive review on the evidence-based approach to failure to thrive in Indigenous Australians. In the same book, there are comprehensive reviews on the social determinants and health problems of Australian Aboriginal child health but obesity is not discussed in detail.

SUMMARY

High-quality evidence for benefit from preventative or intervention strategies for indigenous children on obesity and undernutrition is lacking. For obesity, exercise and diet, alone or combined , are shown in nonindigenous children to confer some benefit with regard to preventing weight gain and weight loss but the generalizability and transfer of evidence on exercise and diet to indigenous communities is uncertain. The single large intervention study in indigenous children for obesity prevention did not show any difference in the outcome of BMI between the intervention groups and the controls. In selected children, pharmacotherapy may have a limited place in conjunction with diet and exercise but, as with surgical intervention, any such approach needs to be taken with great caution.

For undernutrition, there is some evidence of modest benefit from community-based nutrition and counseling interventions that focus on nutrition behavior change and interventions that are well integrated into primary health care systems; except for where specific nutritional deficiencies have been identified, the evidence for other interventions, such as growth monitoring, is weak or absent; however, programs currently in place, such as nutritional support to children and pregnant mothers, should continue.

More high-quality research in these areas is urgently required but addressing the underlying causes of under nutrition and obesity with poverty alleviation programs, food availability, advertising restrictions, better access to health care, improved education, and measures to combat gender and race discrimination need to be addressed for long-term change to be sustained.

REFERENCES

1. Latner JD, Simmonds M, Rosewall JK, et al. Assessment of obesity stigmatization in children and adolescents: modernizing a standard measure. Obesity (Silver Spring) 2007;15(12):3078–85.
2. Cunningham J, O'Dea K, Dunbar T, et al. Perceived weight versus Body Mass Index among urban Aboriginal Australians: do perceptions and measurements match? Aust N Z J Public Health 2008;32(2):135–8.

3. Victora CG, Morris SS, Barros FC, et al. The NCHS reference and the growth of breast- and bottle-fed infants. J Nutr 1998;128(7):1134–8.
4. Nash A, Corey M, Sherwood K, et al. Growth assessment in infants and toddlers using three different reference charts. J Pediatr Gastroenterol Nutr 2005;40(3):283–8.
5. Nash A, Seckar D, Corey M, et al. Field testing of the 2006 World Health Organization growth charts from birth to 2 years: assessment of hospital undernutrition and overnutrition rates and the usefulness of BMI. JPEN J Parenter Enteral Nutr 2008;32(2):145–53.
6. Guillaume M. Defining obesity in childhood: current practice. Am J Clin Nutr 1999;70(1):126S–30S.
7. Mei Z, Ogden CC, Flegal KM, et al. Comparison of the prevalence of shortness, underweight, and overweight among US children aged 0 to 59 months by using the CDC 2000 and the WHO 2006 growth charts. J Pediatr 2008;153(5):622–8.
8. Summerbell CD, Waters E, Edmunds LD, et al. Interventions for preventing obesity in children. Cochrane Database Syst Rev 2005;(3):CD001871.
9. Chumlea C. Which growth charts are the best for children today? Nutr Today 2007;42(4):148–50, 10.1097/01.NT.0000286151.62967.59.
10. Flegal KM, Tabak CJ, Ogden CL. Overweight in children: definitions and interpretation. Health Educ Res 2006;21(6):755–60.
11. WHO Working Group on Infant Growth. An evaluation of infant growth: the use and interpretation of anthropometry in infants. Bull World Health Organ 1995;73(2):165–74.
12. de Onis M, Onyango AW. The Centers for Disease Control and Prevention 2000 growth charts and the growth of breastfed infants. Acta Paediatr 2003;92(4):413–9.
13. Ogden CL. Defining overweight in children using growth charts. Md Med 2004;5(3):19–21.
14. WHO Multicentre Growth Reference Study Group. WHO child growth standards. Length/height-for-age, weight-for-age, weight-for-length, weight-for-height and body mass index-for-age: methods and development. World Health Organization 2006, ISBN 92 4 154693X.
15. Kain J, Uauy R, Vio F, et al. Trends in overweight and obesity prevalence in Chilean children: comparison of three definitions. Eur J Clin Nutr 2002;56(3):200–4.
16. Yang H, de Onis M. Algorithms for converting estimates of child malnutrition based on the NCHS reference into estimates based on the WHO Child Growth Standards. BMC Pediatr 2008;8:19.
17. Barker DJ, Osmond C, Law CM. The intrauterine and early postnatal origins of cardiovascular disease and chronic bronchitis. J Epidemiol Community Health 1989;43(3):237–40.
18. Barker DJ, Winter PD, Osmond C, et al. Weight in infancy and death from ischaemic heart disease. Lancet 1989;2(8663):577–80.
19. Barker DJ. The fetal and infant origins of adult disease. BMJ 1990;301(6761):1111.
20. Barker DJ, Osmond C, Golding J. Height and mortality in the counties of England and Wales. Ann Hum Biol 1990;17(1):1–6.
21. Coggon D, Margetts B, Barker DJ, et al. Childhood risk factors for ischaemic heart disease and stroke. Paediatr Perinat Epidemiol 1990;4(4):464–9.
22. Adair LS, Martorell R, Stein AD, et al. Size at birth, weight gain in infancy and childhood, and adult blood pressure in 5 low- and middle-income-country cohorts: when does weight gain matter? Am J Clin Nutr 2009;89(5):1383–92.

23. Barros AJ, Victoria CG, Santos IS, et al. Infant malnutrition and obesity in three population-based birth cohort studies in Southern Brazil: trends and differences. Cad Saude Publica 2008;24(Suppl 3):S417–26.
24. Victora CG, Sibbritt D, Horta BL, et al. Weight gain in childhood and body composition at 18 years of age in Brazilian males. Acta Paediatr 2007;96(2):296–300.
25. Gigante DP, Victoria CG, Horta BL, et al. Undernutrition in early life and body composition of adolescent males from a birth cohort study. Br J Nutr 2007;97(5):949–54.
26. Singh AS, Mulder C, Twisk JW, et al. Tracking of childhood overweight into adulthood: a systematic review of the literature. Obes Rev 2008;9(5):474–88.
27. Singh GR, Hoy WE. The association between birthweight and current blood pressure: a cross-sectional study in an Australian Aboriginal community. Med J Aust 2003;179(10):532–5.
28. Wang Z, Hoy WE. Body mass index and mortality in aboriginal Australians in the Northern Territory. Aust N Z J Public Health 2002;26(4):305–10.
29. Sayers SM, Mackerras D, Singh G, et al. In an Aboriginal birth cohort, only child size and not birth size, predicts insulin and glucose concentrations in childhood. Diabetes Res Clin Pract 2004;65(2):151–7.
30. Sellers EA, Singh GR, Sayers SM. Large waist but low body mass index: the metabolic syndrome in Australian Aboriginal children. J Pediatr 2008;153(2):222–7.
31. Bucens IK, Reid A, Sayers SM. Risk factors for reduced lung function in Australian Aboriginal children. J Paediatr Child Health 2006;42(7-8):452–7.
32. Mackerras DE, Reid A, Sayers SM, et al. Growth and morbidity in children in the Aboriginal Birth Cohort Study: the urban-remote differential. Med J Aust 2003;178(2):56–60.
33. Daniels SR, Jacobson MS, McCrindle BW, et al. American Heart Association Childhood Obesity Research Summit Report. Circulation 2009;119(15):e489–517.
34. Olshansky SJ, Passaro DJ, Hershow RC, et al. A potential decline in life expectancy in the United States in the 21st century. N Engl J Med 2005;352(11):1138–45.
35. Gibbs WW. Obesity: an overblown epidemic? Sci Am 2005;292(6):70–7.
36. Acton KJ, Burrows NR, Moore K, et al. Trends in diabetes prevalence among American Indian and Alaska native children, adolescents, and young adults. Am J Public Health 2002;92(9):1485–90.
37. Salonen MK, Kajantie E, Osmond C, et al. Role of childhood growth on the risk of metabolic syndrome in obese men and women. Diabete Metab 2009;35(2):94–100.
38. Qiao Q, Gao W, Zhang L, et al. Metabolic syndrome and cardiovascular disease. Ann Clin Biochem 2007;44(Pt 3):232–63.
39. Anderson I, Crengles S, Kamaka ML, et al. Indigenous health in Australia, New Zealand, and the Pacific. Lancet 2006;367(9524):1775–85.
40. Wang Z, Hoy WE. Is the Framingham coronary heart disease absolute risk function applicable to Aboriginal people? Med J Aust 2005;182(2):66–9.
41. Victora CG, Barros FC, Horta BL, et al. Short-term benefits of catch-up growth for small-for-gestational-age infants. Int J Epidemiol 2001;30(6):1325–30.
42. Victora CG, Barros FC. Commentary: the catch-up dilemma–relevance of Leitch's 'low-high' pig to child growth in developing countries. Int J Epidemiol 2001;30(2):217–20.

43. Victora CG, Adair L, Fall C, et al. Maternal and child undernutrition: consequences for adult health and human capital. Lancet 2008;371(9609):340–57.
44. Monteiro PO, Victora CG. Rapid growth in infancy and childhood and obesity in later life—a systematic review. Obes Rev 2005;6(2):143–54.
45. AIHW, Australian Institute of Health and Welfare. International group for indigenous health measurement, Canberra 2006. Cat. no. IHW 26. Canberra: AIHW.
46. Fremantle E, Zutynski YA, Mahajan D, et al. Indigenous child health: urgent need for improved data to underpin better health outcomes. Med J Aust 2008;188(10): 588–91.
47. Brewster DR. Failure to thrive. In: Couzos S, Murray R, editors. Aboriginal primary health care: an evidence-based approach. 3rd edition. Melbourne: Oxford University Press; 2008. p. 265–307.
48. McDonald EL, Bailie RS, Rumbold AR, et al. Interventions to prevent growth faltering in remote Indigenous communities. Canberra: Australian Primary Health Care Research Institute and Menzies School of Health Research; 2006. Available at: http://www.anu.edu.au/aphcri/Domain/ATSIPHC/Final_25_Bailie.pdf. Accessed June 16, 2009.
49. Van Duzen J, Carter JP, Zwagg RV. Protein and calorie malnutrition among preschool Navajo Indian children, a follow-up. Am J Clin Nutr 1976;29(6):657–62.
50. Story M, Strauss KF, Zephier E, et al. Nutritional concerns in American Indian and Alaska Native children: transitions and future directions. J Am Diet Assoc 1998;98(2):170–6.
51. Story M, Evans M, Fabsitz RR, et al. The epidemic of obesity in American Indian communities and the need for childhood obesity-prevention programs. Am J Clin Nutr 1999;69(4):747S–54S.
52. Eisenmann JC, Katzmarzyk PT, Arnall DA, et al. Growth and overweight of Navajo youth: secular changes from 1955 to 1997. Int J Obes Relat Metab Disord 2000;24(2):211–8.
53. Crawford PB, Story M, Wang MC, et al. Ethnic issues in the epidemiology of childhood obesity. Pediatr Clin North Am 2001;48(4):855–78.
54. Story M, Stevens J, Himes J, et al. Obesity in American-Indian children: prevalence, consequences, and prevention. Prev Med 2003;37(6 Pt 2):S3–12.
55. Partington MW, Roberts N. The heights and weights of Indian and Eskimo school children on James Bay and Hudson Bay. Can Med Assoc J 1969; 100(11):502–9.
56. Coodin FJ, Haworth JC, Sayed JE. Protein-energy malnutrition. Can Med Assoc J 1978;118(7):775.
57. Willows ND. Overweight in first nations children: prevalence, implications, and solutions. J Aboriginal Health 2005;2(1):76–86.
58. Willows ND, Johnson MS, Ball GD. Prevalence estimates of overweight and obesity in Cree preschool children in northern Quebec according to international and US reference criteria. Am J Public Health 2007;97(2):311–6.
59. Bryder L. New Zealand's Infant Welfare Services and Maori, 1907–60. Health History 2003;5(2):65–80.
60. Utter J, Scragg R, Schaaf D, et al. Correlates of body mass index among a nationally representative sample of New Zealand children. Int J Pediatr Obes 2007;2(2):104–13.
61. Goulding A, Grant AM, Taylor RW, et al. Ethnic differences in extreme obesity. J Pediatr 2007;151(5):542–4.
62. Ministry of Health. A portrait of health. Key results of the 2006/07 New Zealand health survey. Wellington: Ministry of Health; 2008.

63. Li SQ, Gutheridge SL, Tursan d' Espaignet E, et al. From infancy to young adult-hood: health status in the Northern Territory 2006. Darwin: Department of Health and Community Services; 2007.
64. Ruben AR, Walker AC. Malnutrition among rural aboriginal children in the top end of the Northern Territory. Med J Aust 1995;162(8):400–3.
65. Progress of the Northern Territory Emergency Response Child Health Check Initiative: Health Conditions and Referrals. Aboriginal and Torres Strait Islander Health and Welfare Unit, Australian Institute of Health and Welfare and Office for Aboriginal and Torres Strait Islander Health, Australian Government Depart-ment of Health and Ageing, 26 May 2008. 2008.
66. Cunningham J, Mackerras D. Occasional paper, overweight and obesity, Indig-enous Australians. Canberra (Australia): Australian Bureau of Statistics, ABS; 1994. Catalogue No. 4702.2.
67. O'Dea JA. Gender, ethnicity, culture and social class influences on child-hood obesity among Australian schoolchildren: implications for treatment, pre-vention and community education. Health Soc Care Community 2008;16(3): 282–90.
68. Lee AH, Gracey M, Wang K, et al. Under-nutrition affects time to recurrence of gastroenteritis among Aboriginal and non-Aboriginal children. J Health Popul Nutr 2006;24(1):17–24.
69. Morris PS. Randomised controlled trials addressing Australian aboriginal health needs: a systematic review of the literature. J Paediatr Child Health 1999;35(2): 130–5.
70. Brewster DR. Critical appraisal of the management of severe malnutrition: 1. Epidemiology and treatment guidelines. J Paediatr Child Health 2006;42(10): 568–74.
71. Wadsworth ME. Inequalities in child health. Arch Dis Child 1988;63(4):353–5.
72. McDonald EL, Jacobson MF, et al. Preventing growth faltering among Australian Indigenous children: implications for policy and practice. Med J Aust 2008; 188(8 Suppl):S84–6.
73. Brewster DR. Critical appraisal of the management of severe malnutrition: 4. Implications for Aboriginal child health in northern Australia. J Paediatr Child Health 2006;42(10):594–5.
74. Brewster DR. Critical appraisal of the management of severe malnutrition: 2. Dietary management. J Paediatr Child Health 2006;42(10):575–82.
75. Brewster DR. Critical appraisal of the management of severe malnutrition: 3. Complications. J Paediatr Child Health 2006;42(10):583–93.
76. Doak CM, Visscher TL, Renders CM, et al. The prevention of overweight and obesity in children and adolescents: a review of interventions and programmes. Obes Rev 2006;7(1):111–36.
77. Doak CM, Heitmann BM, Summerbell C, et al. Prevention of childhood obesity; what type of evidence should we consider relevant? Obes Rev 2009;10(3): 350–6.
78. Kamath CC, Vickers KS, Ehrlich A, et al. Clinical review: behavioral interventions to prevent childhood obesity: a systematic review and metaanalyses of random-ized trials. J Clin Endocrinol Metab 2008;93(12):4606–15.
79. Oude Luttikhuis H, Baur L, Jansen H, et al. Interventions for treating obesity in children. Cochrane Database Syst Rev 2009;(1):CD001872.
80. McGovern L, Johnson JN, Paulo R, et al. Clinical review: treatment of pediatric obesity: a systematic review and meta-analysis of randomized trials. J Clin En-docrinol Metab 2008;93(12):4600–5.

81. Love-Osborne K, Sheeder J, Zeitler P. Addition of metformin to a lifestyle modification program in adolescents with insulin resistance. J Pediatr 2008;152(6): 817–22.
82. Kirk S, Scott BJ, Daniels SR. Pediatric obesity epidemic: treatment options. J Am Diet Assoc 2005;105(5 Suppl 1):S44–51.
83. Colquitt J, Clegg A, Loveman E, et al. Surgery for morbid obesity. Cochrane Database Syst Rev 2005;(4):CD003641.
84. Buchwald H, Avidor Y, Braunwald E, et al. Bariatric surgery: a systematic review and meta-analysis. JAMA 2004;292(14):1724–37.
85. WHO Obesity: preventing and managing the global epidemic. Report of a WHO consultation. World Health Organ Tech Rep Ser 2000;894:i–xii, 1–253.
86. Nestle M, Jacobson MF. Halting the obesity epidemic: a public health policy approach. Public Health Rep 2000;115(1):12–24.
87. Reilly JJ. Obesity in childhood and adolescence: evidence based clinical and public health perspectives. Postgrad Med J 2006;82(969):429–37.
88. Reilly JJ, Wilson ML, Summerbell CD, et al. Obesity: diagnosis, prevention, and treatment; evidence based answers to common questions. Arch Dis Child 2002; 86(6):392–4.
89. Araujo CL, Victora CG, Hallal PC, et al. Breastfeeding and overweight in childhood: evidence from the Pelotas 1993 birth cohort study. Int J Obes (Lond) 2006;30(3):500–6.
90. Victora CG, Barros F, Lima RC, et al. Anthropometry and body composition of 18 year old men according to duration of breast feeding: birth cohort study from Brazil. BMJ 2003;327(7420):901.
91. Gillman MW, Rifas-Shiman SL, Camargo CA Jr, et al. Risk of overweight among adolescents who were breastfed as infants. JAMA 2001;285(19):2461–7.
92. Owen CG, Martin RM, Whincup PH, et al. The effect of breastfeeding on mean body mass index throughout life: a quantitative review of published and unpublished observational evidence. Am J Clin Nutr 2005;82(6): 1298–307.
93. Caballero B, Clay T, Davis SM, et al. Pathways: a school-based, randomized controlled trial for the prevention of obesity in American Indian schoolchildren. Am J Clin Nutr 2003;78(5):1030–8.
94. Gittelsohn J, Davis SM, Steckler A, et al. Pathways: lessons learned and future directions for school-based interventions among American Indians. Prev Med 2003;37(6 Pt 2):S107–12.
95. Summerbell CD, Ashton V, Campbell KJ, et al. Interventions for treating obesity in children. Cochrane Database Syst Rev 2003;(3):CD001872.
96. Padwal R, Li SK, Lau DC. Long-term pharmacotherapy for obesity and overweight. Cochrane Database Syst Rev 2004;(3):CD004094.
97. Maziak W, Ward KD, Stockton MB. Childhood obesity: are we missing the big picture? Obes Rev 2008;9(1):35–42.
98. Steele CB, Cardinez CJ, Richardson LC, et al. Surveillance for health behaviors of American Indians and Alaska Natives-findings from the behavioral risk factor surveillance system, 2000-2006. Cancer 2008;113(5 Suppl):1131–41.
99. Huhman M, Berkowitz JM, Wong FL, et al. The VERB campaign's strategy for reaching African-American, Hispanic, Asian, and American Indian children and parents. Am J Prev Med 2008;34(6 Suppl):S194–209.
100. DeLong AJ, Larson NI, Story M, et al. Factors associated with overweight among urban American Indian adolescents: findings from Project EAT. Ethn Dis 2008;18(3):317–23.

101. Adams AK, Harvey H, Brown D. Constructs of health and environment inform child obesity prevention in American Indian communities. Obesity (Silver Spring) 2008;16(2):311–7.

102. American Indian teens: project EAT for healthier living. Ethn Dis 2008;18(3):389.

103. LaRowe TL, Wubben DP, Cronin KA, et al. Development of a culturally appropriate, home-based nutrition and physical activity curriculum for Wisconsin American Indian families. Prev Chronic Dis 2007;4(4):A109.

104. Teufel-Shone NI. Promising strategies for obesity prevention and treatment within American Indian communities. J Transcult Nurs 2006;17(3):224–9.

105. Ng C, Marshall D, Willows ND. Obesity, adiposity, physical fitness and activity levels in Cree children. Int J Circumpolar Health 2006;65(4):322–30.

106. Saksvig BI, Gittelsohn J, Harris SB, et al. A pilot school-based healthy eating and physical activity intervention improves diet, food knowledge, and self-efficacy for native Canadian children. J Nutr 2005;135(10):2392–8.

107. Carrel A, Meinen A, Garry C, et al. Effects of nutrition education and exercise in obese children: the Ho-Chunk Youth Fitness Program. WMJ 2005;104(5):44–7.

108. Harnack L, Himes JH, Anliker J, et al. Intervention-related bias in reporting of food intake by fifth-grade children participating in an obesity prevention study. Am J Epidemiol 2004;160(11):1117–21.

109. Harvey-Berino J, Rourke J. Obesity prevention in preschool native-American children: a pilot study using home visiting. Obes Res 2003;11(5):606–11.

110. Thompson JL, Davis SM, Gittelsohn J, et al. Patterns of physical activity among American Indian children: an assessment of barriers and support. J Community Health 2001;26(6):423–45.

111. Story M, Stevens J, Evans M, et al. Weight loss attempts and attitudes toward body size, eating, and physical activity in American Indian children: relationship to weight status and gender. Obes Res 2001;9(6):356–63.

112. Harvey-Berino J, Wellman A, Hood V, et al. Preventing obesity in American Indian children: when to begin. J Am Diet Assoc 2000;100(5):564–6.

113. Hood DA, Elliott RB. A comparative study of the health of elite Maori and Caucasian children in Auckland. N Z Med J 1975;81(535):242–3.

114. Chang AB, Torzillo PJ, Boyce NC, et al. Zinc and vitamin A supplementation in Indigenous Australian children hospitalised with lower respiratory tract infection: a randomised controlled trial. Med J Aust 2006;184(3):107–12.

Lower Respiratory Tract Infections

Anne B. Chang, MBBS, FRACP, PhD[a,b,c,d,*],
Christina C. Chang, MBBS, FRACP[e], K. O'Grady, PhD[a],
P.J. Torzillo, MBBS, FRACP[f,g]

KEYWORDS

- Acute lower respiratory infection
- Indigenous/nonindigenous comparison
- Bronchiolitis • Pneumonia

BACKGROUND AND BURDEN OF DISEASE

Indigenous populations living in affluent countries bear a high burden of ill health from acute and chronic respiratory disease.[1–3] Acute lower respiratory infections (ALRIs) unfortunately remain a persistently dissonant health issue in Indigenous communities in developed countries. In Australia, ALRIs account for the greatest number of hospitalizations in young Indigenous children younger than 5 years and are the commonest cause of preventable deaths in infants.[4,5] In the period 2005 to 2006, the ALRI-associated hospitalization rate for Indigenous infants was 3.2 times more than that for non-Indigenous Australian infants (201.7/1000 vs 62.6/1000).[5] Although there are limited data from urban settings, the ALRI attack rate in Australian Aboriginal children is much higher in poor, remote populations. It is likely that poverty and remoteness are the key drivers rather than indigeneity itself. Hospitalization rates for respiratory infections in American Indian/Alaska Native (AI/AN) children in the United States

Work supported by Australian NHMRC grant 545216, Royal Children's Hospital Foundation, Brisbane and Queensland Smart State Funds.

[a] Child Health Division, Menzies School of Health Research, Charles Darwin University Darwin, Rocklands Drive, Tiwi, NT 0811, Australia

[b] Queensland Children's Respiratory Centre, Royal Children's Hospital, Herston, Brisbane, Queensland 4029, Australia

[c] Queensland Children's Medical Research Institute, Royal Children's Hospital, Herston Road, Herston 4029, Brisbane, Australia

[d] Poche Centre, University of Sydney, Camperdown, NSW 2006, Australia

[e] Department of Infectious Diseases, Alfred Hospital, Monash University, Commercial Road, Melbourne 3004, Australia

[f] Nganampa Health Council, Wilkinson Street, Alice Springs, NT 0871, Australia

[g] Royal Prince Alfred Hospital, University of Sydney, Missen Road, Camperdown, NSW 2050, Australia

* Corresponding author. Queensland Children's Respiratory Centre, Royal Children's Hospital, Herston, Brisbane, Queensland 4029, Australia.

E-mail address: annechang@ausdoctors.net (A.B. Chang)

were almost double that for the rest of the population (116.1/1000 vs 63.2/1000) from 1999 to 2001,[6] and ALRI has been formally identified by the American Academy of Pediatrics as one of the many remaining health disparities disadvantaging AI/AN communities.[7] ALRIs accounted for almost 75% of AI/AN infant infectious disease hospitalizations in the United States.[8] The same preponderance of ALRI in Indigenous children is also seen in New Zealand and Canada.[9,10]

The importance of acute respiratory illnesses is reflected not only in morbidity and mortality but also in long-term consequences, especially when recurrent. This article outlines the sequelae of ALRIs, preventative measures, and management of the 2 most common and important causes of ALRI, bronchiolitis and pneumonia, in Indigenous children. Readers are referred elsewhere for management of laryngo-tracheo-bronchitis (croup)[11] for which treatment is relatively simple through use of oral corticosteroids. Indigenous children do not have an increased incidence of croup, and the illness severity and management is similar to croup in non-Indigenous children.

CONSEQUENCES OF LOWER RESPIRATORY TRACT INFECTION IN INDIGENOUS CHILDREN

The antecedents of a substantial amount of chronic respiratory disease occur during early childhood.[12] Low birth weight and preexisting small lungs are important determinants of future lung function, and there is increasing evidence that pulmonary events in early life impact on adult pulmonary function.[13–16] Parenchymal lung growth in the first 2 years of life occurs by increasing alveoli number,[17] thus events such as severe ALRIs during this critical period may incur long-term negative effects leading to adult pulmonary dysfunction.[13,16] Indeed it has been shown that young Indigenous children with ALRIs are at risk of later respiratory morbidity.[18] Risk factors for bronchiectasis in Indigenous children include recurrent hospitalization for ALRIs and severity of previous ALRIs (measured by length of stay and requirement for oxygen during hospitalization).[19] In Alaskan children, previous bronchiolitis has been shown to be a risk factor for the development of chronic productive cough,[20] the most common symptom of chronic suppurative lung disease and bronchiectasis.[21] Infections by adenovirus, mycoplasma, and other respiratory viruses may also result in bronchiolitis obliterans, with or without bronchiectasis.[22]

PREVENTATIVE MEASURES FOR RESPIRATORY ILLNESSES

In addressing prevention of acute respiratory illness, the undeniable importance of the social determinants of health is recognized but cannot be adequately addressed here. Health is intertwined with every aspect of life: education, human rights, social justice, the environment, economy, and employment. Redressing health equity through action on the social determinants of health has been recently advocated by the World Health Organization (WHO).[23] A Canadian study on pneumonia and influenza identified that low education, being Aboriginal, behavioral factors (daily smoking and heavy drinking), environmental factors (passive smoking, poor housing, temperature), and health care factors (influenza vaccination) were all significantly associated with increased rates in different age- and gender-specific models.[24]

Specific (as opposed to socioeconomic-educational) primary prevention measures for respiratory disease are only briefly discussed here, and broadly categorized into (1) promoting normal lung development and (2) removing risk factors for development of respiratory disease. Both share common intervention features presented herein. These factors have limited randomized controlled trial (RCT) evidence, and it is highly unlikely such studies will ever be ethically performed. Nevertheless, it is recommended that the factors listed here are implemented for population health (Recommendation GRADE[25]: strong; Evidence: low to moderate).

- Avoidance of in utero and environmental tobacco smoke exposure. Tobacco smoke exposure is a major issue affecting Indigenous children.[3]
- Prevention of low birth weight infants and prematurity. Low birth weight babies are at greater risk of poor health and respiratory illnesses.[26] Contributors to low birth weight include socioeconomic disadvantage, size of parents, age of the mother, number of babies previously born, mother's nutritional status, smoking and alcohol intake, and illness during pregnancy.[5]
- Promotion of breast feeding (preferably exclusive for at least 4 months). Breast feeding has been recurrently shown to be a protective factor for acute respiratory infections and other illnesses.[27]
- Improvement in the living environment, particularly running water, overcrowding, and ventilation.[28,29]
- Appropriate and early treatment of respiratory infections including adequate follow-up, and detection of treatment failure and recurrent infections.
- Avoidance of biomass combustion (particularly indoor cooking fires) and other air pollutants that contribute to acute respiratory infections.[10]
- Promotion of improved nutrition and postnatal growth.
- Complete and timely immunizations, particularly that of yearly influenza vaccinations, for which uptake is currently poor despite being recommended in national guidelines in North America and Australia for children from 6 months of age.
- Improved parenting. Parenting moderates the effects of poverty and underclass status. Although no data exist on the effect of nurse home visiting programs on infectious diseases, parenting programs has been shown to improve birth weight, breast feeding, and hospitalization.[30,31] Preliminary studies in AI/AN populations using paraprofessionals described efficacy in improving maternal knowledge and infant behavior outcomes, thus suggesting parenting interventions may be useful in such communities.[32]

BRONCHIOLITIS
Background and Epidemiology

Bronchiolitis, the most common ALRI in young children,[33,34] is characterized by extensive inflammation of the airways accompanied by increased mucous production and necrosis of airway epithelial cells. Bronchiolitis is primarily caused by infection of the respiratory epithelial cells by viruses. Respiratory syncytial virus (RSV) is the major causative agent, but other viruses (eg, adenovirus, influenza, parainfluenza, human metapneumovirus, rhinovirus) and newly discovered viruses are also implicated. Bacteria such as *Simkania negevensis* (a *Chlamydia*-like microbe) has been implicated in Canadian Inuit infants.[35]

In pediatrics, bronchiolitis is a clinical diagnosis characterized by tachypnea, wheeze, or crepitations in infants following a preceding upper respiratory illness.[33] The upper age limit for a clinical diagnosis of bronchiolitis differs between countries; in Australia the upper limit accepted is usually 12 months, in the United States 24 months.[36] The clinical syndrome is nevertheless similar, as it is a clinical diagnosis based on typical history and examination findings, with no specific confirmatory or exclusionary diagnostic test or gold standard.[37]

The prevalence or severity of bronchiolitis is greater in Indigenous children than in non-Indigenous children in Australia, United States, Canada, and New Zealand.[26,27,38,39] In a regional Australian center, the bronchiolitis-associated hospitalization incidence in

Indigenous infants was 190 per 1000 infants.[40] Among United States Indigenous infants, the overall bronchiolitis-associated hospitalization rate was 61.8 per 1000 (in comparison, the 1995 rate among all United States infants was 34.2 per 1000).[38] Several studies have described being Indigenous as an independent risk factor for hospitalization from bronchiolitis,[26,27] but a retrospective Australian study found this did not hold in RSV hospitalizations, once socioeconomic risks factors were taken into account.[34] More consistently described sociodemographic and environmental risk factors for bronchiolitis include birth to a young mother, being born in the first half of the RSV season, tobacco exposure, lower maternal socioeconomic status, low birth weight, male gender, crowding, prematurity, chronic lung disease/congenital heart disease, and lack of breast feeding.[27,41]

Important Differences Between Bronchiolitis in Indigenous and Non-Indigenous Infants

In addition to the higher incidence of bronchiolitis in Indigenous infants, Indigenous children have higher rates of coexistent clinical pneumonia,[39] and negative postbronchiolitis consequences.[20] The former is thought to result from aspiration of nasal secretions[42] which, in these children, contains large bacterial load.[43] This load potentially overwhelms the local lung defenses (mucosal and innate immunity) already impaired by the viral infection.[44,45] In Indigenous children, bacterial (*Streptococcus pneumoniae*, nontypeable *Haemophilus influenzae*, *Moraxella catarrhalis*) colonization of the nasopharynx occurs earlier (as early 2 weeks of age) and heavier than in non-Indigenous children.[43,46] Some children are susceptible to bacterial infections during, or shortly after, a viral respiratory tract infection.[47] Viral-bacterial interactions are more likely to occur when the upper airway respiratory epithelium is densely colonized with respiratory pathogens or with repeated infections.[44] Australian Indigenous infants (24%) with bronchiolitis have a higher readmission rate for bronchiolitis within 6 months of discharge of the index infection than non-Indigenous infants (19%), but this difference is not statistically significant.[39]

Management of Bronchiolitis in Indigenous Children

The principles of managing bronchiolitis in Indigenous children are similar to that of the general population. Guidelines[11,33,48] are widely available, and key management issues when evaluating an infant with bronchiolitis are:

- Assessment of severity of illness (oxygen status, ability to feed, signs of respiratory distress, hydration status).
- Assessment of risks of increased severity and thus lower threshold for hospitalization.

The majority of children can be managed at home and asked to re-present if severity increases. Adoption of the following steps is recommended:

- Indications for hospitalization include pulse oximetry saturation (SpO_2) from 92% to 94%, poor feeding, dehydration, history of apnea, presence of moderate respiratory distress (chest recession, respiratory rate >70/min). (GRADE: high; Strength of evidence: moderate.)
- Other considerations for hospitalization include transportation difficulty, challenging social circumstances, pattern of illness (such as rapidity of illness severity), presence of significant comorbidity (chronic neonatal lung disease, prematurity, congenital heart disease). (GRADE: low; Strength of evidence: low.)

- Oxygen therapy when SpO$_2$ is less than 93% with respiratory distress. (GRADE: high; Strength of evidence: moderate.) It is uncertain at what exact SaO$_2$ supplemental oxygen should be initiated, and guidelines vary between 90% and 94%. Initiation and weaning of oxygen should take into account the clinical context including degree of respiratory distress, presence of comorbidity, feeding difficulty, apnea, and oxygen availability.
- Nasogastric feeds or intravenous fluids should be implemented when the child is dehydrated, safe oral feeding cannot be maintained, or risk of aspiration is high. (GRADE: high; Strength of evidence: low.)
- Nebulized hypertonic (3%) saline should be considered as it may reduce the length of hospital stay and improve the clinical severity.[49] (GRADE: high; Strength of evidence: high.)
- Bronchodilators (α-adrenergic or β-adrenergic agents, ipratropium) and corticosteroids should not be used routinely.[50,51] (GRADE: weak; Strength of evidence: moderate.)

Inhaled bronchodilators may be tried under close monitoring in selected individuals such as those with recurrent wheeze, a family history of asthma, or previous response to bronchodilators. A Cochrane review found a transient improvement in clinical score may occur in some children treated with bronchodilators, but the clinical relevance is unclear.[50] A recent trial described reduction in hospitalization in those receiving nebulized adrenaline combined with oral dexamethasone (1 mg/kg on day 1 followed by 0.6 mg/kg daily for 5 days).[52] Potential side effects should also be considered.

- Chest physiotherapy should not be used as it increases morbidity.[53] (GRADE: strong; Strength of evidence: moderate.)
- Corticosteroids[54] or leukotriene receptor antagonists[55] do not influence the presence of postbronchiolitis symptoms and should not be routinely used. (GRADE: strong; Strength of evidence: moderate to low.)
- Use of palizumab and infection control measures are well described.[33,48] The application of these are similar in both Indigenous and non-Indigenous infants, and thus is not discussed here.

Additional management considerations in Indigenous children are:

- Antibiotics are not routinely recommended in bronchiolitis but may be used in Indigenous children suspected of concomitant bacterial pneumonia. Further, it is often difficult to establish a diagnosis of pneumonia in a child with bronchiolitis. Antibiotic use should be guided by local resistance patterns of common pathogens.[33,56] (GRADE: weak; Strength of evidence: low).
- Chest radiographs, not generally recommended in bronchiolitis, may be considered in Indigenous children specifically when bronchiolitis is recurrent or pneumonia suspected. (GRADE: weak; Strength of evidence: low.)
- Indigenous children should be reviewed post episode to ensure symptoms resolve for risk of chronic wet cough and readmission risk.[20,39]

PNEUMONIA
Background and Epidemiology

Pneumonia kills more children globally than AIDS, malaria, and measles combined, yet little attention is given to pneumonia.[57] Over 2 million children die each year from pneumonia worldwide.[57] Pneumonia in Indigenous children occurs in various contexts for example, community, hospital acquired, immunodeficient children, and so forth, and the management differs in these different settings. This article is restricted to community-acquired pneumonia (CAP) in otherwise healthy children older than 2 months. Children with immunodeficiency (congenital or acquired) and those with specific predisposition to pneumonia such as sickle cell anemia, human immunodeficiency virus (HIV), and malaria are not discussed here. Infants aged 2 months or younger with pneumonia require hospitalization[58] and often have a different etiology, and thus are also not discussed in this article. Tuberculosis, an important infection in Indigenous populations, is also not described here, and readers are referred to other sources.[59]

Estimates of pneumonia incidence vary depending on definition. Clinical definitions, developed in the 1970s for use in resource poor countries,[60] were primarily aimed at determining which children presenting with breathing problems required antibiotics. Subsequent research has aimed at refining these algorithms and improving their sensitivity and specificity.[61] More recently the WHO established a radiological definition[62] primarily for research purposes, in particular to measure the impact of vaccine trials on pneumonia outcomes, which has limited clinical use. Clinical definitions remain important in CAP not requiring hospitalization (for which chest radiographs and investigations are not routinely recommended),[63] as well as in remote Indigenous populations for whom management is dependent on algorithms, as it is in many regions of resource-poor countries. In this article, for practicality the authors define pneumonia based on clinical symptoms and signs (**Box 1**).

Despite these constraints of definition there is substantial evidence that the burden of pneumonia is high in Indigenous populations. Studies from the late 1980s documented extremely high rates of invasive pneumococcal disease (and high rates of pneumonia) in American Indian and remote Australian Aboriginal children.[64,65] Hospitalization rates for AI/AN infants with pneumonia in the United States were 54.7 per 1000 children in the period 1999 to 2001 and, while trending downwards,[6] remain a major health disparity for AI/AN communities.[7] In New Zealand, Maori children hospitalized with pneumonia

---

Box 1
Definitions used for pneumonia

Clinical definition of pneumonia

Symptoms: Fever (>38.5 axilla) and cough or difficult breathing; and,

Signs: breathing >50/min for infants age 2 months up to 1 year; breathing >40/min for children age 1 to 5 years.

In resource-poor settings, pneumonia is diagnosed (WHO guidelines), based only on cough and tachypnea, that is, although fever is often present it is not an essential requirement for administration of antibiotics.

Definitions of severity

Nonsevere pneumonia: Symptoms and signs of pneumonia plus no chest indrawing, grunting, or "danger signs."

Severe pneumonia: Difficult breathing, plus any general danger sign or chest indrawing or grunting in a calm child.

"Danger signs" for children age 2 months to 5 years: Unable to drink or breastfeed, vomiting, convulsions, lethargy, or unconsciousness.

Data from Pneumonia the forgotten killer of children. 2006. Geneva: The United Nations Children's Fund (UNICEF)/World Health Organization (WHO); 2006; BTS guidelines for the management of community acquired pneumonia in childhood. Thorax 2002;57(Suppl 1):I1–I24.

have more severe pneumonia than children of European descent,[66] and double the annual hospitalization rate at 6.7 versus 2.7 per 1000.[9] Western Australian Indigenous children younger than 2 years had a 13.5 times increased risk of hospitalization for pneumonia in the period 1990 to 2000.[67] In Newfoundland and Labrador, Canada, the hospitalization rate due to pneumonia for the Innu/Inuit communities was 11.6 compared with 3.0 per 1000 population for non-Aboriginal communities, with infants bearing the highest rates (93.4 per 1000 population).[68] Other Canadian studies have also reported increased rates (3.6 to 5 times) of CAP and ALRI in Indigenous Canadians of other regions compared with non-Indigenous Canadians.[68]

Etiology of Pneumonia

Establishing the causative pathogen(s) in pneumonia remains a major challenge, due predominantly to the great variation in sensitivity and specificity of different tests for bacteria and viruses. Blood cultures have low sensitivity in pneumonia, especially when antibiotics have already been administered. Lung aspirates are rarely done because of concern about complications. Sputum examination is particularly difficult in children and contamination by upper airway colonization makes interpretation problematic. Antigen detection techniques for pneumococcus are improving, but their utility in populations with dense bacterial colonization of the nasopharynx has not been established. Viral detection is difficult to interpret because high rates are reported in asymptomatic children.[69] In addition, existing data on etiology are dominated by hospital-based populations with severe disease. The impact of vaccines on reducing pneumonia burden suggest that *S. pneumoniae* is a leading cause of childhood pneumonia in Indigenous children, as it is in developing countries.[64,65] *H. influenzae* type b, a previous major cause of pneumonia in developing countries, has been reduced by immunization. Non-serotypeable *H. influenzae* may be an important pathogen in these populations, but the evidence is very limited. *Staphylococcus aureus* is also an important but less frequently identified organism; community-acquired multiresistant *S. aureus* resulting in a necrotizing fulminant pneumonia has emerged,[70] and is of particular concern for the spread in indigenous communities with poor living conditions. Viral agents include RSV, adenovirus, parainfluenza virus, rhinovirus, influenza virus, human bocavirus, and human metapneumovirus.[71] Some pathogenic agents of pneumonia are age related; mycoplasma is more common in older children whereas viral agents predominate in the very young.[63] Some studies suggest that viral etiologies are more likely in the presence of wheeze.[63] Mixed infections are also commonly reported[62,72,73] and viral-bacterial coinfections are likely to be more important in Indigenous children, as described earlier. A study of Aboriginal children with ALRI in Central Australia found 48% of cases had evidence of an acute viral infection.[73] In a recent Brazilian study[72] using sensitive diagnostic methods, 23% of the 143 children with CAP had mixed viral-bacterial infection.

Important Differences Between Pneumonia in Indigenous and Non-Indigenous Children

In addition to the increased rates to pneumonia and ALRI, Indigenous children have an increased frequency of repeated hospitalizations for pneumonia and development of chronic suppurative lung disease,[18,74] increased likelihood of coinfection or viral-bacterial interactions (speculated rather then proven), and differential impact of routine vaccinations.[75,76] In Australia, New Zealand, and the United States, repeated pneumonias in Indigenous children have been described and linked with the development of bronchiectasis.[74,77,78] Western Australian children born between 1990 and 2000 were 3 times more likely than other children to have multiple admissions for pneumonia.[67]

Routine conjugate pneumococcal and *H. influenzae* type b (Hib) vaccinations have reduced invasive disease related to these organisms in Indigenous and non-Indigenous children.[75,76,79] However, despite high rates of Hib vaccine coverage, *H influenzae* type b disease rates among rural Alaskan Native children younger than 5 years remains higher than in non-Native Alaskan and other United States children.[75] In the circumpolar region, serotype replacement with nonvaccine serotypes has resulted in a reemergence of invasive disease for both *Haemophilus* and pneumococcal infection.[76,79] A study in American Indian children described a substantial reduction in invasive pneumococcal disease from conjugate pneumococcal vaccine.[80] However, in the Alaskan Yukon Delta, while the use of palivizumab prophylaxis may be responsible for a decrease in the RSV hospitalization rate among premature infants, non-RSV pneumonia hospitalizations have not declined since the introduction of the pneumococcal conjugate vaccine (PCV).[81] Despite evidence of decreased pneumonia rates in the United States and other developed countries after introduction of PCV, at present, the long-term effect of PCV on pneumonia rates in Indigenous populations remain uncertain.

Management

In Indigenous children the determinants of management are primarily remoteness, availability of medical resources, ease of access to hospital, and family resources rather than indigeneity alone. In regions with developed country resources, most children with CAP can be managed in the community, and the role of the community doctor includes[63]:

(a) to identify that the child has pneumonia;
(b) to assess the severity and select those who require referral to a hospital or evacuation from a remote site;
(c) to provide information/management advice on temperature control and fluids;
(d) to identify and provide medical treatment where necessary; and
(e) to monitor progress and follow-up.

Assessment

In the management of pneumonia, the priorities include early recognition of a sick child and seeking appropriate care. Only about 20% of caregivers in developing countries recognize difficult or fast breathing as signs of pneumonia, and only about half of the children with pneumonia are taken to an appropriate provider.[57] Poorer children, rural children, and children with poorly educated mothers more often lack appropriate care.[57] These findings from developing countries are likely to be particularly relevant to Indigenous children in remote locations. Thus, education of caregivers on the "danger signs" of a sick child may be an important part of the community approach to the reduction of mortality and morbidity from pneumonia.

The Integrated Management of Childhood Illness (IMCI),[82] which includes that of pneumonia, developed by the WHO, is a broad strategy that includes several complementary interventions at first-level health facilities and in communities. This case management approach has been shown to reduce pneumonia mortality in a meta-analysis.[83] In remote regions of developed countries, without radiography or laboratory facilities, an adapted IMCI approach may be useful. An important example of adapting IMCI is in the assessment of severity of pneumonia (see **Box 1**). Detection of hypoxemia is an important component of the assessment and part of a case management strategy. No single clinical sign best predicts presence of hypoxia, and in resource-poor settings this is best predicted by a combination of signs including respiratory rate (>40/min when age 2–11 months, >50/min age 12–59 months), inability to feed, altered mental status, central cyanosis, and head nodding.[84] In developed countries portable pulse oximeters allow accurate assessment of oxygenation. However, these signs are indicative of the severity of pneumonia.

Treatment

Antibiotics In principle, knowledge of local resistance patterns should assist in the choice of empiric and directed antibiotic therapy (summarized in **Table 1**). Narrow-spectrum antibiotics should be used wherever possible. In general, amoxycillin is the preferred initial antimicrobial of choice in nonsevere pneumonia; 3 to 5 days of amoxycillin therapy (50 mg/kg/d in 2 divided doses) should be used in children age 2 months up to 5 years.[58,63] Other original studies, however, used higher doses (80–90 mg/kg/d).[101] Thus the authors recommend between 50 and 90 mg/kg/d in 2 doses. Although some studies have recommended that children with wheeze should not receive antibiotics,[93] a recent multicenter placebo-controlled RCT in 1671 children younger than 5 years showed that children randomized to placebo (compared with amoxycillin) had higher morbidity and clinical failure (adjusted odds ratio = 1.28).[94] The choice of alternatives to amoxycillin should be guided by activity against *S. pneumoniae* and *H. influenzae* as well as safety. In developing countries, cotrimoxazole has been widely used but its use is driven strongly by cost advantage. The majority of studies have been performed in children younger than 5 years, and there is little high-grade evidence for older children (see **Table 1**).

Short courses (3 days) of antibiotics have been shown to be as efficacious as 5 days.[86] A problem with these studies is that adequate follow-up was not performed with respect to risk of symptoms of bronchiectasis such as chronic wet cough. The studies were not primarily designed for equivalence in current standards whereby the noninferiority margin for outcomes is prespecified.[102] In children older than 5 years, erythromycin is an alternative first-dose antibiotic treatment in view of increasing rates of *Mycoplasma* pneumonia.[63]

When pneumonia is severe and hospital referral not possible, intramuscular penicillin is recommended for treatment of severe pneumonia. When injection is not available, high-dose oral amoxycillin could be given to children with severe pneumonia.[101] Children with very severe pneumonia should receive injectable ampicillin plus gentamicin,[103] although some centers prefer ceftriaxone, which has not been examined in a similar way to ampicillin and gentamicin. Complications of pneumonia are increasingly described; these include parapneumonic effusions, empyema, bronchiolitis obliterans, among others. All these complications require hospital management, which is beyond the scope of this article.

Oxygen Oxygen therapy is beneficial in reducing mortality in hypoxic children[84] and should be used when the SpO_2 is 92% or less.[63] Any child requiring oxygen should be transferred to a hospital. While awaiting transfer, oxygen is routinely best delivered by nasal prongs and any child requiring more than 1.5 L/min requires an alternative delivery mechanism such as a face mask.

Other therapies Children with wheeze and fast breathing or lower chest in-drawing should be given a trial of rapid-acting inhaled bronchodilator before they are classified as pneumonia and prescribed antibiotics.[93] However, if coexistent symptoms and signs of pneumonia are present, amoxycillin should be given.[94] Adjunctive measures include provision of adequate nutrition, micronutrient supplements, and antipyretics when appropriate. Signs of malnutrition should be addressed in all children, as this increases the risk of death due to pneumonia. Children with CAP should continue feeding. Those unable to feed, have persistent vomiting, or are dehydrated require

Table 1
Recommendations for the clinical management of acute pneumonia in Indigenous children

'Intervention'	Recommendation	Recommendation Grade[25]	Quality of Supporting Evidence[85]
General			
Case management	Use a case management strategy (see text)	Strong	High[83]
Assessment of severity	Assess severity of pneumonia using respiratory rate, presence of chest in-drawing, SpO_2, ability to feed	Strong	Moderate[57,63]
Transfer to hospital	Child should be admitted into hospital if: • Hypoxic: $SpO_2 \leq 92\%$ • Severe pneumonia symptoms/sign present; OR • Family is unable to supervise or observe sick child • Significant comorbidities present	Strong	Moderate to high[63]
Community management for nonsevere pneumonia			
Antibiotics	<5 years • First line: amoxycillin (50–90 mg/kg/d in 2 doses) for 3–5 days • Alternative: cefaclor	Strong Weak	High[86,87] Low
	5 years and over: • First line: amoxycillin (50–90 mg/kg/d in 2 doses) for 3–5 d or erythromycin or a macrolide • Alternative: cefaclor	Weak Weak	Low Low
Antibiotics if fails to improve	If persistent tachypnea, consider transfer to hospital for alternative diagnosis. However if pneumonia present and no indications for hospitalization, use amoxil-clavulanic acid (80–90 mg/kg/d in 2 doses) or add erythromycin or a macrolide	Weak	Low
Oxygen	Use oxygen if SpO_2 is $\leq92\%$ and transfer child to hospital	Strong	Moderate[63]
Feeding and fluids	Feeding should be continued unless there is a risk of aspiration Fluid intake should be maintained but not increased	Strong Weak	Low Low[88]
Micronutrients			
Zinc	Not recommended for universal use	Strong	Moderate[89]

Vitamin A	Not recommended for nonmeasles pneumonia	Strong	High[90,91]
Vitamin C	Not recommended for universal use	Weak	Moderate[92]
Any	For all micronutrients, their use may be considered if malnutrition present, or deficiency of micronutrients suspected	Weak	Low
Bronchodilators	Use salbutamol as a trial (600 µg) if wheeze is present	Weak	Low[93]
	Consider adding amoxycillin even if wheeze is present or if symptoms and signs of pneumonia coexist	Weak	Moderate[94]
Antipyretics	Antipyretics are not routinely recommended unless there are additional reasons (pain, discomfort from fever, risk of febrile seizures, etc). However if tachypnea is significant, antipyretics can reduce tachypnea from fever and thus should be considered	Weak	Low
Antivirals	Consider influenza viral therapies in children with proven influenza pneumonia	Weak	Moderate[95,96]
Radiology	Routine CXR is not universally indicated in mild pneumonia	Weak	Moderate[97]
	Perform CXR if recurrent pneumonia	Weak	Moderate[18]
Chest physiotherapy	Chest physiotherapy is not recommended	Strong	High[98]
Blood tests	Routine blood tests for mild pneumonia are not recommended	Weak	Low
Follow-up of progress			
Clinical	Review the child at 24 and 48 hours, and assess for improvement or deterioration (hospitalize if indications present)	Strong	Low
	Review child at 5–7 d or until total resolution of symptoms	Strong	Moderate[18]
Radiological	Routine follow-up radiograph is not universally indicated.	Weak	Low
	Follow-up radiograph is recommended for those with recurrent pneumonia	Strong	Moderate[18,99]
Further investigations	Refer children with persistent symptoms and/or abnormal radiological features for further investigation to evaluate for an underlying respiratory problem	Strong	Moderate[18,100]
Preventative factors	Review for presence of risk factors and implement preventative measures such as vaccination (see text for preventative factors)	Strong	(see text)

Management in the hospital is discussed in the text.
Abbreviation: CXR, chest radiograph.

hospitalization.[63] Intake of fluids should be maintained but not increased.[88] Micronutrient supplementation in children without evidence of deficiency is not recommended.[89,90,92] Chest physiotherapy in the acute period is not recommended. As an adjunctive treatment to standard care, chest physiotherapy does not hasten clinical resolution of children hospitalized with acute pneumonia, and may prolong duration of coughing and rhonchi.[98] Specific antiviral agents (such as neuraminidase inhibitors and rimantadine for influenza) are available, and have been shown to reduce the mean duration of illness.[95] However, their cost and benefit ratios are yet to be determined.

Review Children started on antibiotics require daily review. Treatment failure is defined in IMCI as the development of lower chest-wall in-drawing, central cyanosis, grunting while calm, any "danger signs," or a persistently raised respiratory rate at 72 hours (48 hours in an area of high HIV prevalence). In developed countries these signs would mandate urgent referral and assessment in hospital. Treatment failure may be due to a range of problems, which include poor adherence, development of complication such as empyema, and wrong diagnosis (eg, asthma or tuberculosis). It is important that treatment failure in this setting is not assumed to mean that antibiotic resistance is the mechanism. However, it is likely in this setting that alternative antimicrobials will be introduced with hospital admission; especially for older children macrolides may be added to cover the possibility of mycoplasma, chlamydia, or possibly legionella.

Hospital management Standardized hospitalized management is recommended, and readers are referred to the British Thoracic Society (BTS) guidelines for the evidence.[63]

- Choose antibiotics in accordance with age and local drug susceptibility data. Oxygen should be utilized in those with hypoxemia to maintain SpO_2 92% or greater. Those unable to maintain oxygenation with supplemental oxygen require transfer to intensive care. (GRADE: strong; Strength of evidence: moderate.)
- Continue feeding child unless there is persistent vomiting or risk of aspiration with severe tachypnea or dyspnea. Intravenous fluids may be required in those who are dehydrated or who are unable to feed. If intravenous fluids are required, use 80% maintenance unless dehydrated.[63] (GRADE: strong; Strength of evidence: moderate to low.)
- Obtain standard tests (chest radiograph, blood cultures, nasopharyngeal aspirate, full blood count, electrolytes). The evidence for this is low but it is recommended that these standard tests are performed in those severe enough to require hospitalization. (GRADE: strong; Strength of evidence: low.)
- Chest physiotherapy is not recommended. (GRADE: strong; Strength of evidence: high.[98])
- Children requiring oxygen therapy should be regularly monitored (continuously if very severe, minimum 4 hourly). (GRADE: strong; Strength of evidence: low.)
- Children who fail to respond (persistent fever or symptoms/signs) require evaluation for complications of pneumonia (eg, empyema, pleural effusion). (GRADE: strong; Strength of evidence: low.)
- As noted in the management of CAP, routine use of micronutrients is not recommended.
- Preventative measures for pneumonia should be explored and attended to (see earlier discussion).

Follow-up All children with pneumonia require regular review until all symptoms and signs resolve. Children with repeated episodes of lower respiratory infections or persistent symptoms should raise consideration of an underlying predisposing

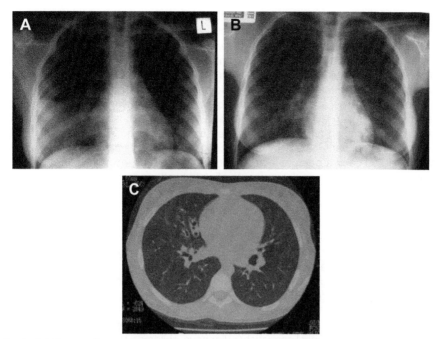

Fig. 1. (*A*) Chest radiograph of a child who presented with acute pneumonia, showing lobar pneumonia in the right middle and lower lobes. Additionally the left lower lobe has abnormal markings. (*B*) Follow-up chest radiograph of the child 2 months after hospitalization for the pneumonia episode. (*C*) High-resolution computed tomography scan of the child, showing right middle lobe bronchiectasis 3 months after the pneumonia episode described in *A*. The child also had left lower lobe bronchiectasis (not shown).

medical condition such as bronchiectasis, and congenital or acquired immunodeficiency states. Given the known increased incidence of bronchiectasis in Indigenous children in Australia,[74] New Zealand,[77] and the United States,[78] it is strongly recommended that all children with pneumonia are followed until all symptoms (especially wet cough) resolve. In some children, pneumonia may be the first presentations of an underlying chronic lung disease such as bronchiectasis (**Fig. 1**A–C). Untreated protracted bacterial bronchitis is likely a precursor to chronic suppurative lung disease and bronchiectasis.[21]

In general, there is no consensus on the use of follow-up chest radiography in children with pneumonia, although it is recommended for children with lobar pneumonia.[63] A small study demonstrated that predischarge chest radiographs were predictive of chronic respiratory morbidity when they showed no or minimal resolution.[18] Radiological features predictive of future bronchiectasis include persistent atelectasis, parenchymal densities, and linear markings on multiple episodes.[18,100] Finally, follow-up of the illness episode should be taken as an opportunity to counsel the family on key prevention issues and aspects of general child health.

SUMMARY

Bronchiolitis and pneumonia account for the majority of the ALRI burden in young children. These diseases are indicators of the socioeconomic and health disparities that persist between Indigenous and non-Indigenous children in developed countries. RSV is the major causative agent of bronchiolitis, and *S. pneumoniae* and *H. influenzae* are important etiological agents in pneumonia. Coinfection and concomitant clinical syndromes in Indigenous children are common.

The early detection, diagnosis, and management of these diseases in Indigenous children are critical to improving outcomes and to minimizing the consequent development of bronchiectasis and other chronic lung disorders. The prevention of repeat infections should be a clinical and public health priority. Ongoing surveillance of disease and regular review of management guidelines is critical, given increasing concerns surrounding antibiotic resistance and the changing epidemiology of both viral and bacterial pathogens. Any measures to reduce the burden of disease in Indigenous children cannot operate independently of the social, economic, and environmental factors that are key determinants of child health in these populations.

REFERENCES

1. Australian Health Ministers' Advisory Council 2. Aboriginal and Torres Strait Islander Health Performance Framework report. Canberra: AHMAC; 2008.
2. Estey EA, Kmetic AM, Reading J. Innovative approaches in public health research: applying life course epidemiology to aboriginal health research. Can J Public Health 2007;98:444–6.
3. Smylie J, Adomako P, editors. Indigenous children's health report. Available at: http://www.stmichaelshospital.com/crich/indigenous_childrens_health_report.php; 2009. Accessed April 22, 2009.
4. Li SQ, Guthridge SL, d'Espaignet ET, et al. From infancy to young adulthood: health status in the Northern Territory 2006. Darwin: Department of Health and Community Services; 2007.
5. ABS. The health and welfare of Australia's Aboriginal and Torres Strait Islander Peoples. Canberra: Australian Bureau of Statistics; 2008. ABS Catalogue No. 4704.0.
6. Peck AJ, Holman RC, Curns AT, et al. Lower respiratory tract infections among American Indian and Alaska native children and the general population of U.S. Children. Pediatr Infect Dis J 2005;24:342–51.
7. Brenneman G, Rhoades E, Chilton L. Forty years in partnership: the American Academy of Pediatrics and the Indian Health Service. Pediatrics 2006;118: e1257–63.
8. Holman RC, Curns AT, Cheek JE, et al. Infectious disease hospitalizations among American Indian and Alaska native infants. Pediatrics 2003;111: E176–82.
9. Grant CC, Scragg R, Tan D, et al. Hospitalization for pneumonia in children in Auckland, New Zealand. J Paediatr Child Health 1998;34:355–9.
10. Kovesi T, Gilbert NL, Stocco C, et al. Indoor air quality and the risk of lower respiratory tract infections in young Canadian Inuit children. CMAJ 2007;177:155–60.
11. Everard ML. Acute bronchiolitis and croup. Pediatr Clin North Am 2009;56: 119–33.
12. Galobardes B, McCarron P, Jeffreys M, et al. Medical history of respiratory disease in early life relates to morbidity and mortality in adulthood. Thorax 2008;63:423–9.
13. Tennant PWG, Gibson JG, Pearce MS. Lifecourse predictors of adult respiratory function: results from the Newcastle Thousand Families Study. Thorax 2008;63: 823–30.

14. Maritz G, Probyn M, De MR, et al. Lung parenchyma at maturity is influenced by postnatal growth but not by moderate preterm birth in sheep. Neonatology 2008; 93:28–35.
15. Snibson K, Harding R. Postnatal growth rate, but not mild preterm birth, influences airway structure in adult sheep challenged with house dust mite. Exp Lung Res 2008;34:69–84.
16. Dharmage SC, Erbas B, Jarvis D, et al. Do childhood respiratory infections continue to influence adult respiratory morbidity? Eur Respir J 2009;33:237–44.
17. Balinotti JE, Tiller CJ, Llapur CJ, et al. Growth of the lung parenchyma early in life. Am J Respir Crit Care Med 2009;179:134–7.
18. Chang AB, Masel JP, Boyce NC, et al. Respiratory morbidity in central Australian Aboriginal children with alveolar lobar abnormalities. Med J Aust 2003;178: 490–4.
19. Valery PC, Torzillo PJ, Mulholland EK, et al. A hospital-based case-control study of bronchiectasis in Indigenous children in Central Australia. Pediatr Infect Dis J 2004;23:902–8.
20. Singleton RJ, Redding GJ, Lewis TC, et al. Sequelae of severe respiratory syncytial virus infection in infancy and early childhood among Alaska Native children. Pediatrics 2003;112:285–90.
21. Chang AB, Redding GJ, Everard ML. Chronic wet cough: protracted bronchitis, chronic suppurative lung disease and bronchiectasis. Pediatr Pulmonol 2008; 43:519–31.
22. Chang AB, Masel JP, Masters B. Post-infectious bronchiolitis obliterans: clinical, radiological and pulmonary function sequelae. Pediatr Radiol 1998;28:23–9.
23. CSDH. Closing the gap in a generation: health equity through action on the social determinants of health. Final report of the Commission on Social Determinants of Health. Geneva: World Health Organization; 2008.
24. Crighton EJ, Elliott SJ, Moineddin R, et al. A spatial analysis of the determinants of pneumonia and influenza hospitalizations in Ontario (1992–2001). Soc Sci Med 2007;64:1636–50.
25. Guyatt GH, Oxman AD, Kunz R, et al. Going from evidence to recommendations. BMJ 2008;336:1049–51.
26. Grimwood K, Cohet C, Rich FJ, et al. Risk factors for respiratory syncytial virus bronchiolitis hospital admission in New Zealand. Epidemiol Infect 2008;136:1333–41.
27. Koehoorn M, Karr CJ, Demers PA, et al. Descriptive epidemiological features of bronchiolitis in a population-based cohort. Pediatrics 2008;122:1196–203.
28. Torzillo PJ, Pholeros P. Household infrastructure in Aboriginal communities and the implications for health improvement. Med J Aust 2002;176:502–3.
29. Hennessy TW, Ritter T, Holman RC, et al. The relationship between in-home water service and the risk of respiratory tract, skin, and gastrointestinal tract infections among rural Alaska natives. Am J Public Health 2008;98:2072–8.
30. Bennett C, Macdonald GM, Dennis J, et al. Home-based support for disadvantaged adult mothers. Cochrane Database Syst Rev 2007;(3):CD003759.
31. Olds DL, Kitzman H, Hanks C, et al. Effects of nurse home visiting on maternal and child functioning: age-9 follow-up of a randomized trial. Pediatrics 2007; 120:e832–45.
32. Walkup JT, Barlow A, Mullany BC, et al. Randomized controlled trial of a paraprofessional-delivered in-home intervention for young reservation-based American Indian mothers. J Am Acad Child Adolesc Psychiatry 2009;48:591–601.
33. Subcommittee on Diagnosis and Management of Bronchiolitis. Diagnosis and management of bronchiolitis. Pediatrics 2006;118:1774–93.

34. Reeve CA, Whitehall JS, Buettner PG, et al. Predicting respiratory syncytial virus hospitalisation in Australian children. J Paediatr Child Health 2006;42:248–52.

35. Greenberg D, Banerji A, Friedman MG, et al. High rate of Simkania negevensis among Canadian Inuit infants hospitalized with lower respiratory tract infections. Scand J Infect Dis 2003;35:506–8.

36. Calogero C, Sly PD. Acute viral bronchiolitis: to treat or not to treat-that is the question. J Pediatr 2007;151:235–7.

37. Bordley WC, Viswanathan M, King VJ, et al. Diagnosis and testing in bronchiolitis: a systematic review. Arch Pediatr Adolesc Med 2004;158:119–26.

38. Lowther SA, Shay DK, Holman RC, et al. Bronchiolitis-associated hospitalizations among American Indian and Alaska Native children. Pediatr Infect Dis J 2000;19:11–7.

39. Bailey EJ, Maclennan C, Morris PS, et al. Risks of severity and readmission of Indigenous and non-Indigenous children hospitalised for bronchiolitis. J Paediatr Child Health 2009 Sep 14 [Epub ahead of print].

40. Bolisetty S, Wheaton G, Chang AB. Respiratory syncytial virus infection and immunoprophylaxis for selected high-risk children in Central Australia. Aust J Rural Health 2005;13:265–70.

41. Bulkow LR, Singleton RJ, Karron RA, et al. Risk factors for severe respiratory syncytial virus infection among Alaska native children. Pediatrics 2002;109: 210–6.

42. Thach BT. Some aspects of clinical relevance in the maturation of respiratory control in infants. J Appl Physiol 2008;104:1828–34.

43. Stubbs E, Hare K, Wilson C, et al. *Streptococcus pneumoniae* and noncapsular *Haemophilus influenzae* nasal carriage and hand contamination in children: a comparison of two populations at risk of otitis media. Pediatr Infect Dis J 2005;24:423–8.

44. Didierlaurent A, Goulding J, Hussell T. The impact of successive infections on the lung microenvironment. Immunology 2007;122:457–65.

45. Didierlaurent A, Goulding J, Patel S, et al. Sustained desensitization to bacterial Toll-like receptor ligands after resolution of respiratory influenza infection. J Exp Med 2008;205:323–9.

46. Leach AJ, Boswell JB, Asche V, et al. Bacterial colonization of the nasopharynx predicts very early onset and persistence of otitis media in Australian aboriginal infants. Pediatr Infect Dis J 1994;13:983–9.

47. Pettigrew MM, Gent JF, Revai K, et al. Microbial interactions during upper respiratory tract infections. Emerg Infect Dis 2008;14:1584–91.

48. Baumer JH. SIGN guideline on bronchiolitis in infants. Arch Dis Child Educ Pract Ed 2007;92:ep149–51.

49. Zhang L, Mendoza-Sassi RA, Wainwright C, et al. Nebulized hypertonic saline solution for acute bronchiolitis in infants. Cochrane Database Syst Rev 2008;(4):CD006458.

50. Gadomski A, Bhasale A. Bronchodilators for bronchiolitis. Cochrane Database Syst Rev 2006;(3):CD001266.

51. Hartling L, Wiebe N, Russell KF, et al. Epinephrine for bronchiolitis. Cochrane Database Syst Rev 2004;(1):CD003123.

52. Plint AC, Johnson DW, Patel H, et al. Epinephrine and dexamethasone in children with bronchiolitis. N Engl J Med 2009;360:2079–89.

53. Perrotta C, Ortiz Z, Figuls M. Chest physiotherapy for acute bronchiolitis in paediatric patients between 0 and 24 months old. Cochrane Database Syst Rev 2007;(1):CD004873.

54. Blom-Danielle JM, Ermers M, Bont L, et al. Inhaled corticosteroids during acute bronchiolitis in the prevention of post-bronchiolitic wheezing. Cochrane Database Syst Rev 2007;(1):CD004881.
55. Bisgaard H, Flores-Nunez A, Goh A, et al. Study of montelukast for the treatment of respiratory symptoms of post-respiratory syncytial virus bronchiolitis in children. Am J Respir Crit Care Med 2008;178:854–60.
56. Bloomfield P, Dalton D, Karleka A, et al. Bacteraemia and antibiotic use in respiratory syncytial virus infections. Arch Dis Child 2004;89:363–7.
57. Pneumonia the forgotten killer of children. 2006. Geneva: The United Nations Children's Fund (UNICEF)/World Health Organization (WHO); 2006.
58. Grant GB, Campbell H, Dowell SF, et al. Recommendations for treatment of childhood non-severe pneumonia. Lancet Infect Dis 2009;9:185–96.
59. Ranganathan SC, Sonnappa S. Pneumonia and other respiratory infections. Pediatr Clin North Am 2009;56:135–56, xi.
60. Shann F, Hart K, Thomas D. Acute lower respiratory tract infections in children: possible criteria for selection of patients for antibiotic therapy and hospital admission. Bull World Health Organ 2003;81:301–5.
61. Mulholland EK, Simoes EA, Costales MO, et al. Standardized diagnosis of pneumonia in developing countries. Pediatr Infect Dis J 1992;11:77–81.
62. Atkinson M, Yanney M, Stephenson T, et al. Effective treatment strategies for paediatric community-acquired pneumonia. Expert Opin Pharmacother 2007; 8:1091–101.
63. BTS guidelines for the management of community acquired pneumonia in childhood. Thorax 2002;57(Suppl 1):I1–24.
64. Torzillo PJ, Hanna JN, Morey F, et al. Invasive pneumococcal disease in central Australia. Med J Aust 1995;162:182–6.
65. Cortese MM, Wolff M, Meido-Hill J, et al. High incidence rates of invasive pneumococcal disease in the White Mountain Apache population. Arch Intern Med 1992;152:2277–82.
66. Grant CC, Pati A, Tan D, et al. Ethnic comparisons of disease severity in children hospitalized with pneumonia in New Zealand. J Paediatr Child Health 2001;37: 32–7.
67. Burgner D, Richmond P. The burden of pneumonia in children: an Australian perspective. Paediatr Respir Rev 2005;6:94–100.
68. Alaghehbandan R, Gates KD, MacDonald D. Hospitalization due to pneumonia among Innu, Inuit and non-Aboriginal communities, Newfoundland and Labrador, Canada. Int J Infect Dis 2007;11:23–8.
69. Zalm MM, van Ewijk BE, Wilbrink B, et al. Respiratory pathogens in children with and without respiratory symptoms. J Pediatr 2008 Sep 27 [Epub ahead of print].
70. Sawicki GS, Lu FL, Valim C, et al. Necrotising pneumonia is an increasingly detected complication of pneumonia in children. Eur Respir J 2008;31:1285–91.
71. Bonzel L, Tenenbaum T, Schroten H, et al. Frequent detection of viral coinfection in children hospitalized with acute respiratory tract infection using a real-time polymerase chain reaction. Pediatr Infect Dis J 2008;27:589–94.
72. Nascimento-Carvalho CM, Ribeiro CT, Cardoso MR, et al. The role of respiratory viral infections among children hospitalized for community-acquired pneumonia in a developing country. Pediatr Infect Dis J 2008;27:939–41.
73. Torzillo P, Dixon J, Manning K, et al. Etiology of acute lower respiratory tract infection in Central Australian Aboriginal children. Pediatr Infect Dis J 1999;18:714–21.
74. Chang AB, Masel JP, Boyce NC, et al. Non-CF bronchiectasis-clinical and HRCT evaluation. Pediatr Pulmonol 2003;35:477–83.

75. Singleton R, Hammitt L, Hennessy T, et al. The Alaska *Haemophilus influenzae* type b experience: lessons in controlling a vaccine-preventable disease. Pediatrics 2006;118:e421–9.

76. Bruce MG, Deeks SL, Zulz T, et al. International circumpolar surveillance system for invasive pneumococcal disease, 1999–2005. Emerg Infect Dis 2008;14:25–33.

77. Edwards EA, Metcalfe R, Milne DG, et al. Retrospective review of children presenting with non cystic fibrosis bronchiectasis: HRCT features and clinical relationships. Pediatr Pulmonol 2003;36:87–93.

78. Singleton RJ, Morris A, Redding G, et al. Bronchiectasis in Alaska Native children: causes and clinical courses. Pediatr Pulmonol 2000;29:182–7.

79. Bruce MG, Deeks SL, Zulz T, et al. Epidemiology of *Haemophilus influenzae* serotype a, North American Arctic, 2000–2005. Emerg Infect Dis 2008;14:48–55.

80. O'Brien KL, Moulton LH, Reid R, et al. Efficacy and safety of seven-valent conjugate pneumococcal vaccine in American Indian children: group randomised trial. Lancet 2003;362:355–61.

81. Singleton RJ, Bruden D, Bulkow LR, et al. Decline in respiratory syncytial virus hospitalizations in a region with high hospitalization rates and prolonged season. Pediatr Infect Dis J 2006;25:1116–22.

82. Department of Child and Adolescent Health and Development (CAH). Handbook: IMCI integrated management of childhood illness. Geneva: World Health Organisation; 2005.

83. Sazawal S, Black RE. Meta-analysis of intervention trials on case-management of pneumonia in community settings. Lancet 1992;340:528–33.

84. Ayieko P, English M. In children aged 2–59 months with pneumonia, which clinical signs best predict hypoxaemia? J Trop Pediatr 2006;52:307–10.

85. Guyatt GH, Oxman AD, Kunz R, et al. What is "quality of evidence" and why is it important to clinicians? BMJ 2008;336:995–8.

86. Haider BA, Saeed MA, Bhutta ZA. Short-course versus long-course antibiotic therapy for nonsevere community-acquired pneumonia in children aged 2 months to 59 months. Cochrane Database Syst Rev 2008;(2):CD005976.

87. Kabra SK, Lodha R, Pandey RM. Antibiotics for community acquired pneumonia in children. Cochrane Database Syst Rev 2006;(3):CD004874.

88. Guppy MP, Mickan SM, Del Mar CB. Advising patients to increase fluid intake for treating acute respiratory infections. Cochrane Database Syst Rev 2005;(4):CD004419.

89. Chang AB, Torzillo PJ, Boyce NC, et al. Zinc and Vitamin-A supplementation in Indigenous children hospitalised with episodes of lower respiratory tract infection: a randomised controlled trial. Med J Aust 2006;184:107–12.

90. Ni J, Wei J, Wu T. Vitamin A for non-measles pneumonia in children. Cochrane Database Syst Rev 2005;(3):CD003700.

91. Brown N, Roberts C. Vitamin A for acute respiratory infection in developing countries: a meta-analysis. Acta Paediatr 2004;93:1437–42.

92. Hemila H, Louhiala P. Vitamin C for preventing and treating pneumonia. Cochrane Database Syst Rev 2007;(1):CD005532.

93. Hazir T, Qazi S, Nisar YB, et al. Assessment and management of children aged 1-59 months presenting with wheeze, fast breathing, and/or lower chest indrawing; results of a multicentre descriptive study in Pakistan. Arch Dis Child 2004;89:1049–54.

94. Awasthi S, Agarwal G, Kabra SK, et al. Does 3-day course of oral amoxycillin benefit children of non-severe pneumonia with wheeze: a multicentric randomised controlled trial. PLoS ONE 2008;3:e1991.

95. Matheson NJ, Harnden AR, Perera R, et al. Neuraminidase inhibitors for preventing and treating influenza in children. Cochrane Database Syst Rev 2007;(1):CD002744.

96. Alves Galvão MG, Rocha Crispino Santos MA, Alves da Cunha AJL. Amantadine and rimantadine for influenza A in children and the elderly. Cochrane Database Syst Rev 2008;(1):CD002745.

97. Swingler GH, Zwarenstein M. Chest radiograph in acute lower respiratory infections in children. Cochrane Database Syst Rev 2003;(1).

98. Paludo C, Zhang L, Lincho CS, et al. Chest physical therapy for children hospitalised with acute pneumonia: a randomised controlled trial. Thorax 2008;63: 791–4.

99. Chang AB, Grimwood K, Macguire G, et al. Management of bronchiectasis and chronic suppurative lung disease (CSLD) in Indigenous children and adults from rural and remote Australian communities. Med J Aust 2008;189:386–93.

100. Redding GJ, Singleton RJ, Lewis T, et al. Early radiographic and clinical features associated with bronchiectasis in children. Pediatr Pulmonol 2004;37:297–304.

101. Hazir T, Fox LM, Nisar YB, et al. Ambulatory short-course high-dose oral amoxicillin for treatment of severe pneumonia in children: a randomised equivalency trial. Lancet 2008;371:49–56.

102. Snapinn SM. Noninferiority trials. Curr Control Trials Cardiovasc Med 2000;1: 19–21.

103. Asghar R, Banajeh S, Egas J, et al. Chloramphenicol versus ampicillin plus gentamicin for community acquired very severe pneumonia among children aged 2–59 months in low resource settings: multicentre randomised controlled trial (SPEAR study). BMJ 2008;336:80–4.

Chronic Respiratory Symptoms and Diseases Among Indigenous Children

Gregory J. Redding, MD[a,b,*],
Catherine A. Byrnes, MBChB, FRACP, GCCE[c]

KEYWORDS

- Indigenous • Cough • Wheeze • Bronchiectasis
- Asthma • Children

There is a paucity of data about chronic respiratory diseases among different indigenous populations of children. Reports by the World Health Organization about childhood respiratory infections and surveys such as the International Study of Asthma and Allergies in Children (ISAAC) focus on prevalence of disease in geographic regions rather than among cultures.[1,2] Indigenous groups vary with regard to geography, socioeconomic status, local customs, health care resources, nutritional status, immunization rates, and concurrent epidemics, eg, tuberculosis and HIV disease.[3–5] "Indigenous" as a descriptor belies the heterogeneity among cultures, languages, and belief systems that impact perceptions of disease and treatments. For example, there are more than 250 language groups among Australian aboriginal and Torres Strait Islanders, and there are 562 separate federally recognized American Indian, Alaska native, and Native Hawaiian tribes in the United States.[4] The aboriginal peoples in Canada represent themselves as belonging to one of several groups, First Nations, Inuit, or Metis, and comprise more than 50 distinct groups each with their own language and traditional land base.[4] Maori society is structured around kinships and territories.[6,7] Similarly, "indigenous" does not necessarily imply rural or remote residence nor categorically reduced access to medical care. In 2006, 84% of Maori people lived in urban areas of New Zealand; 31%

This work is supported in part by a grant from the Maternal Child Health Bureau (Grant No. T72MC000007).

[a] Department of Pediatrics, University of Washington School of Medicine, WA, USA
[b] Pulmonary Division, Seattle Children's Hospital, Mail Stop: A-5937, 4800 Sand Point Way NE, Seattle, WA 98105, USA
[c] Department of Paediatrics, Starship Children's Hospital, Park Road, Grafton Private Bag 92024, Auckland 1142, New Zealand
* Corresponding author. Pulmonary Division, Seattle Children's Hospital, Mail Stop: A-5937, 4800 Sand Point Way NE, Seattle, WA 98105.
E-mail address: gredding@u.washington.edu (G.J. Redding).

of Australian aboriginal people reside in cities.[8,9] In the United States and Canada, fewer than half of American Indians and First Nations people live on reservations.[10,11] However, it is true that mean income is lower, unemployment rates are higher, and family size is larger, and household crowding is greater among multiple indigenous groups in several countries.[4,8,11–13] Consequently, acute respiratory infections and chronic respiratory diseases in children from indigenous groups are usually several fold more common than among nonindigenous counterparts in the same region.[14–17]

The purpose of this article is to describe the prevalence of chronic respiratory symptoms and conditions among selected indigenous populations to illustrate important differences compared with their nonindigenous peers. The article also reviews the evidence for treatments of chronic respiratory conditions common to children of indigenous groups including health programs for asthma that are culturally oriented. Grading of evidence for therapies using the guidelines of the Grade Working Group is uniformly low owing to lack of randomized control trials (RCTs) for the chronic conditions discussed, the young age at which these conditions occur, and the extrapolation to indigenous children.[18] Importantly, there are no treatments that are specifically indicated or contraindicated for children from indigenous cultures with chronic respiratory disease. Many indigenous groups make use of traditional healing practices and traditional healers for their care. Such practices are beyond the scope of this article but must be addressed in a collaborative and coordinated manner. Where published national and international guidelines for care exist, such as with asthma, the reader is referred to those documents for review.

The authors readily acknowledge that information herein does not address each indigenous group in the world and that extrapolations of this evidence are inevitably necessary until more specific data are published. A major issue regarding a review of any health parameters in indigenous peoples, including children, is the poor collection of ethnicity data that have been used by health care facilities over the decades. In Canada, for example, there has been little opportunity until recent years for individuals to identify themselves as being from an indigenous group in vital registration, health care use, and surveillance data. In addition, these opportunities have been almost nonexistent for certain subgroups of the population such as First Nation peoples without status, Metis, and urban-dwelling aboriginal children. Yet in the 2006 census data almost 1.2 million Canadians reported an aboriginal identity: 60% as "North American Indian," 33% as Metis, and 4% as Inuit.[10] Aboriginal and Torres Strait Islander Australians were originally classified under "flora and fauna" until a referendum of 1967.[19] From 1981, the censuses in Australia have included a question (and the same question over the years) to identify indigenous peoples.[20] In New Zealand before the 1986 Census, identifying as Māori required that the individual be "persons of greater than half Maori blood." In 1988 this changed to a social construct definition of ethnicity as determined by the Department of Statistics, Ministry of Health, which was subsequently incorporated into the births and deaths ethnicity data collection in 1995.[21,22] These issues have limited the ability to properly collect health data, as they relate to different indigenous groups and similar issues are likely to confound the collection of indigenous peoples health data worldwide. Readers are encouraged to explore local data related to specific groups to intervene in pertinent ways.

PREVALENCES AND PATTERNS OF CHRONIC RESPIRATORY SYMPTOMS IN INDIGENOUS CHILDREN

Several surveys have been published that describe the importance of chronic respiratory diseases among children of indigenous groups.[23–29] The surveys vary with date and time interval queried and in scale, ranging from several villages to entire nations. The most extensive information is derived from children of American Indian/Alaska Native (AI/AN), Canadian First Nation (including Metis and Inuit groups), Australian Aborigine/Torres Strait Islanders (AA/TSI), and Aotearoa/New Zealand Maori populations. Information about these groups has resulted in part from the juxtaposition of modern health care technology, epidemiologic capabilities, and indigenous groups within the same geographic regions.

Serious acute respiratory infections cause more death and hospitalizations among indigenous children than their age-matched counterparts.[13,16,17,30] The greatest impact of these infections is felt by indigenous children 0 to 4 years of age.[13,16,24,31] Clinical symptoms of persistent lung injury produced early in life by acute lower respiratory tract infections (LRTIs) include recurrent wheeze and persistent productive and nonproductive cough. These sequelae, listed as clinical diagnoses in **Box 1**, may occur after a single serious infection, such as adenovirus[32,33] or pneumococcal pneumonia,[29,34] or following recurrent viral infections, as described among Alaskan Yupik and Canadian Inuit children.[25,35] Recurrent wheezing following severe LRTIs wanes over years in both indigenous and nonindigenous populations following respiratory syncytial virus (RSV) infections.[36,37] Data depicting this natural history among Alaskan Yupik children hospitalized for RSV when younger than 2 years old and age-matched and village-matched controls who were not hospitalized are illustrated in **Fig. 1**. In this series, both chronic productive cough (22%) and wheeze (43%) were common among native Alaska native children 5 years after hospitalization for RSV. Wheezing following RSV was not related to atopy as measured by serum IgE levels or radioallergosorbent (RAST) testing to inhalant allergens.[36] In a cross-sectional survey using a modified ISAAC questionnaire, 40% of Alaska native middle school children had chronic respiratory symptoms as depicted in **Fig. 2**.[26] Chronic productive cough was self-reported in 26% of all surveyed children and in more than half of all symptomatic children, with and without concomitant asthma symptoms. This contrasts with data from 2400 Seattle middle school children using the same survey, which found that chronic productive cough was self-reported in only 7% of respondents. In another series, 6% of 550 Canadian Inuit children 6 to 13 years old reported wheezing but 20% had chronic cough.[25]

Lung injury following acute LRTIs may be adversely influenced by persistent exposure to environmental pollutants and irritants that further predispose young children to chronic cough or wheeze. Practices such as indoor open biomass burning still pose a significant risk for recurrent respiratory infections in young children and are common among indigenous groups residing in developing countries.[38,39] During severe episodes of air pollution, an increase in both the general rate of mortality and respiratory mortality in children, and perinatal mortality occurs.[40,41] The respiratory illnesses sensitive to increased pollutants in children include upper respiratory tract infections, acute bronchitis, cough, asthma, and pneumonia but there are no specific data regarding indigenous children.[42–47] However, higher levels of exposure to other environmental contaminants in infants of indigenous families has been suggested in a number of small studies using cord blood measurement.[48,49]

Box 1
Common chronic respiratory illnesses
Recurrent postviral wheeze
Asthma
Chronic productive cough/Protracted bacterial bronchitis
Bronchiectasis

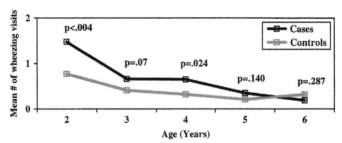

Fig. 1. Mean number of health clinic visits with wheezing per child from age 2 to 6 years of age in children hospitalized with respiratory syncytial virus (RSV) as infants (cases) and age-matched controls who were not hospitalized at <2 years of age. Cases (hospitalized with RSV) are depicted by the dark line and control by the lighter line. *Data from* Singleton RJ, Redding GJ, Lewis TC, et al. Sequelae of severe respiratory syncytial virus infection in infancy and early childhood among Alaska Native children. Pediatrics 2003;112:285–90.

More data are available from surveys regarding prenatal and postnatal passive exposure to tobacco smoke and active tobacco use late in childhood. These indicate that indigenous groups have higher rates of smoke exposure at multiple times during lung development (**Table 1**). Prenatal smoking has increased among pregnant AI/AN, AA/TSI, and Maori women compared with their nonindigenous counterparts, and they are less likely to stop during pregnancy.[50–54] Prenatal smoke exposure is associated with smaller conducting airway caliber and recurrent wheezing after birth.[55] Postnatal passive tobacco smoke exposure is also more common among indigenous groups, including AI/AN, First Nations, AA/TSI, and Maori parents, with family smoking rates exceeding 75% in multiple surveys.[25,31,56,57] Children exposed passively to tobacco smoke have increased cough, wheeze, respiratory infections, and severity of asthma.[58,59] Finally, active smoking is very common among indigenous youth and more so than among age-matched nonindigenous youth, particularly if there is a smoker in the family (**Table 1**).[56,60,61]

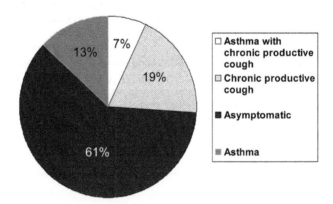

(n = 466); 1997 data. *Mean age = 13 ± 1.4 years

Fig. 2. Prevalence of chronic asthma like symptoms and chronic cough among middle school Alaska Native children using a modified ISAAC survey. *Data from* Lewis TC, Stout JW, Martinez P, et al. Prevalence of asthma and chronic respiratory symptoms among Alaska Native children. Chest 2004;125:1665–73.

Table 1
Tobacco smoke exposure among indigenous populations

Group	No. Surveyed	Rate	Method	Data
Prenatal smoking prevalence				
AI/AN[51]	359	21%	PRAMS	2000
First Nation (Canada)[10]	22,178	48%	RHS	2002
Maori (NZ)[50]	77	54%	Survey	2003
Aboriginal/TSI (Aust)[8]	10,439	51%	NATSIHS	2001–04
Passive smoke exposure				
Inuit (Canada)[25]	594	72%	PFT study	1997
First Nations (Canada)[57]	36	79%	School survey	2004
AI/AN[60]	336	75%	School survey	2006
Alaskan Native (US)[36]	208	46%	RSV study	2000
Aboriginal/TSI (Aust)[8]	217,815	68%	NATSIHS	2004
Maori (NZ)[56]	8,632	64%	NY10SS	2007
Active tobacco smoking (Current smoking or within the last 30 days) (Youth and adolescents)				
Inuit (Canada)[25]	594	32%	PFT study	1997
First Nation (Canada) (12–14 y)[10]	4,860	29%	RHS	2002
Oji-Creek, First Nations (15–19 y)[61]	236	82%	Survey	2005
AI/AN (12–17 y)[124]	6,052	21%	NSDUH	2006
AI/AN (11–18 y)[60]	336	37%	AICTP survey	2006
Maori (NZ) (14–15 y)[56]	8,632	32/17%	NY10SS	2007

Abbreviations: AI/AN, American Indian/Alaska Native; AICTP, American Indian Community Tobacco Project (US); Aust, Australia; NATSIHS, National Aboriginal and Torres Strait Islander Health Survey (Aust); NSDUH, National Survey on Drug Use and Health (US); NY10SS, National Year 10 Smoking Survey (NZ); NZ, New Zealand; PRAMS, Pregnancy Risk and Monitoring System (US); RHS, First Nations Regional Longitudinal Health Survey (Canada); RSV, Respiratory Syncytial Virus; TSI, Torres Strait Islanders.

The roles of recurrent upper airway infections, aspiration tendencies, and gastro-esophageal reflux following early lung injury have not been studied specifically in indigenous populations. All of these conditions can produce wheeze and cough in previously well children and can aggravate persistent lung disease caused by previous respiratory infections. Rempel and colleagues[62] recently described seven indigenous children with recurrent respiratory symptoms who underwent serial videofluoroscopic swallowing tests that demonstrated clinically silent aspiration that persisted for months after the initial respiratory infections resolved. The prevalence of this condition has not been studied with larger numbers among high-risk indigenous groups and culturally specific feeding practices that might predispose to recurrent aspiration have not been identified.

In the sections below, descriptions of common chronic respiratory conditions reported among but not exclusive to indigenous children are described. Treatment options are also provided and graded based on quality of evidence (**Table 2**).

PROTRACTED BACTERIAL BRONCHITIS, CHRONIC SUPPURATIVE LUNG DISEASE, AND BRONCHIECTASIS

Chronic "wet" or productive cough lasting longer than 3 to 4 weeks in the absence of radiographic evidence of pneumonia, atelectasis, or bronchiectasis has been described as protracted bacterial bronchitis (PBB) in children.[63] PBB is often preceded by an LRTI, is accompanied by wheeze in up to 45% of children, and

Table 2
Grades for treatment options for chronic respiratory symptoms and disease

Treatment	Quality of Evidence	Recommendation	Recommendation Grade
Protracted Bacterial Bronchitis (PBB)			
Oral Antibiotic	Low		
Amoxicillin or Amoxicillin/ Clavulinate		Trial of 2 courses of 4–6 weeks	Probably use
CSLD/bronchiectasis			
Chronic oral antibiotic	Low		
Azithromycin 1–3 times/ week		Trial of 3–6 months	Probably not
Amoxacillin once-twice/day		Outcome specific versus resistance	Probably not
Clarythromycin once/day		Outcome specific versus resistance	Probably not
Short-term oral antibiotic	Moderate		
Amoxicillin		Acute symptom (fever, cough) relief	Probably use
Amoxicillin/clavulinate		7–14 days for acute symptom relief	Probably use
Intravenous antibiotics		7 Day course for pneumonia	Use
Airway clearance			
Alpha dornase inhalation	Moderate	2.5 mg 2×/day	Don't use
Mannitol inhalation	Low	Daily	Probably not
Hypertonic saline (7%)	Low	1–2×/day	Probably not
Chest physiotherapy	Low	1–2×/day	Probably not
Prevention			
Pneumococcal vaccine	Moderate	Age-dependent guidelines	Probably use
Influenza vaccine	Low	Annual	Probably use
Recurrent viral/Postviral wheeze			
Bronchodilator			
Albuterol (nebulizer/MDI)	Moderate	Therapeutic trial with best device	Probably use
Albuterol iptratroprium (nebulizer/MDI)	Low	Therapeutic trial in ED/ Hospital	Probably not
Asthma controller treatment			
Inhaled corticosteroid	Moderate	Treatment trial of acute symptoms	Probably use
Oral corticosteroid	Moderate	Treatment of acute symptoms	Probably use
Montelukast (Age-dependent dose)	Moderate	Treatment trial of acute symptoms	Probably use
Recurrent multi-trigger wheeze			
Bronchodilator			
Albuterol (MDI + spacer/ mask)	Moderate	Treatment of acute symptoms as needed	Use

(continued on next page)

Table 2
(continued)

Treatment	Quality of Evidence	Recommendation	Recommendation Grade
Asthma controller treatment			
Inhaled corticosteroid	High	Treatment trial twice daily × 3 months	Probably use Probably not if <1 year
(MDI + spacer/mask)	Moderate	Treatment trial for acute symptoms	Probably use
Oral corticosteroid	Moderate	Treatment trial once daily for 1 month	Probably use
Montelukast	Moderate	Treatment trial for acute symptoms	Probably use
General prevention measures			
Smoke exposure reduction	Low	Smoke outside/smoking jacket/cessation	Use
Allergen avoidance/ reduction	Low	If no clear relationship of contact and symptoms	Probably not
Use of MDI delivery device	Moderate	Treatment trial with MDI + spacer + mask first	Use
Education Programs (Assessment skills, knowledge)	Moderate	Program tailored to learning style of family	Use

Abbreviations: MDI, metered dose inhaler; ED, emergency department.

responsive to asthma therapy in one-third of patients.[64] Symptoms of PBB often begin during the first 3 years of life and persist for months to years.[64,65] The features of PBB parallel what has been described epidemiologically among indigenous children with chronic "wet" cough without specifically using the same terminology. Evaluation of PBB after an initial 6-week course of antibiotics includes a chest radiograph and in some cases, a high-resolution computerized tomography (HRCT) scan of the chest if the "wet" cough persists or recurs. The chest radiograph in children with PBB usually demonstrates peribronchial thickening.

Children with a chronic "wet" cough who are unresponsive to several extended courses of antibiotics but have no HRCT findings of bronchiectasis are described as having chronic suppurative lung disease (CSLD).[66] CSLD occurred in 20% of aboriginal children hospitalized for lobar pneumonia during the prior 6 months.[29] Whether this condition leads to bronchiectasis in a subset of children remains controversial, although the diagnosis of bronchiectasis has been associated with having a preceding prolonged wet cough for years, and is described as beginning in childhood among those who are diagnosed with bronchiectasis as adults.[34,67–69] However, postinfectious bronchiectasis unrelated to cystic fibrosis is particularly common among certain indigenous children, including Alaska native, Australian aboriginal, and New Zealand's Maori children with rates ranging from 14 to 20 per 1000 children.[29,34,35] These rates of bronchiectasis are 40 times greater than the prevalence of cystic fibrosis among nonindigenous children in Australia.[69,70] Among all 3 indigenous groups, serious LRTIs, presenting as lobar pneumonia or more diffuse pneumonitis but not bronchiolitis, commonly precede the development of bronchiectasis.[29,34,71] The risk of bronchiectasis increases with recurrent pneumonias and LRTIs, suggesting multiple injuries or "hits" predispose to chronic airway damage.[29,71]

Treatment Options

The treatment of PBB is an antibiotic directed toward *Haemophilus influenza* non-type b, *Streptococcus pneumoniae*, and *Moraxella caterrhalis* for a period of 4 to 6 weeks for up to six treatment courses.[64,65] *Pseudomonas* and *Staphylococcus* airway infections have not been described with PBB. Initial improvement in symptoms usually occurs within 2 weeks of starting oral antibiotic therapy and permanent resolution of the cough occurs in the majority of children after 1 to 2 prolonged courses of antibiotics.[64,65] These data are derived from restrospective and prospective case series from two pulmonary referral centers. There are no RCTs of treatment to assess relative risks and benefits. However, fewer than 20% of children with chronic productive cough resolve spontaneously.[63] The need for additional modalities, such as bronchodilator therapy, antacid treatment, or airway mucus clearance techniques for treatment of PBB has not been prospectively addressed.

Treatment of CSLD and postinfectious bronchiectasis are the same. A review of evidence-based treatments for bronchiectasis unrelated to cystic fibrosis (CF) has been published recently in *Pediatric Clinics of North America*.[72] Categories of treatments for postinfectious bronchiectasis are listed in **Box 2**. The outcomes for each treatment option depend in part on the severity and extent of bronchiectasis at initial encounter. Reported outcome measures include lung functions, severity and frequency of respiratory exacerbations, sputum volume, daily symptoms, days of disability, hospitalizations, and quality of life over variable intervals of time. In most instances, RCTs have been conducted in adults with idiopathic bronchiectasis rather than in children. It is unclear to what degree these data can be extrapolated to children as disease severity, airway bacterial pathogens, and comorbid conditions differ among different age groups. Chronic disease management programs, similar to those for children with CF, which regularly assess lung function, lung infection, nutrition, and family adherence to home treatment programs have been proposed for indigenous children with postinfectious bronchiectasis but clinical outcomes resulting from these programs have not been described.

Antibiotics have been used to reduce the bacterial density within the airways, and thereby reduce the inflammatory response, mucus production, and airway destruction characteristic of bronchiectasis. There are no RCTs evaluating the long-term use of

---

Box 2
Treatment strategies for CSLD and postinfectious bronchiectasis

Prevention and reduction of airway infection

Prevention and reduction in airway mucus production

Enhancement of airway mucus clearance

Improvements in sputum rheology

Treatment of reversible airway obstruction

Increase in respiratory muscle strength and endurance

Improved nutrition

Reduction in airway inflammation

Surgical resection of involved areas

antibiotics to treat postinfectious bronchiectasis in children. Macrolide therapy has been used for its antimicrobial, anti-secretagogue, and anti-inflammatory properties.[73] Short-term trials (3–6 months) with azithromycin in adults and with roxithromycin and clarithromycin in children reduced airway reactivity and improved quality of life but did not improve lung functions.[74–76] A 1-week course of amoxicillin reduced expectorated sputum volume and improve lung function in children with bronchiectasis unrelated to CF, suggesting rapid onset of antibiotic effects.[77] No antibiotic therapy protocol has been shown to reduce respiratory exacerbation rates in children with this condition. The ideal drug, dose, dosing frequency, and duration of antibiotic use per treatment course have not been established in children with postinfectious bronchiectasis.

Airway secretions and their rheologic properties can be altered such that sputum is cleared more easily from the airways with coughing. Airway sputum is less viscous and tenacious among indigenous children who have postinfectious bronchiectasis than among children with CF or ciliary defects.[78] Consequently, therapies such as DNAse, which improve airway function in CF, may not be of benefit in children with bronchiectasis from other causes. Of note, O'Donnell and colleagues[79] evaluated the effects of DNAse used for 24 weeks in an RCT among adults with idiopathic bronchiectasis. The treated group had more acute respiratory exacerbations and a greater decline in lung function than did those receiving placebo. Hence, there is currently no indication for DNAase use among children with bronchiectasis unrelated to CF until safety and efficacy are demonstrated. Airway hydration, using inhaled mannitol, improved secretion clearance in a dose-dependent manner among adults with bronchiectasis with short-term use but no studies have been conducted in children with postinfectious bronchiectasis using this agent.[80] Similarly, inhalations of 7% hypertonic saline have reduced exacerbation frequency and improved lung function among patients with CF but have not been studied in children with bronchiectasis unrelated to CF.[81] Chest physiotherapy can be provided using a variety of methods, some of which are age-dependent and require no assistance from another person. Although there are theoretical reasons for possible benefit, none of these techniques have been studied in the short or long term as an RCT in children with postinfectious bronchiectasis; so insufficient evidence exists to specifically recommend their use.

An updated Cochrane review (2009)[67] on the benefits of 23-valent pneumococcal vaccine identified two studies, one in adults and one in children with bronchiectasis unrelated to CF. In the RCT studying adults, those receiving the pneumococcal vaccine had fewer respiratory exacerbations over a 2-year period compared with the untreated group.[82] The children who were studied after receiving the same pneumococcal vaccine experienced elimination of pneumococcus from their sputum but no mention was made of clinical outcomes.[67] The reviewers recommended use of pneumococcal vaccines but acknowledged that more studies are needed to better assess benefits and risks.

There are no RCTs assessing many supportive care measures to treat postinfectious bronchiectasis in childhood. Cochrane reviews have examined the use of bronchodilators, inhaled steroids, nonsteroidal anti-inflammatory agents, leukotriene receptor antagonists, surgical versus medical therapy, and influenza vaccines in children with bronchiectasis unrelated to CF.[67,83–87] In all of these reviews, there is insufficient evidence to ensure that these interventions are of predictable benefit to children with postinfectious bronchiectasis.

RECURRENT WHEEZE AND ASTHMA

Unlike chronic cough, asthma prevalences among indigenous children do not consistently differ from those of their nonindigenous peers. Asthma prevalences among indigenous groups range from 3% among the Mam children of Guatemala to 23% among aboriginal and Torres Strait Islanders in Australia.[14,38] Larger and more recent assessments of asthma prevalence, as listed in **Table 3**, focus on asthma symptoms or household telephone surveys about asthma rather than physiologic or physician-based diagnoses. Prevalences of asthma and asthmalike symptoms among indigenous children have increased significantly since the 1980s, in parallel with the worldwide trends of children in developing countries.[1,88] Among AI/AN children, the prevalence of asthma nationwide between 2001 and 2005 was 13%, similar to all US children.[89] However, among Australian aboriginal children, asthma prevalence exceeds that of nonindigenous children (24.0% vs 21.3% ever asthma and 13.5% vs 11.3% current asthma respectively).[14] AI/AN and Maori children residing in urban settings have a higher prevalence of asthma than indigenous counterparts in rural settings.[27,90] Children of ethnic minority populations in the Unites States have higher rates of asthma if they are born in the United States than if they are born in other countries.[89] These data suggest that place of residence both early and later in life may have a greater impact on asthma prevalence than one's indigenous background.

Asthma hospitalizations among AI/AN children increased through the 1990s and have since declined, similar to all groups of US children younger than 20 years of age (**Fig. 3**).[91] Asthma-related hospitalization rates remain highest among infants younger than 1 year of age and children 1 to 4 years old in both indigenous and nonindigenous groups.[31] However, "asthma" as a diagnosis in infants younger than 1 year old remains problematic and may include diseases of the lower airways other than asthma. Between 2001 and 2005 in the United States, asthma attacks occurred at similar rates among the minority ethnicities surveyed.[89] In Australia, hospitalization rates for asthma in 2004 to 2005 were equivalent for aboriginal children 0 to 14 years

Table 3
Prevalence estimates of asthma among indigenous children

Group	No.	Prevalence, %	Age Group	Method[a]	Date
AI/AN (US)[125]	2288	7	1–17 y	SAIAN	1987
Kawerau Maori (NZ)[28]	708	21	8–13 y	ISAAC	1992
Yupik (Alaska, US)[26]	365	10	10–15 y	ISAAC	1997
Aboriginal/TSI (Aus)	1650	12	0–17 y	ISAAC	1999
AI/AN (US)[89]	489	13	2–17 y	NHIS	2000–05
Aboriginal/TSI (Aust)[126]	1,327	14[a]	3–17 y	ISAAC	2003
Ever asthma[14]	10,439	24	0–17 y	NATSIHS	2004
Current asthma[14]	10,439	13	0–17 y	NATSIHS	2004
Mam (Guatemala)[38]	31	3	4–6 y	ISAAC	2004
First Nations (Canada)[127]	14,170	12	<6 y	ACS	2006
	10,500	16	6–14 y	ACS	2006
Inuit (Canada)[128]	3,800	11	<6 y	ACS	2006
	3,800	5	6–14 y	ACS	2006

Abbreviations: AI/AN, American Indian/Alaska Native; ACS, 2006 Aboriginal Children's Survey (Canada); Aust, Australia; ISAAC, International Study of Asthma and Allergy in Children; NATSIHS, National Aboriginal and Torres Strait Islander Health Survey (Aust); NHIS, National Health Interview Survey (US); NZ, New Zealand; SAIAN, Survey of American Indians and Alaskan Natives (US); TSI, Torres Strait Islanders.
[a] Ranges in asthma prevalence among 5 communities was 3.8%–20.1%.

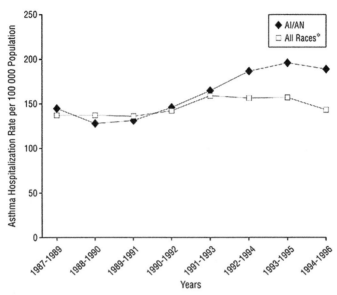

Fig. 3. Hospitalization rates from 1987 to 1996 for AI/AN children compared with all children 0 to 17 years old residing in Washington State. Closed triangles represent hospitalization rates for AI/AN children; open boxes represent national state data for all races of children. *Data from* Liu LL, Stout JW, Sullivan M, et al. Asthma and bronchiolitis hospitalizations among American Indian children. Arch Pediatr Adolesc Med 2000;154:991–96.

of age and their nonindigenous peers.[14] However, in New Zealand, the hospitalization for asthma was twice that for Maori compared with European children.[92]

The prevalence of atopy, as manifested by eczema and allergic rhinitis, varies substantially among nations and is changing over time.[93] The frequency of atopy among different indigenous groups varies greatly as well. Prevalence estimates in the few published series about indigenous children are based on different indices of atopy and these indices may not correlate with one another. Among native Inuit Greenlander children, the prevalence of positive specific IgE antibodies to inhalant allergens increased from 10% in 1988 to 19% in 1998.[94] Among 303 6- to 8-year-old Alaska native children tested in 2005, 20% had a serum IgE greater than 1000 IU/mL.[95] However, RAST tests to inhalant allergens (dust mite, dog, grass, trees, cats) were rarely positive and did not correlate with IgE levels. In 1995, among 550 Inuit children 6 to 13 years of age, only 5% had a positive skin test to at least one inhalant allergen using a similar allergen panel.[25] In direct contrast to these figures, the prevalence of atopy among adolescents of Maori descent 2 decades ago was found to be high (31%) and equal to non-Maori age-matched children.[90] A current birth cohort of 1105 children in New Zealand, including 167 Maori children, is part of a longitudinal study to characterize the emergence of atopy by age 6 years.[96] The study will provide updated comparisons of atopy prevalence between New Zealand's indigenous and overall population of children. These wide variations in atopy among indigenous groups suggest that predispositions to atopy are complex and specific to each indigenous group.

Treatment Options

Wheezing is often episodic but severe in young children following severe LRTIs early in life. Evidence-based guidelines for treatment of these young children are hampered by lack of randomized controlled treatment trials and by lack of consensus about what constitutes "asthma" among the very young. National and international guidelines for the treatment of childhood asthma acknowledge that many of their treatment recommendations for very young children are empiric and extrapolated from studies in older children.

A Cochrane review evaluated the impact of short-acting beta agonist therapy, ie, albuterol, in children younger than 2 years with recurrent wheezing in the absence of acute bronchiolitis.[97] Six RCTs involving 229 children were included in the review but had different outcome variables, different dosing protocols and drug-delivery devices, and were conducted in different settings, eg, home, emergency department, or pulmonary function laboratory.[98–105] Benefits included reductions in respiratory rate, marginal improvements in oxy-hemoglobin saturation, and increased airway conductance, but there were no consistent improvements in symptom scores, maximal expiratory flows at functional residual capacity, or hospital admission rates. The review concluded that although wheezing children younger than 2 years of age can respond to albuterol, the clinical benefit of inhaled beta agonists is unpredictable.

A Cochrane review evaluating the effects of inhaled anticholinergic therapy with ipratropium (six RCTs involving 329 children younger than 2 years of age) found similarly unpredictable short-term and no long-term benefits.[106] The limitation of this review is that it identified RCTs involving young children with primarily acute wheezing or bronchiolitis; no studies specifically involved indigenous children. Ipratropium improved clinical respiratory scores more than placebo, but did not improve respiratory rate, oxy-hemoglobin saturation, nor shorten duration of hospital stay.[107–109] The combination of inhaled albuterol (or fenoterol) and ipratropium reduced the number of inhalation treatments needed by acutely ill wheezing children more than albuterol alone.[108,110] One study comparing nebulized water, sodium cromoglycate, and ipratropium in a blinded 3-month crossover trial among "asthmatic" toddlers showed no difference in daily symptom scores among the treatment groups.[111] Based on these studies, there is no evidence to recommend the use of ipratropium in young children with recurrent wheezing in the outpatient setting.

A recent consensus statement by the European Respiratory Task Force addressed the evidence for treatment of recurrent wheezing in preschool children.[112] It did not specifically address indigenous or minority groups nor postinfectious etiologies for wheezing. The Task Force found that the grade of evidence for these recommendations was uniformly low and that empiric therapeutic trials were reasonable. The Task Force separated preschool wheezing into categories of viral-induced wheeze and multi-trigger wheeze, as children with the latter diagnosis tend to be more responsive to long-term inhaled corticosteroid therapy. A summary of Task Force recommendations and grading of each recommendation is provided as part of **Table 3**. Aside from medications, the authors emphasized reductions in tobacco smoke exposure, educational programs about acute and recurrent childhood wheezing, and suggested use of metered dose inhalers with spacers and tight-fitting masks to deliver inhaled medications in young children.

The age-specific definitions, criteria for diagnosis, prevention, monitoring and treatment options for childhood asthma have been published by many countries and the international community.[113–116] Most guidelines recommend that the plan of care be individualized to the asthmatic child in the context of his or her family and community, and that family concerns be addressed. Models of care that include asthma specialists and community health workers who belong to the indigenous community have been piloted.[117] These models take into consideration the belief systems, barriers to care, and languages that are specific to indigenous families. The following list of beliefs about asthma reported by Navajo families highlight why asthma care must be individualized[118]:

○ Asthma is person specific and its process and course vary among individuals
○ Medicine is more or less compatible with a person's constitution and finding the best asthma medicine results from trial and error
○ It is important to teach an asthmatic child's body how to handle symptoms
○ Asthma results from triggers during times when a child is vulnerable to asthma
○ A child's body is best known by the child and treatment should be directed by the one who knows the child's body best

These beliefs are not specific to Navajo people nor necessarily applicable to all. However, they impact how families manage asthma in each culture. **Fig. 4** illustrates the age of children at which Navajo families transferred responsibility for asthma care to the child as a result of these beliefs.[118]

There have been several recent Cochrane Reviews pertaining to culture-specific asthma care. One published in 2009 described three randomized controlled trials of culturally specific asthma education programs involving more than 250 children of Puerto Rican, African American, and Indian subcontinent heritage.[119] Asthma education was provided in family-specific dialects pertaining to asthma assessment and monitoring, drug-delivery techniques, and medications that was culturally relevant. Compared to usual care, these programs produced significant improvements in Asthma Quality of Life scores and asthma knowledge scores among children.[120] However reductions in asthma exacerbations or visits to emergency departments

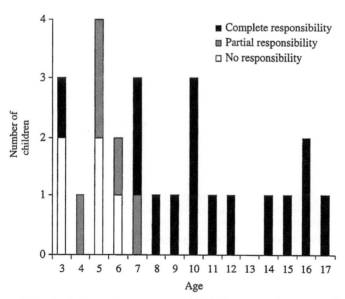

Fig. 4. Ages of Navajo children with asthma at which they assume responsibility for their asthma care. Open areas represent children with no responsibility for self-management and black portions represent number of children completely responsible for management of their own asthma. *Data from* Van Sickle D, Wright AL. Navajo perceptions of asthma and asthma medications: clinical implications. Pediatrics 2001;108:E11.

for asthma care occurred in only one of the three studies.[120–122] An additional study evaluated the impact of involving an indigenous health care worker in a childhood asthma management program.[123] The study included both intervention and control groups but was not blinded. Asthma knowledge scores of the children were better but asthma exacerbation rates were no different between the two groups. Both Cochrane Reviews underscored the need for more studies to evaluate culturally specific approaches to asthma care in children.

SUMMARY

Chronic respiratory symptoms and diseases are common among indigenous children in many countries. They often represent the sequelae of acute LRTIs that may be aggravated by environmental factors, eg, tobacco smoke exposure. Public health measures to reduce passive and active tobacco smoke exposure and indoor pollution, and prevent recurrent infections through immunizations, running water, and reduced crowding will reduce the incidence and burden of chronic respiratory diseases in these groups. No treatments of any respiratory diseases have been studied specifically as to how they affect indigenous children. Randomized controlled trials to assess current treatment options in these populations are needed. Culturally oriented disease management systems have been piloted and show promise in several countries. More surveys about the prevalence of these disorders worldwide are needed to impact more than the populations that have been studied.

ACKNOWLEDGMENTS

The authors thank Ms Holly Kaopuiki for her assistance with preparation of this manuscript.

REFERENCES

1. Asher MI, Montefort S, Bjorksten B, et al. Worldwide time trends in the prevalence of symptoms of asthma, allergic rhinoconjunctivitis, and eczema in childhood: ISAAC phases one and three repeat multicountry cross-sectional surveys. Lancet 2006;368:733–43.
2. World Health Organization. The World Health Organization Report 2005. Available at: http://www.who.int/whr/en. Accessed July 2008.
3. Peat JK, Veale A. Impact and aetiology of respiratory infections, asthma and airway disease in Australian Aborigines. J Paediatr Child Health 2001;37: 108–12.
4. Smylie J, Adomako P. Indigenous children's health report: health assessment in action. Toronto: Centre for Research on Inner City Health, St. Michael's Hospital; 2009.
5. Zar HJ. Pneumonia in HIV-infected and HIV-uninfected children in developing countries: epidemiology, clinical features, and management. Curr Opin Pulm Med 2004;10:176–82.
6. Orange C. The Treaty of Waitangi. Wellington, New Zealand: Allen and Unwin in association with Port Nicholson Press; 1987.
7. Walker R. Ka Whawhai Tonu Matou: Struggle without end. Auckland, New Zealand: Penguin Books; 1990.
8. Australian Bureau of Statistics. Population distribution, aboriginal and Torres Strait Islander Australians; 4705.02006.

9. Statistics New Zealand. QuickStats about Maori. Census 2006. Wellington, New Zealand: Statistics New Zealand; 2007.

10. Statistics Canada. Aboriginal peoples in Canada in 2006: Inuit, Metis, and First Nations, 2006 Census. Ottawa, Canada: Ministry of Industry; 2008. Cat. No. 7-558-XIE. 2006.

11. U.S. Census Bureau, Census Public Law. 94–171.

12. Statistics Canada. Aboriginal children's survey 2006. Catalogue number 89-634-XIE. Ottawa, Canada: Statistics Canada; 2009.

13. Robson B, Cormack D, Cram F. Social and economic indicators: Hauora Maori standards of health IV. Wellington, New Zealand: Te Ropu Rangahau Hauora a Eru Pomare; 2007.

14. Australian Centre for Asthma Monitoring. Asthma in Australia. Canberra, Australia: Australian Institute of Health and Welfare; 2008. p (AIHW Asthma Series No. 3 AIHW Cat. No. ACEM 14). Available at: http://www.aihw.gov.au/publications/index.cfm/title/10584. Accessed Mar 12, 09.

15. Carville KS, Lehmann D, Hall G, et al. Infection is the major component of the disease burden in aboriginal and non-aboriginal Australian children. Pediatr Infect Dis J 2007;26:210–6.

16. Holman RC, Curns AT, Cheek JE, et al. Infectious disease hospitalizations among American Indian and Alaska Native infants. Pediatrics 2003;111: e176–82.

17. Moore H, Burgner D, Carville K, et al. Diverging trends for lower respiratory infections in non-aboriginal and aboriginal children. J Paediatr Child Health 2007;43:451–7.

18. Grade Working Group. Education and debate—grading quality of evidence and strength of recommendations. BMJ 2007;328:1–8.

19. Freemantle J, Officer K, McAullay D, et al. Australian Indigenous Health—Within an international context. Darwin: Cooperative Research Centre for Aboriginal Health; 2007.

20. Ross K. A Occasional paper: population issues, Indigenous Australia 1996. Australian Bureau of Statistics, Canberra. Cat. No. 4708.0; 1999.

21. Robson B, Reid P. Ethnicity matters: Maori perspectives. Wellington, New Zealand: Statistics New Zealand; 2001.

22. Thomas DR. Assessing ethnicity in New Zealand health research. N Z Med J 2001;114:86–8.

23. Glasgow NJ, Goodchild EA, Yates R, et al. Respiratory health in aboriginal and Torres Strait Islander children in the Australian Capital Territory. J Paediatr Child Health 2003;39:534–9.

24. Harris SB, Glazier R, Eng K, et al. Disease patterns among Canadian aboriginal children. Can Fam Physician 1998;44:1869–77.

25. Hemmelgarn B, Ernst P. Airway function among Inuit primary school children in far northern Quebec. Am J Respir Crit Care Med 1997;156:1870–5.

26. Lewis TC, Stout JW, Martinez P, et al. Prevalence of asthma and chronic respiratory symptoms among Alaska Native children. Chest 2004;125:1665–73.

27. Poulos LM, Toelle BG, Marks GB. The burden of asthma in children: an Australian perspective. Paediatr Respir Rev 2005;6:20–7.

28. Shaw R, Woodman K, Crane J, et al. Risk factors for asthma symptoms in Kawerau children. N Z Med J 1994;12:387–91.

29. Valery PC, Torzillo PJ, Mulholland K, et al. Hospital-based case-control study of bronchiectasis in indigenous children in Central Australia. Pediatr Infect Dis J 2004;23:902–8.

30. Torzillo PJ, Hanna JN, Morey F, et al. Invasive pneumococcal disease in central Australia. Med J Aust 1995;162:182–6.
31. Singleton RJ, Holman RC, Cobb N, et al. Asthma hospitalizations among American Indian and Alaska Native people and for the general US population. Chest 2006;130:1554–62.
32. Castro-Rodriguez JA, Daszenies C, Garcia M, et al. Adenovirus pneumonia in infants and factors for developing bronchiolitis obliterans: a 5-year follow-up. Pediatr Pulmonol 2006;41:947–53.
33. Colom AJ, Teper AM, Vollmer WM, et al. Risk factors for the development of bronchiolitis obliterans in children with bronchiolitis. Thorax 2006;61:503–6.
34. Edwards EA, Asher MI, Byrnes CA. Paediatric bronchiectasis in the twenty-first century: experience of a tertiary children's hospital in New Zealand. J Paediatr Child Health 2003;39:111–7.
35. Singleton R, Morris A, Redding G, et al. Bronchiectasis in Alaska Native children: causes and clinical courses. Pediatr Pulmonol 2000;29:182–7.
36. Singleton RJ, Redding GJ, Lewis TC, et al. Sequelae of severe respiratory syncytial virus infection in infancy and early childhood among Alaska Native children. Pediatrics 2003;112:285–90.
37. Stein RT, Sherrill D, Morgan WJ, et al. Respiratory syncytial virus in early life and risk of wheeze and allergy by age 13 years. Lancet 1999;354:541–5.
38. Schel MA, Hessen JO, Smith KR, et al. Childhood asthma and indoor woodsmoke from cooking in Guatemala. J Expo Anal Environ Epidemiol 2004;14:s110–7.
39. Torres-Duque C, Maldonado D, Perez-Padilla R, et al. Biomass fuels and respiratory diseases: a review of the evidence. Proc Am Thorac Soc 2008;5:577–90.
40. Anderson HR, Pounce de Leon A. Air pollution and daily mortality in London: 1987–1992. Br Med J 1996;312:665–9.
41. Bates DV. The effects of air pollution on children. Environ Health Perspect 1995;103:49–53.
42. Aunan K. Exposure -response functions for health effects of air pollutants based on epidemiological findings. Risk Anal 1996;16:693–709.
43. Braun-Fahriander C, Vuille JC, Sennhauser FH, et al. Respiratory health and long-term exposure to air pollutants in Swiss schoolchildren. SCARPOL Team. Swiss study on childhood allergy and respiratory symptoms with respect to air pollution, climate and pollen. Am J Respir Crit Care Med 1997;155:1042–9.
44. Dockery DW, Speizer FE. Effects of inhaled particles on respiratory health of children. Am Rev Respir Dis 1989;139:587–94.
45. Jaakkola JJ, Paunio M, Virtanen M, et al. Low-level air pollution and upper respiratory infections in children. Am J Public Health 1991;82:896–7.
46. Nicolai T. Air pollution and respiratory disease in children: what is the clinically relevant impact? Pediatr Pulmonol Suppl 1999;18:9–13.
47. Ostro B, Broadwin R, Green S, et al. Fine particulate air pollution and mortality in nine California counties: results from CALFINE. Environ Health Perspect 2006;114:29–33.
48. Dewailly E, Nantel A, Bruneau S, et al. Breast milk contamination by PCDDs, PCDFs and PCBs in Arctic Quebec: a preliminary assessment. Chemosphere 1992;25:1245–79.
49. Van Oostdam J, Donaldson SG, Feeley M, et al. Human health implications of environmental contaminants in Arctic Canada: a review. Sci Total Environ 2005;351–352:165–246.
50. McLeod D, Pullon S, Cookson T. Factors that influence changes in smoking behaviour during pregnancy. N Z Med J 2003;116:1–8.

51. Phares TM, Morrow B, Lansky A, et al. Surveillance for disparities in maternal health-related behaviors—selected states, Pregnancy Risk Assessment Monitoring System (PRAMS), 2000–2001. MMWR Surveill Summ 2004;53:1–13.
52. Scott S, Fogarty C, Day S, et al. Smoking rates among American Indian women giving birth in Minnesota. A call to action. Minn Med 2005;88:44–9.
53. Tong VT, Jones JR, Dietz PM, et al. Trends in smoking before, during, and after pregnancy—Pregnancy Risk Assessment Monitoring System (PRAMS), United States, 31 sites, 2000–2005. MMWR Surveill Summ 2009;58:1–29.
54. Wills RA, Coory MD. Effect of smoking among indigenous and non-indigenous mothers on preterm birth and full-term low birthweight. Med J Aust 2008;189:490–4.
55. Stocks J, Dezateux C. The effect of parental smoking on lung function and development during infancy. Respirology 2003;8:266–85.
56. Scragg R, Glover M. Parental and adolescent smoking: does the association vary with gender and ethnicity? N Z Med J 2007;120:1–11.
57. Sin DD, Sharpe HM, Cowie RL, et al. Spirometric findings among school-aged First Nations children on a reserve: a pilot study. Can Respir J 2004;11:45–8.
58. Landau LI. Parental smoking: asthma and wheezing illnesses in infants and children. Paediatr Respir Rev 2001;2:202–6.
59. Peat JK, Keena V, Harakeh Z, et al. Parental smoking and respiratory tract infections in children. Paediatr Respir Rev 2001;2:207–13.
60. Forster JL, Brokenleg I, Rhodes KL, et al. Cigarette smoking among American Indian youth in Minneapolis-St. Paul. Am J Prev Med 2008;35:449–56.
61. Retnakaran R, Hanley AJ, Connelly PW, et al. Cigarette smoking and cardiovascular risk factors among aboriginal Canadian youths. CMAJ 2005;11:885–9.
62. Rempel GR, Borton BL, Kumar R. Aspiration during swallowing in typically developing children of the First Nations and Inuit in Canada. Pediatr Pulmonol 2006;41:912–5.
63. Marchant JM, Masters IB, Taylor SM, et al. Utility of signs and symptoms of chronic cough in predicting specific cause in children. Thorax 2006;61:694–8.
64. Donnelly D, Critchlow A, Everard ML. Outcomes in children treated for persistent bacterial bronchitis. Thorax 2007;62:80–4.
65. Marchant JM, Gibson PG, Grissell TV, et al. Prospective assessment of protracted bacterial bronchitis: airway inflammation and innate immune activation. Pediatr Pulmonol 2008;43:1092–9.
66. Chang AB, Redding GJ, Everard ML. Chronic wet cough: protracted bronchitis, chronic suppurative lung disease and bronchiectasis. Pediatr Pulmonol 2008; 43:519–31.
67. Chang CC, Singleton RJ, Morris PS, et al. Pneumococcal vaccines for children and adults with bronchiectasis. Cochrane Database Syst Rev 2009;(2):CD006316.
68. Kolbe J, Wells AU. Bronchiectasis: a neglected cause of respiratory morbidity and mortality. Respirology 1996;1:221–5.
69. Twiss J, Metcalfe R, Edwards E, et al. New Zealand national incidence of bronchiectasis "too high" for a developed country. Arch Dis Child 2005;90:737–40.
70. Massie RJ, Olsen M, Glazner J, et al. Newborn screening for cystic fibrosis in Victoria: 10 years' experience (1989–1998). Med J Aust 2000;172:584–7.
71. Redding G, Singleton R, Lewis T, et al. Early radiographic and clinical features associated with bronchiectasis in children. Pediatr Pulmonol 2004; 37:297–304.
72. Redding GJ. Bronchiectasis in children. Pediatr Clin North Am 2009;56:157–71.
73. Bush A, Rubin BK. Macrolides as biological response modifiers in cystic fibrosis and bronchiectasis. Semin Respir Crit Care Med 2003;24:737–47.

74. Cymbala AA, Edmonds LC, Bauer MA, et al. The disease-modifying effects of twice-weekly oral azithromycin in patients with bronchiectasis. Treat Respir Med 2005;4:117–22.

75. Koh YY, Lee MH, Sun YH, et al. Effect of roxithromycin on airway responsiveness in children with bronchiectasis: a double-blind, placebo-controlled study. Eur Respir J 1997;10:994–9.

76. Yalcin E, Kiper N, Ozcelik U, et al. Effects of claritromycin on inflammatory parameters and clinical conditions in children with bronchiectasis. J Clin Pharm Ther 2006;31:49–55.

77. Cole PJ, Roberts DE, Davies SF, et al. A simple oral antimicrobial regimen effective in severe chronic bronchial suppuration associated with culturable *Haemophilus influenzae*. J Antimicrob Chemother 1983;11:109–13.

78. Redding GJ, Kishioka C, Martinez P, et al. Physical and transport properties of sputum from children with idiopathic bronchiectasis. Chest 2008;134: 1129–34.

79. O'Donnell AE, Barker AF, Ilowite JS, et al. Treatment of idiopathic bronchiectasis with aerosolized recombinant human DNase I. rhDNase Study Group. Chest 1998;113:1329–34.

80. Daviskas E, Anderson SD, Gomes K, et al. Inhaled mannitol for the treatment of mucociliary dysfunction in patients with bronchiectasis: effect on lung function, health status and sputum. Respirology 2005;10:46–56.

81. Elkins MR, Robinson M, Rose BR, et al. A controlled trial of long-term inhaled hypertonic saline in patients with cystic fibrosis. N Engl J Med 2006;354:229–40.

82. Furumoto A, Ohkusa Y, Chen M, et al. Additive effect of pneumococcal vaccine and influenza vaccine on acute exacerbation in patients with chronic lung disease. Vaccine 2008;26:4284–9.

83. Chang CC, Morris PS, Chang AB. Influenza vaccine for children and adults with bronchiectasis. Cochrane Database Syst Rev 2007;(3):CD006218.

84. Corless JA, Warburton CJ. Leukotriene receptor antagonists for non-cystic fibrosis bronchiectasis. Cochrane Database Syst Rev 2000;(4):CD002174.

85. Corless JA, Warburton CJ. Surgery versus non-surgical treatment for bronchiectasis. Cochrane Database Syst Rev 2000;(4):CD002180.

86. Halfhide C, Evans HJ, Couriel J. Inhaled bronchodilators for cystic fibrosis. Cochrane Database Syst Rev 2005;(4):CD003428.

87. Kapur N, Chang AB. Oral non steroid anti-inflammatories for children and adults with bronchiectasis. Cochrane Database Syst Rev 2007;(4):CD006427.

88. Zar HJ, Ehrlich RI, Workman L, et al. The changing prevalence of asthma, allergic rhinitis and atopic eczema in African adolescents from 1995 to 2002. Pediatr Allergy Immunol 2007;18:560–5.

89. Brim SN, Rudd RA, Funk RH, et al. Asthma prevalence among US children in underrepresented minority populations: American Indian/Alaska Native, Chinese, Filipino, and Asian Indian. Pediatrics 2008;122:e217–22.

90. Shaw RA, Crane J, O'Donnell TV. Asthma symptoms, bronchial hyperresponsiveness and atopy in a Maori and European adolescent population. N Z Med J 1991; 8:175–9.

91. Liu LL, Stout JW, Sullivan M, et al. Asthma and bronchiolitis hospitalizations among American Indian children. Arch Pediatr Adolesc Med 2000;154:991–6.

92. Ellison-Loschmann L, King R, Pearce N. Regional variations in asthma hospitalisations among Maori and non-Maori. N Z Med J 2004;30:U745.

93. Williams H, Stewart A, von Mutius E, et al. Is eczema really on the increase worldwide? J Allergy Clin Immunol 2008;121:947–54.

94. Krause T, Koch A, Friborg J, et al. Frequency of atopy in the Arctic in 1987 and 1998. Lancet 2002;360:691–2.

95. Redding GJ, Singleton RJ, DeMain J, et al. Relationship between IgE and specific aeroallergen sensitivity in Alaskan native children. Ann Allergy Asthma Immunol 2006;97:209–15.

96. Epton MJ, Town GI, Ingham T, et al. The New Zealand Asthma and Allergy Cohort Study (NZA2CS): assembly, demographics and investigations. BMC Public Health 2007;7:26.

97. Chavasse RJPG, Seddon P, Bara A, et al. Short acting beta2-agonists for recurrent wheeze in children under two years of age. Cochrane Database Syst Rev 2002;(2):CD002873.

98. Bentur L, Canny GJ, Shields MD, et al. Controlled trial of nebulized albuterol in children younger than 2 years of age with acute asthma. Pediatrics 1992;89:133–7.

99. Chavasse RJ, Bastian-Lee Y, Richter H, et al. Inhaled salbutamol for wheezy infants: a randomised controlled trial. Arch Dis Child 2000;82:370–5.

100. Clarke JR, Aston H, Silverman M. Delivery of salbutamol by metered dose inhaler and valved spacer to wheezy infants: effect on bronchial responsiveness. Arch Dis Child 1993;69:125–9.

101. Fox GF, Marsh MJ, Milner AD. Treatment of recurrent acute wheezing episodes in infancy with oral salbutamol and prednisolone. Eur J Pediatr 1996;155:512–6.

102. Kraemer R, Frey U, Sommer CW, et al. Short-term effect of albuterol, delivered via a new auxiliary device, in wheezy infants. Am Rev Respir Dis 1991;144:347–51.

103. Kraemer R, Graf Bigler U, Casaulta Aebischer C, et al. Clinical and physiological improvement after inhalation of low-dose beclomethasone dipropionate and salbutamol in wheezy infants. Respiration 1997;64:342–9.

104. Prahl P, Petersen NT, Hornsleth A. Beta 2-agonists for the treatment of wheezy bronchitis? Ann Allergy 1986;57:439–41.

105. Prendiville A, Green S, Silverman M. Airway responsiveness in wheezy infants: evidence for functional beta adrenergic receptors. Thorax 1987;42:100–4.

106. Everard M, Bara A, Kurian M, et al. Anticholinergic drugs for wheeze in children under the age of two years. Cochrane Database Syst Rev 2005;(3):CD001279.

107. Mallol J, Barrueto L, Girardi G, et al. Use of nebulized bronchodilators in infants under 1 year of age: analysis of four forms of therapy. Pediatr Pulmonol 1987;3: 298–303.

108. Mallol J, Barrueto L, Girardi G, et al. Bronchodilator effect of fenoterol and ipratropium bromide in infants with acute wheezing: use of MDI with a spacer device. Pediatr Pulmonol 1987;3:352–6.

109. Wang EE, Milner R, Allen U, et al. Bronchodilators for treatment of mild bronchiolitis: a factorial randomised trial. Arch Dis Child 1992;67:289–93.

110. Naspitz CK, Sole D. Treatment of acute wheezing and dyspnea attacks in children under 2 years old: inhalation of fenoterol plus ipratropium bromide versus fenoterol. J Asthma 1992;29:253–8.

111. Henry RL, Hiller EJ, Milner AD, et al. Nebulised ipratropium bromide and sodium cromoglycate in the first two years of life. Arch Dis Child 1984;59:54–7.

112. Brand PLP, Baraldi E, Bisgaard H, et al. Definition, assessment and treatment of wheezing disorders in preschool children: an evidence-based approach. Eur Respir J 2008;32:1096–110.

113. Bateman ED, Hurd SS, Barnes PJ, et al. Global strategy for asthma management and prevention: GINA executive summary. Eur Respir J 2008;31:143–78.

114. Becker A, Lemiere C, Berube D, et al. Summary of recommendations from the Canadian Asthma Consensus Guidelines, 2003. CMAJ 2005;173:S3–11.

115. British Thoracic Society, Scottish Intercollegiate Guidelines Network. British guideline on the management of asthma. Thorax 2003;58(Suppl 1):i1–94.

116. National Heart, Lung, and Blood Institute National Asthma Education and Prevention Program. Expert panel report 3: guidelines for the diagnosis and management of asthma. Bethesda (MD): National Heart, Lung and Blood Institute; 2007.

117. Chang AB, Shannon C, O'Neil MC, et al. Asthma management in indigenous children of a remote community using an indigenous health model. J Paediatr Child Health 2000;36:249–51.

118. Van Sickle D, Wright AL. Navajo perceptions of asthma and asthma medications: clinical implications. Pediatrics 2001;108:E11.

119. Bailey E, Cates CJ, Kruske SG, et al. Culture-specific programs for children and adults from minority groups who have asthma. Cochrane Database Syst Rev 2009;(1):CD006580.

120. Moudgil H, Marshall T, Honeybourne D. Asthma education and quality of life in the community: a randomised controlled study to evaluate the impact on white European and Indian subcontinent ethnic groups from socioeconomically deprived areas in Birmingham, UK. Thorax 2000;55:177–83.

121. Canino G, Vila D, Normand SL, et al. Reducing asthma health disparities in poor Puerto Rican children: the effectiveness of a culturally tailored family intervention. J Allergy Clin Immunol 2008;121:665–70.

122. La Roche MJ, Koinis-Mitchell D, Gualdron L. A culturally competent asthma management intervention: a randomized controlled pilot study. Ann Allergy Asthma Immunol 2006;96:80–5.

123. Chang AB, Taylor B, Masters IB, et al. Indigenous healthcare worker involvement for indigenous adults and children with asthma. Cochrane Database Syst Rev 2007;(4):CD006344.

124. Substance Abuse and Mental Health Services Administration (SAMHSA). 2005 National survey on drug use and health: detailed tables. Rockville (MD): USDHHS; 2007.

125. Stout JW, Sullivan M, Liu LL, et al. Asthma prevalence among American Indian and Alaska Native children. Public Health Rep 1999;114:257–61.

126. Valery PC, Purdie DM, Chang AB, et al. Assessment of the diagnosis and prevalence of asthma in Australian indigenous children. J Epidemiol 2003;56: 629–35.

127. First Nations Information Governance Committee. First Nations Regional Longitudinal Health Survey (RHS) 2002/03: results for adults, youth and children living in First Nations communities. 2nd edition. Ottawa, Canada: Assembly of First Nations; 2007. Available at: http://www.rhs-ers.ca/english/pdf/rhs2002-03reports/rhs2002-03-technicalreport-afn.pdf. Accessed February 28, 2009.

128. Statistics Canada. The Health of Inuit Children: Report 2001. Inuit in Canada: Findings from the Aboriginal Peoples Survey—Survey of Living Conditions in the Arctic. Available at: http://www.statcan.gc.ca/bsolc/olc-cel/olc-cel?catno=89-627-XIE&lang=eng#Formatdisp.

Acute and Persistent Diarrhea

Keith Grimwood, MB ChB, FRACP, MD[a,b,c,*],
David A. Forbes, MBBS, FRACP[d,e,f]

KEYWORDS

• Diarrhea • Enteropathy • Indigenous • Aboriginal
• Child • Management

GLOBAL DIARRHEAL DISEASE BURDEN

Infectious diarrhea remains one of the leading causes of childhood morbidity and mortality worldwide. It results from infection of the intestinal tract by a wide range of enteric pathogens that can disrupt intestinal function. The resulting symptom complex of diarrhea is characterized by an increased number of loose or watery (≥ 3 in 24 hours) stools. The term dysentery is used when blood, mucus, and white blood cells are present in the stool. The annual global burden of infectious diarrhea is enormous, involving 3 to 5 billion cases and nearly 2 million deaths, with the latter accounting for almost 20% of all deaths in children younger than 5 years.[1] Of these diarrhea-related deaths, acute watery diarrhea is responsible for 35%; dysentery, for 20%; and persistent or chronic diarrhea, 45%.[2] Most deaths are in young children from rural regions of developing countries where there is limited access to safe drinking water, sewage disposal, and health care, and reduced opportunities for personal sanitation, hygiene, and safe food preparation. In this setting, repeated episodes of enteric

[a] Queensland Paediatric Infectious Diseases Laboratory, Queensland Children's Medical Research Institute, Royal Children's Hospital, Herston Road, Herston, Brisbane, Queensland, Australia 4029
[b] Discipline of Paediatrics and Child Health, University of Queensland, Royal Children's Hospital, Herston Road, Herston, Brisbane, Queensland, Australia 4029
[c] Department of Infectious Disease, Royal Children's Hospital, Herston Road, Herston, Brisbane, Queensland, Australia 4029
[d] School of Paediatrics and Child Health, University of Western Australia, GPO Box D184, Perth, Western Australia, Australia 6840
[e] Paediatric Medicine Clinical Care Unit, Princess Margaret Hospital, Roberts Road, Subiaco, Perth, Western Australia, Australia 6008
[f] Gastroenterology, Princess Margaret Hospital, Roberts Road, Subiaco, Perth, Western Australia, Australia 6008
* Corresponding author. Queensland Paediatric Infectious Diseases Laboratory, Queensland Children's Medical Research Institute, Royal Children's Hospital, Herston Road, Herston, Brisbane, Queensland, Australia 4029.
E-mail address: keith_grimwood@health.qld.gov.au (K. Grimwood).

Pediatr Clin N Am 56 (2009) 1343–1361
doi:10.1016/j.pcl.2009.09.004
0031-3955/09/$ – see front matter
pediatric.theclinics.com

infection can contribute to malnutrition by interfering with nutrient absorption. As these episodes usually occur during the first few years of life, a period critical for physical growth and brain development, they can be followed by impaired linear growth, intellectual function, and school performance.[3]

In industrialized countries, where medical access is more readily available and modern standards of water quality, personal hygiene, sanitation, and food safety exist, deaths from diarrheal illness have decreased dramatically.[4] However, sporadic diarrheal illness remains an important cause of morbidity, second only to respiratory infections as the most common cause of childhood infectious disease resulting in health-care attendance.[5–8] Most episodes are caused by enteric viruses and are self-limited in nature, rarely resulting in persistent diarrhea, malnutrition, or death in a previously healthy child. Nevertheless, socially disadvantaged Indigenous children living in western industrialized countries experience high rates of severe diarrheal disease and, in some communities, the pattern of morbidity resembles that seen in developing countries.

BURDEN IN INDIGENOUS CHILDREN IN INDUSTRIALIZED SOCIETIES

In the United States, high rates of acute diarrheal disease are observed in American Indian (AI) and Alaskan Native (AN) infants residing in reservations or remote locations lacking adequate sanitation. **Table 1** summarizes 2 separate studies spanning 25 years conducted by the Centers for Disease Control and Prevention.[9,10] During the early 1980s, the annual incidence of diarrhea-associated hospitalization for AI/AN infants younger than 12 months living in or near reservations was 1148 per 10,000 infants, which was more than 3 times that of other infants residing in the United States.[9] However, by the 1990s, the annual incidence in AI/AN infants had fallen to 275 cases per 10,000 infants. Rates of hospitalization for diarrhea in older AI/AN children were also similar to that of the general US population. At the same time, the

Table 1
Annual diarrhea-associated hospitalization incidence rates among US children younger than 5 years for 3 time periods between 1980 and 2004

	1980–1982			1993–1995			2000–2004		
	IHS[a]	US[b]	Rate Difference (%)	IHS	US[b]	Rate Difference (%)	IHS	US[c]	Rate Difference (%)
Age: <1y	1148	348	230	275	192	43	263	155	70
1–4y	81	78	4	36	64	-44	29	60	-52
Total	236	136	74	71	89	-20	66	79	-16

Age-specific incidence rates are per 10,000 children.
[a] Indian Health Service hospital discharge data; rate estimates were calculated from the 1996 IHS user population.[8]
[b] Rate estimates were calculated from the National Hospital Discharge Survey and the 1981 and 1994 national census data, respectively.[8]
[c] National rate estimates for the US population were calculated from the 2003 Kids Inpatient Database and the 2003 national census data.[9]
Data from Holman RC, Parashar UD, Clarke MJ, et al. Trends in diarrhea-associated hospitalizations among American Indian and Alaskan Native Children, 1980–1995. Pediatrics 1999;103:e11; with permission and *from* Singleton RJ, Holman RC, Yorita KL, et al. Diarrhea-associated hospitalizations and outpatient visits among American Indian and Alaska Native children younger than five years of age, 2000–2004. Pediatr Infect Dis J 2007;26:1006–13.

median time spent in hospital for AI/AN children decreased significantly from 4 days in 1980 to 1982 to just 2 days in 1993 to 1995. Possible causes for this substantial decline in hospitalization rates include improved provision of safe drinking water, construction of sanitation facilities, increased coverage of measles vaccination, and introduction of oral glucose-electrolyte rehydration therapy into the routine management of acute infectious diarrhea.

Table 1 also shows that since the 1990s, there has been little improvement in hospitalization rates for AI/AN infants with diarrhea, which remain almost twice that of other US infants.[10] Furthermore, diarrhea-associated outpatient visits for AI/AN infants are also more than twice that of the general infant population (2956 and 1312 per 10,000, respectively). The higher rates of infectious diarrhea-related morbidity amongst AI/AN infants are attributed to continuing limited access to safe water supply and inadequate sanitation in some communities and to more severe rotavirus-related diarrhea.[10,11] Despite the high rate of health care utilization by AI/AN infants, diarrheal episodes are short, persistent diarrhea is uncommon, and malnutrition is rarely encountered.[11]

Diarrheal disease is also common among children in Australian Aboriginal communities, reflecting overcrowding and difficulties with sanitation and hygiene.[12] The most robust data for Aboriginal children are collected at the state level,[4,13,14] and these demonstrate sustained and disproportionately high rates of hospitalization for acute diarrheal illnesses.[15] First recognized as a major health problem in the 1950s, episodes of infectious diarrhea in Aboriginal children were severe, with high rates of dehydration, hypokalemia, lactose intolerance, and prolonged hospital admission because of accompanying malnutrition, heavy intestinal parasitic infestation, and malabsorption.[16] Even by the 1970s, hospital case fatality rates in Western Australia were approximately 5%, although these declined steeply during the next decade.[16,17] Nevertheless, hospitalization rates for acute diarrhea were 16 to 20 times higher for infants and 12 to 15 times higher for children aged 1 to 5 years than for non-Aboriginal children of the same ages.[18] Moreover, bed usage rates were 40 to 50 times greater in Aboriginal infants and 30 to 40 times greater in those aged 1 to 5 years than in similarly aged non-Aboriginal children.

During the last 2 decades there have been several initiatives to improve Aboriginal child health, including better housing, sanitation, and water supply, improved access to health care, enhanced surveillance, and concerted health and hygiene promotion campaigns. Deaths are now rare and during the 1990s, hospital admission rates in Western Australia for aboriginal infants and children with infectious diarrhea declined 20% to 30% (**Fig. 1**). Nevertheless, hospitalization rates for acute diarrhea in Aboriginal children remain 7 to 8 times higher than their non-Aboriginal peers.[4,14] The disparity in hospitalization rates is greatest for Aboriginal infants where, for example, annual admission rates in the late 1990s in the Northern Territory of Australia exceeded 3330 cases per 10,000 infants, which is 16 times greater than that encountered for the non-Aboriginal infant population from that region.[19] Furthermore, 38% of Aboriginal children hospitalized for acute diarrhea are subsequently readmitted with another diarrheal episode, a rate that is almost 3 times higher than for other children.[20,21]

Aboriginal children hospitalized for infectious diarrhea still have high rates of malnutrition (12%–50%), lactose intolerance (8%–27%), severe iron deficiency anemia (5%–8%), and other coinfections (25%–50%), such as lower respiratory tract infections, otitis media, urinary tract infections, or scabies.[13,19–23] Diarrhea severity, comorbid conditions, and difficulties with arranging transport, often to remote settlements, contribute to the length of time in hospital, which on average is about twice that of non-Aboriginal children (4.8 vs 2.2 and 8.9 vs 3.9 days in Western Australia and the Northern Territory, respectively).[13,19] The highest rates of hospital admission and other

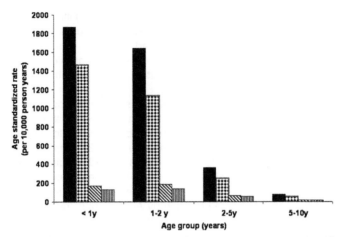

Fig. 1. Age-standardized gastroenteritis hospitalization rates, Western Australia, 1994 and 2000. Aboriginal 1994; Aboriginal 2000; non-Aboriginal 1994; non-Aboriginal 2000. (*Adapted from* Gracey M, Cullinane J. Gastroenteritis and environmental health among Aboriginal infants and children from Western Australia. J Paediatr Child Health 2003;39:427–31; with permission.)

comorbid conditions are found in Aboriginal infants and children from remote rural regions of Northern Australia, where disparities in housing quality, environmental and personal hygiene, sanitation, household crowding, and access to high quality food and to health care are most evident.

Other Indigenous populations living in western industrialized countries also have high rates of childhood diarrhea from an early age. For example, First Nations and Inuit infants from remote settlements in northern Canada had 3 times the rate of rotavirus infection during the first 6 months of life compared with infants from urban Winnipeg.[24] High rates of diarrheal disease are reported amongst New Zealand's Maori children, although more recently the incidence of diarrheal illness has been greatest amongst immigrant Polynesian infants living in the most socioeconomically deprived suburbs of New Zealand's largest cities.[25,26]

PATHOGENS

The most frequently detected enteric pathogens in Indigenous communities are displayed in **Table 2**. These organisms are similar to those causing diarrhea in children from developing countries. Multiple pathogens are often isolated from individual patients, reflecting the effects of overcrowding, inadequate sanitation, and poor personal hygiene. The predominant enteric pathogens can vary by region, by season, and with time. Older studies may therefore no longer reliably predict the major causes of infectious diarrhea in some Indigenous communities. Where improvements in drinking water and personal and environmental hygiene have taken place, there should be decreased illness from bacterial and parasitic agents.[9] Similarly, rotavirus vaccines are likely to further reduce episodes of severe diarrhea in infants and young children, where for example, in Australia, rural Aboriginal children have had the greatest disease burden.[27,28] Indeed, shortly after their introduction, rotavirus vaccines protected immunized Aboriginal infants from a rotavirus outbreak simultaneously affecting several remote settlements in Central Australia.[29] Finally, modern molecular

Table 2
Enteric pathogens associated with diarrhea in Indigenous children from North America, Australia and New Zealand

Viral	Bacterial	Parasitic
Rotavirus	Nontyphoidal Salmonella	Giardia
Norovirus	Campylobacter	Cryptosporidium
Enteric adenovirus	Shigella	Strongyloides
	Diarrheagenic *Escherichia coli*[a]	

[a] Predominantly (1) enteroaggregative or EAEC; (2) enteropathogenic or EPEC; and (3) enterotoxigenic or ETEC pathotypes.

diagnostic techniques have shown that previously difficult-to-detect gastrointestinal pathogens, such as noroviruses, play an important etiologic role in acute diarrhea amongst disadvantaged populations.[30]

In tropical Northern Australia, the pattern of diarrheal disease is similar to many developing countries, with peak prevalence of bacterial and parasitic infections during the warm, wet season and rotavirus outbreaks during the cooler, dry months of the year. Dysentery is uncommon and most affected children present with acute watery diarrhea. The most frequently isolated enteric pathogens from hospitalized Aboriginal children are rotavirus (27%), enteroaggregative *Escherichia coli* (EAEC; 29%), enteropathogenic *E coli* (EPEC; 17%), nontyphoidal *Salmonella* spp (11%), enterotoxigenic *E coli* (ETEC; 11%), *Cryptosporidium parvum* (7%), and *Strongyloides stercoralis* (7%).[16,31,32] At the community level, the predominant pathogens associated with diarrhea are rotavirus (12%), nontyphoidal *Salmonella* (13%), *Shigella* spp (5%), ETEC (15%), and *C parvum* (8%), and *S stercoralis* (1%).[16,33,34] In Australia's Northern Territory, the burden from rotavirus disease is particularly high, with notifications for Aboriginal children younger than 5 years almost 3 times that of non-Aboriginal children from the same region (2.75 vs 0.98 per year), and hospitalization duration is also about 3 times that recorded for non-Aboriginal children.[28,35] In addition, rotavirus notifications begin at a younger age for Aboriginal children, where 56% are younger than 1 year and 24%, younger than 6 months. Comparable figures for non-Aboriginal children are 31% and 7%, respectively. As observed previously, in AI/AN children, unpredictable and explosive outbreaks of rotavirus diarrhea can happen simultaneously in several remote settlements, resulting in severe illness in susceptible individuals.[36,37] Noroviruses are an important cause of diarrhea in urban Australian children[38] and, given their global importance, they are also likely to play an important role in diarrheal disease in Aboriginal children living in tropical Australia.[7]

Multiple enteric pathogens are frequently isolated from Aboriginal children.[16,32–34] Nontyphoidal *Salmonella* spp, *Giardia* spp., diarrheagenic *E coli* and *Campylobacter* spp are found in 12% to 45% of asymptomatic children living in remote, rural Aboriginal settlements.[32–34] These organisms are transmitted from person-to-person or in food and water contaminated by human or animal feces. Detection of these pathogens reflects the overcrowding, inadequate water supply and personal hygiene, and poor sanitation that persist in these communities.[19]

PERSISTENT DIARRHEA AND ENTEROPATHY

Persistent diarrhea is defined as diarrhea that begins acutely, but persists for more than 14 days. Cases of persistent diarrhea occur predominantly in children younger than 3 years. Poor nutrition is a risk factor and an outcome of persistent diarrhea.[39] Consequently, there is a vicious cycle of infection, malabsorption, and malnutrition leading to stunted growth and cognitive impairment in some children.[3,39] Although noninfectious causes, such as celiac disease, food protein-related enteropathies, and rare congenital causes of intractable diarrhea need to be considered, most cases in the developing world and amongst disadvantaged Indigenous children living in industrialized countries are likely to result from repeated enteric infections. Although still not fully understood, multiple consecutive infections can lead to small-bowel mucosal injury with blunting of the villi, cellular infiltration of the lamina propria, and loss of epithelial barrier and absorptive functions, which can persist into adulthood.[39–42] Undernutrition delays epithelial cell repair, and secondary carbohydrate malabsorption from reduced production of disaccharidase enzymes prolongs the diarrheal symptoms and has an adverse effect on growth. Pathogens that are frequently isolated in persistent diarrhea include EAEC, EPEC, and *Cryptosporidium* spp, although *Giardia, Cyclospora*, and *Strongyloides* spp may also be important, especially in malnourished or immunocompromised children.[39]

Persistent diarrhea is not commonly reported in Aboriginal children. This has been attributed to prolonged breastfeeding and prompt treatment of diarrhea with low-osmolarity lactose-free milk formula.[32] Nevertheless, in Northern and Central Australia more than one-third of Aboriginal children without gastrointestinal symptoms have abnormal intestinal permeability, with evidence of impaired barrier function and decreased absorptive function as markers of underlying partial villous atrophy and intestinal inflammation.[19,23,32] Others have observed that the stools of young Aboriginal children from remote communities are frequently loose and unformed, suggesting the acceptance of persistent loose stools as normal in children from isolated Indigenous communities.[34] A recent health survey from Western Australia found that 6% of Aboriginal children had recurring episodes of diarrhea, with prevalence doubling amongst those living in remote rural settlements.[43] Although cow's milk protein intolerance does not appear to be an important cause of enteropathy in Aboriginal children, pathogens associated with small-bowel enteropathy, such as *Cryptosporidium* and *Strongyloides* may cause severe acute diarrheal episodes and contribute to malnutrition and reduced "catch-up" growth between episodes of diarrhea.[23,32] Although *Brachyspira* spp have been identified in Aboriginal children with persistent diarrhea and poor growth, whether they play a genuine pathogenic role is still uncertain.[44] Coinfections with rotavirus and diarrheagenic *E coli* strains can also result in more severe disease.[32,45] Acute enteric infections, superimposed on underlying enteropathy, are thought to lead to further reductions in brush-border disaccharidase levels so that breast or cow's milk results in osmotic diarrhea, dehydration, acidosis, and hypokalemia.[46] Thus, repeated and frequent subclinical enteric infections associated with poor environmental hygiene can lead to an underlying enteropathy with impaired growth and, on occasions, episodes of severe gastroenteritis in young children.

MANAGEMENT
Assessment

Children presenting with acute diarrhea should be assessed quickly to determine whether they have infectious diarrhea. Next, the nature (watery or bloody dysenteric stools) and duration of the diarrhea, the presence and degree of dehydration, and the existence of associated conditions, such as pneumonia or malnutrition, must be established. Bile-stained vomiting, severe abdominal pain, tenderness, distension, or masses suggest a surgical cause, whereas high fever, pallor, drowsiness, signs of circulatory impairment or respiratory distress inconsistent with the history of vomiting or diarrhea should raise the possibility of sepsis, pneumonia, urine infection or other serious illness. Malnourished Aboriginal children with diarrhea are at greater risk of dehydration, acidosis, and hypokalemia and are more likely to harbor multiple enteric pathogens or have other comorbidities than well-nourished non-Aboriginal children with gastroenteritis.[16,19,23,47]

A systematic review of 13 studies (1246 participants) found that prolonged capillary refill time greater than 2 seconds, skin turgor greater than 2 seconds, and abnormal respiratory pattern, alone or together, were the best individual signs for predicting 5% dehydration in children.[48] Signs appear at about 3% dehydration, and children can be categorized as having mild-to-moderate dehydration if they are about 5% dehydrated (range; 3%–8%) and having severe dehydration if they are dehydrated by 9% or more. There is no direct evidence of when serum electrolytes should be measured in a child with diarrhea. Nevertheless, if feasible, children requiring intravenous rehydration should have their serum electrolytes measured.[49] Furthermore, because rates of hypokalemia can exceed 60% in Aboriginal children hospitalized with diarrhea, these children should also have their serum electrolytes and glucose measured, especially if they are malnourished, have impaired conscious state or seizures, are younger than 3 months, or are dehydrated or suffering from persistent diarrhea.[50] Similarly, when dysentery is present, stools should be examined for enteric pathogens and, if diarrhea is persistent, the stools should be tested for reducing sugars.[51]

Treatment

Treatment recommendations and evidence are summarized in **Table 3**. The pillars of clinical management of acute diarrhea are (1) correction of any dehydration and electrolyte and acid-base disturbance, (2) maintenance of nutrition, (3) treatment of associated conditions, and (4) prudent use of antimicrobial agents. Much of the evidence for managing and preventing infectious diarrhea in **Tables 3** and **4** comes from studies conducted at large tertiary pediatric hospitals or community-based trials in developing regions of the world. In contrast, there are relatively few studies involving Indigenous children from industrialized countries.

A Cochrane review of 17 randomized controlled trials (RCTs; 1811 participants with acute gastroenteritis) found that there were no clinically important differences between oral glucose-electrolyte solutions and intravenous (IV) fluid therapy for managing children with mild-to-moderate dehydration from different countries or in different states of nutrition.[52] For every 25 children receiving oral rehydration therapy, one will fail and require IV fluid replacement. A systematic review and meta-analysis reached similar conclusions.[53,54] Best results were achieved with low osmolarity (eg, sodium [Na] 60, potassium [K] 20, chloride [Cl] 50, citrate 10, glucose 86 mmol/L; osmolarity 226 mOsm/L) oral rehydration solutions. Cereal-based oral rehydration solutions offer theoretical advantages, but these benefits may be negated by early feeding, and further studies are required to define their role in the management of non-cholera gastroenteritis.[55] Although, nasogastric tubes allow continuous administration of oral rehydration fluids for children with persistent vomiting, they may not be acceptable in some cultures.[56] Rehydration can usually be achieved within 4 to 6 hours. Overall, oral rehydration therapy for acute diarrhea in young children is safer and associated with lower costs, fewer hospital admissions, and less time spent in health care facilities.[57] Contraindications to oral rehydration include severe dehydration, impaired conscious state, paralytic ileus, severe hypokalemia, alternative diagnoses, such as

Table 3
Recommendations for the clinical management of acute and persistent diarrhea in Indigenous children

Intervention	Recommendation	Grading of Recommendation[106]	Quality of Supporting Evidence[107]
Oral glucose-electrolyte fluid	Use low-osmolarity oral rehydration solution over 4–6h to correct mild-to-moderate dehydration	Strong	High
Intravenous isotonic fluids	Use to correct severe dehydration over 3–4h or when oral rehydration therapy is contraindicated	Strong	High
Antiemetics	Not recommended	Weak	Low
Antidiarrheal agents	Not recommended	Strong	High
Early feeding, including breastfeeding	Recommended	Strong	Moderate
Lactose-free formula	Recommended for those with malnutrition, severe or persistent diarrhea, and if high rates of enteropathy exist	Strong	High
Micronutrients:			
Zinc	Recommended for those with malnutrition, severe or persistent diarrhea, and if high rates of enteropathy exist	Weak	Low
Vitamin A	Not recommended	Strong	Low
Probiotics	Not recommended	Strong	Moderate
Antimicrobials			
Acute watery diarrhea (noncholera)	Recommended only for giardiasis	Strong	High
Dysentery	Recommended only for select pathogens	Strong	Moderate
Persistent diarrhea	Recommended only for select pathogens	Strong	Moderate

Table 4
Recommendations for the prevention of acute and persistent diarrhea in Indigenous children

Intervention	Recommendation	Grading of Recommendation[105]	Quality of Supporting Evidence[106]
High standards of environmental hygiene			
Clean water	Recommended	Strong	Moderate
High-level sanitation	Recommended	Strong	Low
Personal hygiene	Recommended	Strong	Moderate
Breastfeeding	Recommended	Strong	Moderate
Micronutrients			
Zinc	Not recommended	Strong	Low
Vitamin A	Not recommended	Strong	Very low
Rotavirus vaccines	Recommended	Strong	Moderate

surgical abdomen or sepsis, and some preexisting medical conditions, such as short gut syndrome, cyanotic heart disease, or renal impairment.[50,51]

Children who have severe dehydration, other contraindications to oral rehydration solutions, or failed oral glucose-electrolyte solution treatment require IV fluid resuscitation with isotonic fluids, preferably Ringer's lactate solution (Na 130, K 4, Cl 109, lactate 28 mmol/L).[40,58] Evidence is limited to cohort studies, but IV rehydration can be safely accomplished within 4 hours and this includes Aboriginal children with acidosis and hypokalemia complicating their diarrheal illness.[50,59] Although IV normal saline can be used to rapidly restore the circulation of severely dehydrated children, it is important to start oral rehydration fluids as soon as the children are able to drink, so as to replenish their depleted electrolytes, especially potassium. Risks associated with rapid IV fluid administration include electrolyte disturbance and fluid overload from hypotonic IV fluids and overestimating the degree of dehydration. Cardiac failure and hypoglycemia may result if there is severe malnutrition and phlebitis can follow IV cannulation.[60] These risks are minimized by careful clinical assessment and monitoring and avoiding hypotonic IV fluids. If the child is severely malnourished or presenting with hypernatremic dehydration, IV fluid replacement rates are decreased, followed by early introduction of oral rehydration solutions with regular checking of serum glucose and electrolytes.

Vomiting is a common and distressing symptom of acute diarrhea. If severe, it may hinder successful oral rehydration therapy.[27] Adverse effects, including drowsiness and extrapyramidal reactions, have meant that antiemetic agents are not recommended for young children with acute gastroenteritis.[49,51] Ondansetron, a 5-hydroxytryptamine antagonist, is a new class of antiemetic, which is well tolerated by patients with cancer following chemotherapy, including young infants. A recent Cochrane review of 4 RCTs (501 subjects) and a systematic review that included a meta-analysis of 6 RCTs (745 participants) found that ondansetron decreased vomiting in mildly dehydrated children and reduced the risk of receiving IV fluids or admission to hospital by about 50%.[61,62] To prevent one hospitalization, the number needed to treat was 14 (95% confidence interval 9, 44).[62] Ondansetron resulted in increased diarrhea, but this was not deemed clinically important for the study population, which consisted mainly of children presenting to emergency departments at large tertiary pediatric hospitals. Although promising, ondansetron remains expensive, and additional studies demonstrating safety and efficacy in severely dehydrated Indigenous or malnourished children are required before a general recommendation in its favor can be made. Similarly, antidiarrheal agents are not recommended in children because of concerns over safety.[40,51] Loperamide is widely prescribed for adults, but a recent systematic review of 13 RCTs, involving 1788 subjects, found that for a 1 day reduction of diarrhea in mildly dehydrated children, about 2% of those younger than 3 years experienced severe adverse effects, including paralytic ileus, abdominal distension, lethargy, and even death.[63] The main goals for the initial treatment of acute diarrhea should therefore remain the correction of fluid and electrolyte deficits and any acid-base disturbance present.

For 2 decades, early refeeding, including continuation of breastfeeding, has been recommended for children with diarrhea, because it may decrease stool output, shorten the duration of illness, and improve nutrition.[64,65] Surprisingly, there are only limited clinical data supporting this recommendation.[66] The development of lactose intolerance has been of concern,[67] but a meta-analysis of 29 RCTs (2215 subjects) found that when oral rehydration, early refeeding, and reintroduction of milk were an integral part of management, only young children with severe dehydration, malnutrition, or persistent diarrhea benefited from lactose-free formulae.[68] However, lactose intolerance is still an important clinical problem for Indigenous children, especially when an acute infection is superimposed on an underlying enteropathy.[19] In such circumstances, low-osmolarity, lactose-free formula hastens clinical recovery in Aboriginal and AI children[69,70] and should be used when there is severe dehydration, malnutrition, or high rates of enteropathy present.[71]

Zinc has pleiotropic functions, including positive effects on immune and mucosal barrier functions. Although its mechanisms of action are unknown, it reduces the severity and duration of acute and persistent diarrhea in children living in developing countries, where zinc deficiency is common. A Cochrane review of 18 RCTs (6165 participants) and a recent systematic review and meta-analysis of 22 studies (18,199 participants) concluded that zinc administration of 10 to 20 mg/d to infants and children older than 6 months presenting to hospital with acute or persistent diarrhea resulted in almost a 20% reduction in diarrheal frequency and duration.[72,73] In contrast, vitamin A supplementation is not recommended for managing infectious diarrhea. Results from studies of vitamin A supplementation are contradictory. A meta-analysis of 9 RCTs (45,468 subjects) failed to detect any overall benefit.[74] Recent studies from Mexico show that vitamin A and zinc have distinct effects on different enteric pathogens; for example vitamin A seems protective for some E coli pathotypes and norovirus infections, possibly from its regulatory effects upon types 1 and 2 helper cell function.[75,76] Although zinc continues to be prescribed for malnourished Aboriginal children with diarrhea,[77] an RCT from Central Australia found that neither zinc nor vitamin A, alone or in combination, provided short-term benefits for Aboriginal children hospitalized because of diarrhea.[78] However, none of these children were severely dehydrated and only a small proportion had signs of stunting. The roles for both micronutrients in the treatment of acute and persistent diarrhea caused by specific pathogens require further evaluation. Finally, probiotics in acute, childhood, infectious diarrhea appear to have moderate beneficial effects that are strain- and dose-dependent, limited to watery diarrhea, and best seen if administered early in the course of the illness.[79] Further questions over dose, duration, and safety must be addressed before probiotics can be recommended.

As acute watery diarrhea in Indigenous children from industrialized countries is usually self-limiting or caused by viruses, antibiotics do not have an important role in management. An exception is metronidazole for giardiasis. In contrast, for some patients presenting with dysentery or persistent diarrhea, there is evidence that antibiotics may shorten symptom duration and decrease disease transmission when caused by certain pathogens.[39,40,80,81] Nonetheless, indiscriminate antibiotic usage increases the likelihood of persistent diarrhea, is associated with increased rates of antibiotic resistance, and can result in adverse outcomes, such as the hemolytic uremic syndrome in enterohemorrhagic *E coli* infections or prolonging carriage of *Salmonella* spp.[80–82] Decisions to prescribe antibiotics are further complicated by limited access to laboratory facilities, unavailability of specialized tests (eg, molecular probes for diarrheagenic *E coli*), antibiotic resistance, and difficulties obtaining some recommended agents, such as nitazoxanide, for treating persistent cryptosporidiosis or giardiasis. Moreover, enteric pathogens are often found in asymptomatic children living in remote communities, so their presence in diarrheal stools does not always mean that they have a causative role.[32–34] In general, children with dysentery require treatment if *Shigella spp* or *Entamoeba histolytica* are isolated from their stools. The choice is determined by local antibiotic susceptibility patterns, but trimethoprim-sulfamethoxazole, quinolones, (eg, nalidixic acid), or azithromycin for shigellosis and metronidazole for amebic dysentery are the usual choices.[80,81] Antibiotics are unnecessary for self-limited infections caused by nontyphoidal *Salmonella* or *Campylobacter* spp., unless the diarrhea becomes persistent or, for *Salmonella*, if the patient is younger than 3 months, immunocompromised, or shows signs of invasive disease. In addition to oral rehydration therapy, dietary management, and zinc supplementation, Indigenous children with persistent diarrhea may benefit from treating *Giardia, Cyclospora, Strongyloides* and EAEC with agents such as metronidazole, trimethoprim-sulfamethoxazole, ivermectin, or albendazole and azithromycin, respectively.[39,81,83] Although antibiotic treatment of comorbid extraintestinal infections is appropriate, there is little evidence to support empiric antimicrobial therapy for children with persistent diarrhea from no known cause.[82] Earlier enthusiasm for treatment of potential bacterial overgrowth using broad-spectrum nonabsorbable antibiotics,[84] has not been sustained following an RCT from India, which failed to demonstrate either symptom reduction or accelerated recovery.[85]

Prevention

Recommendations and evidence for the prevention of acute and persistent diarrhea in Indigenous children are summarized in **Table 4**. Provision of safe water for drinking and food preparation, safe food handling, sufficient water to allow regular hand washing, and other hygienic practices, including adequate sanitation with secure disposal of human feces, are required to reduce recurrent diarrheal disease, enteropathy, and malnutrition amongst Indigenous populations.[4,16] Recent Cochrane reviews provide a level of support for this approach. An analysis of 5 cluster RCTs involving whole communities (8055 participants) from the low- or middle-income countries of Africa and Asia reported a 32% reduction in diarrheal episodes following the introduction of hand washing education programs.[86] Another review of 30 trials (53,000 participants) also found that interventions to improve the microbiologic quality of the water in countries where infectious diarrhea is endemic, successfully reduced diarrheal disease for all age groups by almost 30%, with interventions at the household proving to be most successful.[87] However, significant heterogeneity, variable study quality, and limited follow-up means the effectiveness of these interventions may vary substantially between communities. Two systematic reviews examined the impact of measures to improve environmental hygiene on the incidence of diarrheal illness. Both commented on continuing limitations in study design. One included 46 studies and a meta-analysis, which found that attention to hand hygiene, sanitation, and water supply and quality reduced diarrhea by about 30%, although no additive effects were observed when single and multiple interventions were compared.[88] The second review selected 19 studies from developing countries and highlighted the complexity of implementing and measuring the effectiveness of hygiene interventions.[89] The investigators concluded that for Aboriginal children living in remote settlements, education and hand washing with soap was likely to have the greatest impact and could lead to a 50% reduction in diarrheal episodes. Just over a decade ago, a survey of Aboriginal people from remote and rural settlements in Western Australia found that 70% lived in substandard housing and 33% of the communities had inadequate water supply and sanitation.[90] Although more government resources for improving infrastructure have later become available, the health inequalities between Aboriginal and non-Aboriginal children remain.[43] Care must be taken to ensure that improving the social determinants of health, such as education, employment, child care, and housing, should also play a central role in policies to decrease malnutrition and burden of disease.[91]

Breastfeeding provides important protection against infectious diarrhea. A meta-analysis of 6 studies (18,162 infants) from developing countries that attempted to address difficulties associated with self-selection, reverse causation, and potential confounding reported that during the first 6 months of life, non–breastfed infants had a 6 fold greater chance of dying from diarrheal disease than infants receiving breast milk.[92] However, protection decreased thereafter, presumably as potentially contaminated solid food and water are introduced into the diet. This is supported by the high diarrhea-related hospitalization and breastfeeding rates observed during the first 2 years of life for Aboriginal infants living in remote and rural communities.[4,16,21,43] Similarly, although exclusive breastfeeding may reduce the risk of severe rotavirus diarrhea by as much as 90%, this protection disappears once it is discontinued or when mixed feeding is introduced.[27,93] In contrast, neither routine vitamin A nor zinc supplementation is recommended for otherwise healthy Indigenous children. The aforementioned meta-analysis and a later-published systematic review for vitamin A supplementation found no evidence for a protective effect against diarrhea.[74,94] Another meta-analysis of 17 RCTs of zinc supplementation in 7660 children younger than 5 years from 10 developing countries found a 15% reduction in diarrheal illness and 25% fewer episodes of persistent diarrhea.[95] These reviews found evidence for publication bias, follow-up was fairly short, and adverse effects and adherence to treatment were not reported. The emergence of data from Mexico suggesting that vitamin A and zinc have different effects on enteric pathogens means further studies are needed in specific populations and communities, taking into account predominant pathogens, age, nutritional state, safety, adherence, and duration of effect.[75,76,96]

Another major approach to diarrhea prevention is immunization. The World Health Organization (WHO) has given the highest priority to the development of new and improved vaccines against rotavirus, *Shigella* spp., ETEC, *Vibrio cholerae* O1 and *Salmonella typhi*. Of these, the most recent major advance is the development and licensure of 2 live-attenuated oral rotavirus vaccines. Their safety and efficacy have been confirmed in large field trials, each involving more than 60,000 infants from Europe, the United States and Latin America.[97,98] One vaccine, RIX4414, (Rotarix, GlaxoSmithKline Biologicals, Rixensart, Belgium), derived from a single human G1P[8] strain relies on inducing homologous and broadly reactive heterotypic immunity for protection, whereas the other, RotaTeq (Merck & Co, Inc, Whitehouse Station, NJ, USA), is a multi-strain G1 to G4,P[8] bovine-human reassortant vaccine, which elicits serotype-specific responses to the most common circulating human rotavirus strains. For both vaccines, protective efficacy for any form of rotavirus diarrhea was 67% to 79% and for severe rotavirus disease, 81% to 100%.[27,99] The WHO is awaiting the results from field trials in Africa and Asia to be published before issuing a global recommendation for rotavirus vaccines (WHO made a global recommendation of including rotavirus vaccines in national immunization programs in June 2009).[100] Meanwhile, early postlicensure surveillance data from the United States and Australia show that the numbers of laboratory-confirmed cases of rotavirus diarrhea have declined by almost 70% and the onset of the rotavirus season has been delayed by 2 to 4 months.[101,102] Data are limited for rotavirus vaccines in Indigenous infants. The previously licensed rhesus-human reassortant rotavirus vaccine, RRV-TV (RotaShield, Wyeth Lederle Vaccines, Philadelphia, PA, USA), provided a protective efficacy of just 69% against severe rotavirus diarrhea in AI infants living in Arizona tribal reservations.[103] More than 500 AI infants received the multi-strain G1-G4,P[8] bovine-human reassortant vaccine, RotaTeq, in the pivotal phase III trial, although no specific safety and efficacy details were provided for AI vaccine recipients.[98] Outbreaks provide another opportunity to determine vaccine effectiveness. In March 2007, the single human G1P[8] strain vaccine, Rotarix, reduced the risk of hospitalization from gastroenteritis in fully immunized Aboriginal infants by 78% during a G9P[8] rotavirus outbreak in Central Australia.[29] However, 2 years later the vaccine appeared less effective for a G2P[4] outbreak, once again involving Aboriginal infants from the same region (Carl Kirkwood, PhD, Melbourne, Australia, personal communication, May 2009). It remains too early to judge whether this outbreak is part of a natural cycle of G2P[4] outbreaks in Central Australia or whether it results from reduced effectiveness of this vaccine.[104] Concerns have been raised previously in Brazil over increased G2P[4] activity since the introduction of Rotarix into the national infant immunization schedule, emphasizing the importance of continuing surveillance to determine the effectiveness of rotavirus vaccine programs and their impact on rotavirus ecology and to inform immunization policies.[105]

SUMMARY

Despite recent improvements, hospitalization rates for infectious diarrhea in disadvantaged Indigenous children remain higher than for other children living in western industrialized societies. This is particularly true for Australian Aboriginal children. The patterns of disease resemble those observed in developing countries, where poor environmental hygiene and overcrowding contribute to high rates of infection and intestinal mucosal injury, leading to malnutrition and, for some children, poor growth, and impaired intellectual function. Judicious use of oral rehydration solutions, early refeeding, dietary management, micronutrients, and selective prescribing of antimicrobial agents can assist recovery for individual episodes. However, it is by implementing equitable social and educational policies to enable self-determination and full community participation in decision making that will have the greatest impact. Only then will sustainable high standards in housing and environmental hygiene be achieved, which when accompanied by easily accessible health care and immunization programs "delivered on time", will help lead to decreased health inequalities for many Indigenous communities.

REFERENCES

1. Boschi-Pinto C, Velebit L, Shibuya K. Estimating child mortality due to diarrhoea in developing countries. Bull World Health Organ 2008;86:710-7.
2. Black RE. Persistent diarrhea in children of developing countries. Pediatr Infect Dis J 1993;12:751-61.
3. Petri WA, Miller M, Binder HL, et al. Enteric infections, diarrhea, and their impact on function and development. J Clin Invest 2008;118:1277-90.

4. Gracey M, Cullinane J. Gastroenteritis and environmental health among Aboriginal infants and children in Western Australia. J Paediatr Child Health 2003;39: 427–31.

5. Vernacchio L, Vezina RM, Mitchell AA, et al. Diarrhea in American infants and young children in the community setting. Incidence, clinical presentation and microbiology. Pediatr Infect Dis J 2006;25:2–7.

6. Barnes GL, Uren E, Stevens KB, et al. Etiology of acute gastroenteritis in hospitalized children in Melbourne, Australia, from April 1980 to March 1993. J Clin Microbiol 1998;36:133–8.

7. Patel MM, Widdowson MA, Glass RI, et al. Systematic literature review of role of noroviruses in sporadic gastroenteritis. Emerg Infect Dis 2008;14:1224–31.

8. Forster J, Guarino A, Parez N, et al. Hospital-based surveillance to estimate the burden of rotavirus gastroenteritis among European children younger than 5 years of age. Pediatrics 2009;123:e393–400.

9. Holman RC, Parashar UD, Clarke MJ, et al. Trends in diarrhea-associated hospitalizations among American Indian and Alaskan Native Children, 1980–1995. Pediatrics 1999;103:e11.

10. Singleton RJ, Holman RC, Yorita KL, et al. Diarrhea-associated hospitalizations and outpatient visits among American Indian and Alaska Native children younger than five years of age, 2000–2004. Pediatr Infect Dis J 2007;26:1006–13.

11. Santosham M, Sack RB, Reid R, et al. Diarrhoeal diseases in the White Mountain Apaches: epidemiologic studies. J Diarrhoeal Dis Res 1995;13:18–28.

12. Currie BJ, Brewster DR. Childhood infections in the tropical north of Australia. J Paediatr Child Health 2001;37:326–30.

13. Gracey M, Lee AH, Yau KK. Hospitalisation for gastroenteritis in Western Australia. Arch Dis Child 2004;89:768–72.

14. Fremantle E, Zurynski YA, Mahajan D, et al. Indigenous child health: urgent need for improved data to underpin better health outcomes. Med J Aust 2008;188: 588–91.

15. Carville KS, Lehmann D, Hall G, et al. Infection is the major component of the disease burden in Aboriginal and non-Aboriginal Australian children. Pediatr Infect Dis J 2007;26:210–6.

16. Gracey M. Diarrhoea in Australian Aborigines. Aust J Public Health 1992;16: 216–25.

17. Gracey M, Bower G. Enteric disease in young Australian Aborigines. Aust N Z J Med 1973;3:576–9.

18. Gracey M, Anderson CM. Hospital admissions for infections of Aboriginal and non-Aboriginal infants and children in Western Australia, 1981–1986. Aust Paediatr J 1989;25:230–5.

19. Kukuruzovic RH, Brewster DR. Small bowel intestinal permeability in Australian Aboriginal children. J Pediatr Gastroenterol Nutr 2002;35:206–12.

20. Lee AH, Flexman J, Wang K, et al. Recurrent gastroenteritis among infants in Western Australia: a seven-year hospital-based cohort study. Ann Epidemiol 2004;14:137–42.

21. Yau KKW, Lee AH, Gracey M. Multilevel modelling of hospitalisations for recurrent diarrhoeal disease in Aboriginal and non-Aboriginal infants and young children in Western Australia. Paediatr Perinat Epidemiol 2005;19:165–72.

22. Skull SA, Ruben AR, Walker AC. Malnutrition and microcephaly in Australian Aboriginal children. Med J Aust 1997;166:412–4.

23. Kukuruzovic R, Brewster DR, Gray E, et al. Increased nitric oxide production in acute diarrhoea is associated with abnormal gut permeability, hypokalaemia

and malnutrition in tropical Australian Aboriginal children. Trans R Soc Trop Med Hyg 2003;97:115–20.

24. Gurwith M, Wenmen W, Gurwith D, et al. Diarrhea among infants and young children in Canada: a longitudinal study in three northern communities. J Infect Dis 1983;147:685–92.

25. Arden-Holmes SL, Lennon D, Pinnock R, et al. Trends in hospitalization and mortality from rotavirus disease in New Zealand infants. Pediatr Infect Dis J 1999;18:614–9.

26. Craig E, Jackson C, Han D. Monitoring the health of New Zealand children and young people: indicator handbook. Auckland, New Zealand: Paediatric Society of New Zealand; 2007. p. 287–290.

27. Grimwood K, Lambert SB. Rotavirus vaccines: opportunities and challenges. Hum Vaccin 2009;5:57–69.

28. Newall AT, MacIntyre R, Wang H, et al. Burden of severe rotavirus disease in Australia. J Paediatr Child Health 2006;42:521–7.

29. Snelling TL, Schultz R, Graham J, et al. Rotavirus and the Indigenous children of the Australian outback: monovalent vaccine effective in a high-burden setting. Clin Infect Dis 2009;49:428–31.

30. Ajjampur SS, Rajendram P, Ramani S, et al. Closing the diarrhoea diagnostic gap in Indian children by the application of molecular techniques. J Med Microbiol 2008;57:1364–8.

31. Assadamongkol K, Gracey M, Forbes D, et al. *Cryptosporidium* in 100 Australian children. Southeast Asian J Trop Med Public Health 1992;23:132–7.

32. Kukuruzovic R, Robins-Browne RM, Anstey NM, et al. Enteric pathogens, intestinal permeability and nitric oxide production in acute gastroenteritis. Pediatr Infect Dis J 2002;21:730–9.

33. Gracey M. Gastro-enteritis in Australian children: studies on the aetiology of acute diarrhoea. Ann Trop Paediatr 1988;8:68–75.

34. Gunzburg S, Gracey M, Burke V, et al. Epidemiology and microbiology of diarrhoea in young Aboriginal children in the Kimberley region of Western Australia. Epidemiol Infect 1992;108:67–76.

35. Schultz R. Rotavirus gastroenteritis in the Northern Territory, 1995–2004. Med J Aust 2006;185:354–6.

36. Santosham M, Yolken RH, Wyatt RG, et al. Epidemiology of rotavirus diarrhea in a prospectively monitored American Indian population. J Infect Dis 1985;152:778–83.

37. Bishop RF, Masendycz PJ, Bugg HC, et al. Epidemiological patterns of rotaviruses causing severe gastroenteritis in young children throughout Australia from 1993 to 1996. J Clin Microbiol 2001;39:1085–91.

38. Kirkwood CD, Clark R, Bogdanovic-Sakran N, et al. A 5-year study of the prevalence and genetic diversity of human caliciviruses associated with sporadic cases of acute gastroenteritis in young children admitted to hospital in Melbourne, Australia (1998–2002). J Med Virol 2005;77:96–101.

39. Ochoa TJ, Salazar-Lindo E, Cleary TG. Management of children with infection-associated persistent diarrhea. Semin Pediatr Infect Dis 2004;15:229–36.

40. Alam NH, Ashraf H. Treatment of infectious diarrhea in children. Paediatr Drugs 2003;5:151–65.

41. Bhutta ZA, Nelson EA, Lee WS, et al. Recent advances and evidence gaps in persistent diarrhea. J Pediatr Gastroenterol Nutr 2008;47:260–5.

42. Campbell DI, Lunn PG, Elia M. Age-related association of small intestinal mucosal enteropathy with nutritional status in rural Gambian children. Br J Nutr 2002;88:499–505.

43. Zubrik SR, Lawrence DM, Silburn SR, et al. The Western Australian Aboriginal child health survey: the health of Aboriginal children and young people. Perth (WA): Telethon Institute for Child Health Research; 2004.

44. Brooke CJ, Riley TV, Hampson DJ. Comparison of prevalence and risk factors for faecal carriage of the intestinal spirochaetes *Brachyspira aalborgi* and *Brachyspira pilosicoli* in four Australian populations. Epidemiol Infect 2006;134: 627–34.

45. Grimprel E, Rodrigo C, Desselberger U. Rotavirus disease: impact of coinfections. Pediatr Infect Dis J 2008;27:S3–S10.

46. Kukuruzovic RH, Haase A, Dunn K, et al. Intestinal permeability and diarrhoeal disease in Aboriginal Australians. Arch Dis Child 1999;81:304–8.

47. Ruben AR, Fisher DA. The casemix system of hospital funding can further disadvantage Aboriginal children. Med J Aust 1998;169(8 Suppl):S6–10.

48. Steiner MJ, DeWalt DA, Byerley JS. Is this child dehydrated? JAMA 2004;291: 2746–54.

49. Elliott EJ. Acute gastroenteritis in children. Br Med J 2007;334:35–40.

50. Brewster DR. Dehydration in acute gastroenteritis. J Paediatr Child Health 2002; 38:219–22.

51. King CK, Glass R, Bresee JS, et al. Managing acute gastroenteritis among children. Oral rehydration, maintenance, and nutritional therapy. MMWR Morb Mortal Wkly Rep 2003;52(RR-16):1–16.

52. Hartling L, Bellemare S, Wiebe N, et al. Oral versus intravenous rehydration for treating dehydration due to gastroenteritis in children. Cochrane Database Syst Rev 2006;(3):CD004390.

53. Bellemere S, Hartling L, Wiebe N, et al. Oral rehydration versus intravenous therapy for treating dehydration due to gastroenteritis in children: a meta-analysis of randomised controlled trials. BMC Med 2004;2:11.

54. Fonseca BK, Holdgate A, Craig JC. Enteral vs intravenous rehydration therapy for children with gastroenteritis. Arch Pediatr Adolesc Med 2004; 158:483–90.

55. Gregorio GV, Gonzales MLM, Dans LF, et al. Polymer-based oral rehydration solution for treating acute watery diarrhoea. Cochrane Database Syst Rev 2009;(2):CD006519.

56. Nager AL, Wang VJ. Comparison of nasogastric and intravenous methods of rehydration in pediatric patients with acute dehydration. Pediatrics 2002;109: 566–72.

57. Atherly-John YC, Cunningham SJ, Crain EF. A randomized trial of oral vs intravenous rehydration in a pediatric emergency department. Arch Pediatr Adolesc Med 2002;156:1240–3.

58. Neville KA, Verge CF, Rosenberg AR, et al. Isotonic is better than hypotonic saline for intravenous rehydration of children with gastroenteritis: a prospective randomised study. Arch Dis Child 2006;91:226–32.

59. Reid SR, Bonadio WA. Outpatient rapid intravenous rehydration to correct dehydration and resolve vomiting in children with acute gastroenteritis. Ann Emerg Med 1996;28:318–23.

60. Ahmed T, Ali M, Ullah MM, et al. Mortality in severely malnourished children with diarrhoea and use of a standardised management protocol. Lancet 1999;353: 1919–22.

61. Alhashimi D, Al-Hashimi H, Fedorowicz Z. Antiemetics for reduced vomiting related to acute gastroenteritis in children and adolescents. Cochrane Database Syst Rev 2009;(2):CD005506.

62. DeCamp LR, Byerley JS, Doshi N, et al. Use of antiemetic agents in acute gastroenteritis. A systematic review and meta-analysis. Arch Pediatr Adolesc Med 2008;162:858–65.
63. Li ST, Grossman DC, Cummings P. Loperamide therapy for acute diarrhea in children. Systematic review and meta-analysis. PLoS Med 2007;4:e98.
64. Duggan C, Nurko S. "Feeding the gut": the scientific basis for continued enteral nutrition during acute diarrhea. J Pediatr 1997;131:801–8.
65. Brown KH, Gastanaduy AS, Saavedra JM, et al. Effect of continued oral feeding on clinical and nutritional outcomes of acute diarrhea in children. J Pediatr 1988; 112:191–200.
66. Dans LF, Gregorio GV, Silvestre MA. Early versus delayed refeeding for children with acute diarrhoea. Cochrane Database Syst Rev 2008;(3):CD007296.
67. Penny ME, Paredes P, Brown KH. Clinical and nutritional consequences of lactose feeding during persistent postenteritis diarrhea. Pediatrics 1989;84:835–44.
68. Brown KH, Peerson JM, Fontaine O. Use of nonhuman milks in the dietary management of young children with acute diarrhea: a meta-analysis of clinical trials. Pediatrics 1994;93:17–27.
69. Mitchell JD, Brand J, Halbisch J. Weight-gain inhibition by lactose in Australian Aboriginal children. A controlled trial of normal and lactose hydrolysed milk. Lancet 1977;(8010):500–2.
70. Santosham M, Foster S, Reid R, et al. Role of soy-based, lactose- free formula during treatment of acute diarrhea. Pediatrics 1985;76:292–8.
71. Kukuruzovic RH, Brewster DR. Milk formulas in acute gastroenteritis and malnutrition: a randomized trial. J Paediatr Child Health 2002;38:571–7.
72. Lazzerini M, Ronfani L. Oral zinc for treating diarrhoea in children. Cochrane Database Syst Rev 2008;(3):CD005436.
73. Lukacik M, Thomas RL, Aranda JV. A meta-analysis of the effects of oral zinc in the treatment of acute and persistent diarrhea. Pediatrics 2008;121:326–36.
74. Grotto I, Mimouni M, Gdalevich M, et al. Vitamin A supplementation and childhood morbidity from diarrhea and respiratory infections: a meta-analysis. J Pediatr 2003;142:297–304.
75. Long KZ, Rosado JL, Montoya Y, et al. Effect of vitamin A and zinc supplementation on gastrointestinal parasitic infections among Mexican children. Pediatrics 2007;120:e846–55.
76. Long KZ, Santos JI, Rosado JL, et al. Impact of vitamin A on selected gastrointestinal pathogen infections and associated diarrheal episodes among children in Mexico City, Mexico. J Infect Dis 2006;194:1217–25.
77. Brewster D. CARPA standard treatment manual reference book. 4th edition. Alice Springs: Central Australian Rural Practitioners Association; 2004.
78. Valery PC, Torzillo PJ, Boyce NC, et al. Zinc and vitamin A supplementation in Australian Indigenous children with acute diarrhoea: a randomised controlled trial. Med J Aust 2005;182:530–5.
79. Szajewska H, Mrukowicz JZ. Use of probiotics in children with acute diarrhea. Paediatr Drugs 2005;7:111–22.
80. Dennehy PH. Acute diarrheal disease in children: epidemiology, prevention and treatment. Infect Dis Clin North Am 2005;19:585–602.
81. Isaacs D. Gastrointestinal infections. In: Elliott E, Gilbert R, Moyer V, et al, editors. Evidence-based pediatric infectious diseases. Oxford: Blackwell Publishing Ltd; 2007. p. 74–101.
82. Abba K, Sinfield R, Hart CA, et al. Antimicrobial drugs for persistent diarrhea of unknown or non-specific cause in children under six in low and middle income

countries: systematic review of randomized controlled trials. BMC Infect Dis 2009;9:24.

83. Escobedo AA, Almirall P, Alfonso M, et al. Treatment of intestinal protozoan infections in children. Arch Dis Child 2009;94:478–82.

84. Hill ID, Mann MD, Househam KC, et al. Use of oral gentamicin, metronidazole, and cholestyramine in the treatment of severe persistent diarrhea in infants. Pediatrics 1986;77:477–81.

85. Bhatnagar S, Bhan MK, Sazawal S, et al. Efficacy of massive dose oral gentamicin therapy in nonbloody persistent diarrhea with associated malnutrition. J Pediatr Gastroenterol Nutr 1992;15:117–24.

86. Ejemot RI, Ehiri JE, Meremikwu MM, et al. Hand washing for preventing diarrhoea. Cochrane Database Syst Rev 2008;(1):CD004265.

87. Clasen TF, Roberts IG, Rabie T, et al. Interventions to improve water quality for preventing diarrhoea. Cochrane Database Syst Rev 2006;(3):CD004794.

88. Fewtrell L, Kaufmann RB, Kay D, et al. Water, sanitation, and hygiene interventions to reduce diarrhoea in less developed countries: a systematic review and meta-analysis. Lancet Infect Dis 2005;5:42–52.

89. McDonald E, Bailie R, Brewster D, et al. Are hygiene and public health interventions likely to improve outcomes for Australian Aboriginal children living in remote communities? A systematic review of the literature. BMC Public Health 2008;8:153.

90. Gracey M, Williams P, Houston S. Environmental health conditions in remote and rural Aboriginal communities in Western Australia. Aust N Z J Public Health 1997;21:511–8.

91. Brewster DR. Critical appraisal of the management of severe malnutrition: 4. Implications for Aboriginal child health in northern Australia. J Paediatr Child Health 2006;42:594–5.

92. Effect of breastfeeding on infant and child mortality due to infectious diseases in less developed countries: a pooled analysis. WHO Collaborative Study Team on the Role of Breastfeeding on the Prevention of Infant Mortality. Lancet 2000;355: 451–5.

93. Clemens J, Rao M, Ahmed F, et al. Breast-feeding and the risk of life-threatening rotavirus diarrhea: prevention or postponement? Pediatrics 1993;92: 680–5.

94. Gogia S, Sachdev HS. Neonatal vitamin A supplementation for prevention of mortality and morbidity in infancy: systematic review of randomised controlled trials. Br Med J 2009;338:b919.

95. Aggarwal R, Sentz J, Miller MA. Role of zinc administration in prevention of childhood diarrhea and respiratory illnesses: a meta-analysis. Pediatrics 2007;119: 1120–30.

96. Scrimgeour AG, Lukaski HC. Zinc and diarrheal disease: current status and future perspectives. Curr Opin Clin Nutr Metab Care 2008;11:711–7.

97. Ruiz-Palacios GM, Perez-Schael I, Velazquez FR, et al. Safety and efficacy of an attenuated vaccine against severe rotavirus gastroenteritis. N Engl J Med 2006; 354:11–22.

98. Vesikari T, Matson DO, Dennehy P, et al. Safety and efficacy of pentavalent human-bovine (WC3) reassortant rotavirus vaccine. N Engl J Med 2006;354: 23–33.

99. Cortese MM, Parashar UD. Prevention of rotavirus gastroenteritis among infants and children. Recommendations of the Advisory Committee on Immunization Practices. MMWR Morb Mortal Wkly Rep 2009;58(RR-2):1–25.

100. WHO. Rotavirus vaccination. Wkly Epidemiol Rec 2009;84:232–6.
101. Staat MA, Fairbrother G, Edwards KM, et al. Delayed onset and diminished magnitude of rotavirus activity – United States, November 2007–May 2008. MMWR Morb Mortal Wkly Rep 2008;57:697–700.
102. Lambert SB, Faux CE, Hall L, et al. Early evidence for direct and indirect effects of the infant rotavirus vaccine program in Queensland. Med J Aust 2009;191: 157–60.
103. Santosham M, Moulton LH, Reid R, et al. Efficacy and safety of high-dose rhesus-human reassortant rotavirus vaccine in Native American populations. J Pediatr 1997;131:632–8.
104. Kirkwood CD, Cannan D, Boniface K, et al. Australian Rotavirus Surveillance Program annual report, 2007/08. Commun Dis Intell 2008;32:425–9.
105. Grimwood K, Kirkwood CD. Human rotavirus vaccines: too early for the strain to tell. Lancet 2008;371:1144–5.
106. Guyatt GH, Oxman AD, Kunz R, et al. GRADE: going from evidence to recommendations. Br Med J 2008;336:1049–51.
107. Atkins D, Best D, Briss PA, et al. Grading quality of evidence and strength of recommendations. Br Med J 2004;328:1490–7.

Glomerulonephritis and Managing the Risks of Chronic Renal Disease

Gurmeet R. Singh, MBBS, DCH, DGO, MD, DNB, MPH&TM, FRACP, PhD[a,b,c,d]

KEYWORDS

- Glomerulonephritis • Poststreptococcal glomerulonephritis
- End-stage renal disease • Chronic kidney disease

GLOMERULONEPHRITIS

Many infectious and noninfectious conditions can lead to the development of glomerulonephritis (GN). The immunologic response of the kidney to an insult results in GN. For example, the kidney's response to infection by streptococcus results in poststreptococcal glomerulonephritis (PSGN), which is the most common and most studied postinfectious disease of the kidney. Although the clinical presentation and histopathology has been thoroughly described, the exact mechanisms that initiate the disease remain unclear despite major advances in knowledge.[1]

Burden of Disease

The causes of GN in Indigenous people in developed countries are similar to those seen in non-Indigenous people, with the exception of PSGN, the rates of which are disproportionately high[2] in Indigenous people. Streptococcal disease, especially that caused by group A β-hemolytic streptococcal (GAS) infection is very common in children. A wide spectrum of diseases, from superficial infections to invasive diseases and postinfectious conditions, such as rheumatic fever and GN, are caused by GAS.[2,3] Worldwide annual estimates of PSGN cases are in the order of 470,000 cases, with 97% in less developed countries.[2] A review of 11 population based studies has derived incident rates of PSGN: median incident rate of 24.3 cases per 100,000 person-years in children in less developed and disadvantaged populations compared with 6 cases per 100,000 person-years for children in developed countries.[2] Estimates

a Child Health Division, Menzies School of Health Research, Charles Darwin University Darwin, PO Box 41096, Casuarina, NT 0810, Australia
b Institute of Advanced Studies, Charles Darwin University, Darwin, Casuarino, NT, Australia
c Northern Territory Clinical School, Flinders University, Adelaide, South Australia.
d James Cooks University, Townville, Queensland, Australia
E-mail address: gurmeet.singh@menzies.edu.au

Pediatr Clin N Am 56 (2009) 1363–1382
doi:10.1016/j.pcl.2009.09.014
0031-3955/09/$ – see front matter © 2009 Elsevier Inc. All rights reserved.

for adults were 2 cases per 100,000 person-years in less developed countries compared with 0.3 per 100,000 person-years in developed countries.[2] Another recent study described a slightly higher incidence of 9.5 to 28.5 cases per 100,000 person-years in developing countries.[4] These rates represent only the clinical cases. Asymptomatic disease is estimated to be 4 to 19 times greater.[4–6] PSGN primarily affects children, aged 2 to 12 years, with clinically detectable cases estimated to be 10% of children with pharyngitis and up to 25% of children with impetigo during epidemics.[7,8] Children account for 50% to 90% of epidemic cases, with 5% to 10% occurring in people older than 40 years and 10% in those younger than 2 years.[4] Males have more symptomatic disease, but this difference is no longer present when symptomatic and asymptomatic cases are considered together.[9] Spontaneous recovery occurs in almost all patients, including those who develop renal insufficiency during the acute phase,[8] with only 1% of all pediatric patients developing chronic renal insufficiency.

Sporadic cases of PSGN occur worldwide. Epidemics are described in "closed" communities, clusters of densely populated dwellings, or areas with poor hygienic conditions, both urban and rural.[10] The changing pattern of PSGN over the last few decades has been described in studies from Florida[11] and Singapore.[12] The overall incidence of PSGN has decreased over the last few decades.[13] The reasons for this decline have not been clearly delineated, but possible reasons are the widespread use of antibiotics, changes in etiologic pathogens, altered susceptibility of the host, better health care delivery, and improved socioeconomic conditions.[11–13] Although epidemic PSGN has decreased dramatically and is almost unknown in the developed world, epidemics of PSGN continue to occur in the developing world, mainly in Africa, the West Indies, and the Middle East, and in Indigenous people living in the developed world.[14] These are especially prevalent in Aboriginal peoples of Australia living in remote communities, settings with a high burden of infectious disease and overcrowding.[14,15] Sporadic cases of acute PSGN occur in the Northern Territory of Australia each year, with outbreaks every 5 to 7 years.[16] PSGN in New Zealand occurs mostly in children of Pacific Island and Maori descent (>85% of cases).[17]

Clinical Presentation

The typical presentation is abrupt onset of acute nephritis occurring 1 to 3 weeks after a streptococcal throat infection and 3 to 6 weeks after skin infection.[1] The nephritis is characterized by edema (seen in 85% of cases), gross hematuria (seen in 40% of cases), and hypertension (seen in 50%–95% of hospitalized cases).The classical presentation feature is coca-cola–colored urine that is the characteristic of homogenous gross hematuria.[18] Other common features are facial puffiness and hypertension secondary to fluid overload and urinary abnormalities, such as albuminuria, and the presence of red cell casts. Within a week or so following onset of symptoms, most patients with PSGN begin to experience spontaneous resolution of fluid retention and hypertension and the urine abnormalities begin to subside, although proteinuria may persist for 6 months[10] to 3 years and microscopic hematuria for 1 to 4 years[10] after the onset of nephritis. Accompanying this clinical picture is laboratory evidence of streptococcal infection, typically increasing antistreptolysin O titers (ASOT) or streptozyme titers following throat infections and anti-DNase B titers following skin infections. Complement levels are decreased; low C3 levels are found in almost all patients with acute PSGN and C4 levels may be slightly low. These low C3 levels usually normalize within 8 weeks after the first sign of PSGN,[19] although up to 12 weeks has been reported.[10] The typical accompanying histopathology is diffuse cellular proliferation in the glomerulus, an exudate containing neutrophils and monocytes, and variable degrees of complement and immunoglobulin deposition. In most cases, hypertension subsides, renal function returns to normal, and all urinary abnormalities eventually disappear.[10]

There is, however, a wide variation in the clinical presentation and in the histopathology associated with PSGN. At the severe end of the spectrum is a rapidly rising azotemia with a rapidly progressive nephritic picture associated with severe cell proliferation, massive exudates, and crescent formation in biopsy specimens. This is seen in less than 5% of PSGN cases.[9] The severity of renal failure tends to be directly related to the degree of proliferation and crescent formation, and about 50% of these patients recover renal function.[20] This type of presentation is more common in the elderly. The mild end of the spectrum, represented by subclinical or asymptomatic GN, is more common. Diligent examination of people with acute, trivial, or self-limited infections caused by a range of organisms, including various bacteria, parasites, or viruses reveal subclinical infection in the form of microscopic hematuria, proteinuria, and pyuria. Histopathology reveals mesangial proliferation with mesangial deposits of C3 and IgG.[9] Asymptomatic household contacts of PSGN cases show subclinical disease 4 to 5 times more commonly than the in acute classical presentation.[5,21] An older study puts the ratio as high as 19:1.[6]

Pathology

Typical glomerular changes include proliferation of mesangial, endothelial, and epithelial cells, inflammatory exudate, and C3 deposition early in the disease process followed by IgG deposition. This immune deposition has been classified into 3 patterns.[22] The "starry sky pattern" represents an irregular and finely granular deposit of C3 and IgG deposition along the glomerular capillary walls and in the mesangium. This occurs early in the course of the disease and is also seen in subclinical cases.[1,22] The "mesangial pattern" has mainly C3 and some IgG in the mesangium. The "garland pattern" shows dense deposits along the capillary walls and is commonly associated with severe proteinuria and a poor prognosis.[1,22]

Pathogenesis

The pathognomonic feature of PSGN is the deposition of immune complexes in the glomerular basement membrane (**Fig. 1**). A proposed sequence of events is that a nephritogenic antigen or antigens lead to the activation of the complement pathway and/or activate plasmin or production of the circulating immune-complexes (**Fig. 2**). These then lead to increased permeability of the glomerular basement membrane, which allows deposition of the immune complexes and leakage of the protein and red blood cells. The nephritogenic antigen is responsible for C3 deposition, recruitment of immune cells, tissue destruction, and IgG deposition that further aggravates tissue injury. Complement activation leads to the release of cytokines, such as C5a, which attract phagocytes, proliferation of intrinsic cells, and formation of a membrane attack complex, which also aggravate the process.

The kidney has a limited number of ways of responding to injury. Similar pathologic signs may be the product of vastly different processes, produced by different imitating processes and different cytokines perpetuating the injury process. The initiation and development of the inflammatory response of the kidney to infection are still poorly understood.

The concept of a nephritogenic strain of GAS was advanced by Seegal and Earle[23] to explain the differences between rheumatic fever and PSGN, both nonsuppurative complications of streptococcal infection, which did not coexist in the same patient,

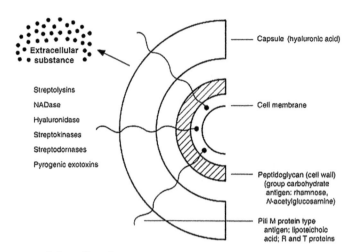

Fig. 1. Structure of the cell wall.

differed in geographic location, in sex incidence (2:1 male:female predominance in PSGN), and in propensity to healing (PSGN) rather than to relapsing attacks (rheumatic fever).[24] Although recognizing that host differences may play a definite role in explaining these contrasting characteristics, they championed a straightforward explanation: the existence of hemolytic streptococcal strains that caused rheumatic fever (hence

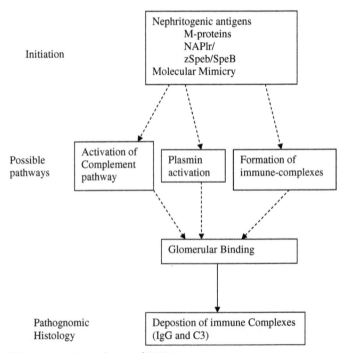

Fig. 2. Possible mechanistic pathway of PSGN.

rheumatogenic strains) and other strains that caused GN (nephritogenic strains). The definitive nephritogenic antigen has not yet been defined, although numerous streptococcal factors have been proposed as triggers. These are M proteins, M-like proteins (homologous host-binding proteins on the surface of the streptococcal organism), and later, glyceraldehyde phosphate dehydrogenase (GADPH) or endostreptosin (nephritis-associated plasmin receptor [NAPlr/Plr]) and streptococcal pyrogenic exotoxin B (zymogen, SPEB) streptokinase.[1,10,25] M proteins are present on the pili of the organism and more than a hundred have been identified so far. Nephritogenic M-proteins are types 1, 2, 4, 3, 25, 49, and 12 following skin infections and types 47, 49, 55, 2, 60, and 57 following throat infections.[1] M-proteins may be nephritogenic by combining with other factors and have been shown to be antigenically cross-reactive with glomerular basement membrane (GBM).[1,9] Similar molecular mimicry has been shown by various streptococcal antigens and various renal structural constituents, such as laminin, collagen, and GBM.[1,9] The varied responses could be explained by differing host factors, including genetic susceptibility.[26] Association with HLA antigens, HLA-DRW4[27] and HLA-DRB1*03011,[28] and with polymorphisms of endothelial nitric oxide synthase gene intron 4a/b have been described,[29] but frequency of alleles does not correlate with severity of disease.

The variety of findings in different studies, some seemingly contradictory, add to the difficulty. Cardinal features of PSGN are proteinuria, hematuria, glomerular hypercellularity, and deposition of C3 and IgG. Variations occur with all these findings not being present at the same time; severe diffuse GN occurs without C3 or IgG deposition or without severe hematuria or proteinuria. On the other hand, gross hematuria can occur with minimal histologic findings. Similar findings can be found with other infectious diseases[9,30] and with other conditions, such as alcoholism, IgA nephropathy, and diabetic nephropathy.[1,9,31]

Treatment

Treatment of PSGN remains supportive. Fluid overload is responsive to diuresis and sodium restriction. Hypertension may be controlled by loop diuretics but may need other antihypertensive agents. Captopril has been shown to be effective[32,33] but should be used with caution in the presence of renal failure and hyperkalemia. Occasionally acute renal failure requires dialysis. Aggressive therapy using pulse methylprednisolone has been used in adults with poor prognostic factors, such as nephritic-range proteinuria, cellular crescents on biopsy, and renal insufficiency.[34] Plasmapharesis and pulse methylprednisolone was successfully used in a 6-year-old girl with garland pattern PSGN.[35] Whether this would benefit all patients with poor prognosis has not been studied. Penicillin treats any persisting streptococcal infection (summarized in **Table 1**).[39]

Prognosis

In keeping with the clinicopathologic picture, the prognosis of PSGN is also extremely variable and largely influenced by clinical presentation and histopathology. Complete recovery, progression of symptoms, or progression to renal failure may follow an episode of PSGN. Persistence of symptoms may represent either a slow recovery, limited injury without further progression, or progression to renal failure. In general, children are believed to have a good prognosis, with most showing complete recovery, whereas a larger proportion of adults with PSGN progress to renal failure. However, some studies have reported persistent urinary abnormalities[9,11,14,17,40] and subtle abnormalities in renal function as defined by reduction in renal functional reserve in patients who had recovered from PSGN without apparent sequelae.[41]

Table 1
Recommendations for the clinical management of PSGN in Indigenous children

'Intervention'	Recommendation	Recommendation Grade	Quality of Supporting Evidence
Transfer to hospital	Child should be admitted into hospital if there is: • hypertension • combination of oliguria, generalized edema and elevation of serum creatinine or potassium	Strong	Low
Treatment	Supportive	Strong	Low
	Fluid restriction	Strong	Low
	Diuretics	Strong	Low
	Antihypertensive medications in presence of hypertension		
	• calcium channel blockers	Strong	Moderate[36]
	• ACE inhibitors	Strong	Moderate[32,33]
Antibiotics	Penicillin to prevent spread of disease	Strong	Moderate[11]
Severe cases	Pulse methylprednisolone	Weak	Moderate[37]
	Plasmapheresis	Weak	Moderate[37]
Community	Preventing spread		
Contacts	Treatment with Penicillin	Strong	Moderate[38]
Skin infections	Treatment with Penicillin	Strong	Moderate[11,12]
Environmental factors	Improvement in socioeconomic conditions, eg, decreasing overcrowding	Strong	Low[12]

Abbreviation: ACE, angiotensin-converting enzyme.

Epidemic cases have a better prognosis than sporadic cases,[17,42] but not always. An outbreak of PSGN in Brazil following an epidemic of *Streptococcus equi zooepidemicus* resulted in a high prevalence of renal abnormalities at a mean follow-up of 5.4 years.[43,44] However, these were mainly adult patients. Elderly people have poorer outcomes as do those with comorbidities, including diabetes and cardiovascular and liver diseases.[1,4] In an Aboriginal population with high rates of end-stage renal disease (ESRD), follow-up of children 6 to 18 years later (mean 14.6 years) following epidemic PSGN showed that risk of overt proteinuria was more than 6 times (95% CI 2.2–16.9) greater than in healthy controls after adjustment of age, sex, and birth weight.[14,45] It is proposed that in this high-risk population, childhood PSGN might be an important risk factor for ESRD.[14,46,47]

Preventing Spread

A case of PSGN has 2 or more of the following clinical manifestations: edema, macroscopic hematuria or count on the dipstick hematuria (defined as blood + + or >) or high diastolic blood pressure (780 mmHg if $\leq$ 13 years, >90 mmHg if >13 years) in the presence of a reduced complement level (C3) and evidence of streptococcal infection. Either elevated ASO or anti-DNase B titers or positive cultures of GAS (from skin sores if they are present, or throat if there are no sores) indicate Streptococal infection.

There is evidence that outbreaks can be halted by treating all children who have any evidence of skin sores with intramuscular benzathine penicillin to stop the transmission of the bacteria in the community.[38] In experimental PSGN, the nephritic process is prevented if penicillin is given within 3 days of the streptococcal infection.[39] Prevention of epidemics requires the control of spread of skin sores and infected scabies.[47] Following the identification of a case, family and household members are screened for the presence of skin sores and scabies and tested for urinary abnormalities. Those with skin manifestations are treated with penicillin. Those with urinary abnormalities undergo complete investigation for PSGN, including testing of urea, electrolytes, C3, ASO, and anti-DNase B and cultures for streptococcal infection.

Prevention of epidemics of PSGN requires a community-level control of skin sores and infected scabies. Promotion of regular washing, especially of children, will prevent spread. Improvement in housing, especially reduction in overcrowding, will hinder spread of infectious disease. The significant decline in PSGN in Singapore children is attributed to improvement in the socioeconomic status and health care system and the urbanization of the country.[12]

The development of a vaccine has been the focus of research for many decades. Three GAS vaccines have been approved for phase 1 human trials and will provide information on serum immunogenicity and safety over the next 5 years.[48] However, it is thought that those systems that induce significant responses at mucosal sites will provide superior vaccines, and as technology to provide mucosal adjuvants and vaccine delivery improves, these will become available.[48]

CHRONIC RENAL DISEASE (CKD)
Magnitude of the Problem

The global prevalence of chronic renal disease (CKD) has increased rapidly in the last 20 to 30 years. This reported prevalence is thought to represent just the tip of the iceberg of covert kidney disease. CKD being a major risk factor for developing cardiovascular disease (CVD) and the enormous cost of treatment are increasingly focusing attention on CKD and its prevention. Well-defined registries for reporting on the uptake of renal replacement therapies (RRT) exist in many countries, such as the United States

(United States Renal Data Systems),[49] Australia and New Zealand (Australia and New Zealand Dialysis and Transplantation Data [ANZDATA]),[50,51] the United Kingdom[52] and Europe.[53] The 2002 classification and staging system called the Kidney Disease Outcome Quality Initiative (KDOQI) is a fairly new concept that has allowed a more uniform reporting of chronic kidney disease across the world and has helped to shift the focus to the earlier stages (**Table 2**).[54] There are several limitations in interpretation of data from these registries. These registries record the uptake of RRT for ESRD. The uptake of RRT does not necessarily equate to an accurate reflection of the incidence of ESRD.[55] The difference between uptake of RRT and the actual incidence of ESRD would be greatest in poorer countries with limited capacity to provide RRTs. The modification of diet in renal disease (MDRD) equation used to stratify CKD was designed to quantify and stratify disease severity, not for diagnosis of kidney disease in those without known disease. There is also disagreement regarding the inclusion of albuminuria in stage 1 and 2 of CKD. Albuminuria is a well-recognized risk factor for CKD but there is controversy over whether albuminuria, and in particular microalbuminuria (including the level of urinary albumin that actually defines microalbuminuria) is a marker of kidney disease and concern that using this definition would greatly inflate the numbers of patients with stage 1 and 2 chronic disease.[56–58] Despite these limitations, the use of a standard definition has helped improve the comparison of disease magnitude in different populations, across genders, ages, and ethnic groups.

Prevalence of earlier stages of CKD is obtained from epidemiologic studies. A systematic review of CKD in 26 studies from the general population in adults 18 years or older has highlighted the following facts.[59] The median prevalence of CKD in patients older than 30 years is 7.2%, in those 64 years or older, varies from 23.4% to 35.8%, and this prevalence was strongly dependent on the equation used to define glomerular filtration rate (GFR). There was a marked variation in prevalence among the study populations. In general, the prevalence of CKD increased with age within the same study population. The prevalence was greater in women than in men regardless of age, but this difference was most marked in middle age. This gender difference was statistically significant only in the Australian Diabetes, Obesity and Lifestyle (AusDiab) study.[60] The prevalence was strongly dependent on the estimating equations, being higher when using the Cockroft-Gault equation than with the MDRD equation.[59] African Americans had a lower prevalence than Caucasians, and, in general, Asians had a fairly high prevalence.[61] Unfortunately, information on prevalence from developing countries is not as regularly or as reliably available, so international comparisons must be based on ESRD rather than CKD.

Aboriginals living in Australia, New Zealand, Canada, and the Unites States have a higher incidence of ESRD than the non-Aboriginal people in these countries. The

Table 2
The KDOQI definition and Staging of CKD[a]

Stage	eGFR (ml/min/1.73m^3)
-	high risk
1	≥90
2	60–89
3	30–59
4	15–29
5	<15 (or dialysis)

Abbreviations: ACR, albumin:creatinine ratio; eGFR, estimated glomerular filtration rate.
[a] Based on eGFR and kidney damage (ACR > 17 mg/g in males,>25 mg/g in females) for >3 months.

ANZDATA reports results for Aboriginal and non-Aboriginal Australians and for the Maori, Pacific Islanders, and "other" New Zealanders.[62] Between the ages of 15 and 64 years, Aboriginal Australians had ESRD rates about twice that of the Maori and Pacific Islanders, who, in turn, had rates 2 to 10 times those of non-Aboriginal Australian and "other" New Zealanders. There was no difference in rates in the 0 to 14 age group, nor in those older than 65 years.[62] Similarly, the rates of ESRD reported from indigenous people from North America and Canada are 2 to 4 times higher than those in non-Aboriginal people.[63,64] Although influenced in a large part by the increasing burden of diabetes, Aboriginal people without diabetes still have a 2- to 3-fold greater risk of developing ESRD compared with the non-Aboriginal people.[63] In contrast, rates of CKD are lower in the United States in minority populations (indigenous, African American, and Mexican American)[64,65] than in the US composite population and slightly lower in First Nations people than non-First Nations people in Alberta, Canada.[63] First Nations people were also younger and more likely to be to have social disadvantage, such as lowest quintiles of household incomes and rural residences.

Data from the United States suggest that for every patient with ESRD, there are more than 200 with overt CKD (stage 3–4) and almost 5000 with covert disease (stage 1–2).[63] Although the burden of disease is quite high in some studies, less than 2% of CKD patients progress to ESRD according to data from the United States.[59,61,66]

Blacks from North America have lower reported rates of CKD but higher ESRD.[65] In Zuni Indians with high rates of ESRD, rates of early CKD (stages 1–2) are higher, but those in later stages (3–4) have lower rates than in the United States composite population.[67] Possible explanations for this seeming paradox are a likelihood of higher acceptance rate for Aboriginal people, improved survival rates in Aboriginal people on dialysis, or rates of unmeasured CKD being higher in Aboriginal people. These scenarios are not substantiated by available data.[68,69] The most likely explanation is a higher risk profile at a given risk of CKD, such as diabetes, severe hypertension, and proteinuria in a setting of lower nephron endowment, resulting in faster kidney function loss and increased likelihood of developing ESRD, a scenario that seems likely from studies in Aboriginal Australians.[46,66,70]

Causes and Risk Factors of ESRD in Children and Young Adults

The main causes of ESRD in children are available from several Pediatric renal registries from developed and developing nations.[71] Comprehensive reports are available from Italy (ItalKid study),[72] the United Kingdom (British Association of Pediatric Nephrology)[73] and the United States (North American Pediatric Renal Transplant Cooperative Study).[74] These data suggest that congenital abnormalities of the kidney and urinary tract are the cause of ESRD in 50%; other congenital and inherited diseases, in 20%; unknown, in 4% to 5%; and GN, in 20%.[71–74] In half the cases, GN is described as focal segmental glomerulosclerosis. GN has decreased as a cause of ERSD in recent years in the developed world.[50,75]

Many of the childhood primary renal diseases do not present with ESRD till later in life. The causes of CKD in young adults is not well characterized. Although pediatric renal registries only have a median age of 16 years (range 12–22 years),[71] adult registries do not adequately describe the causes for the age range of 25 to 30 years. The ESRD caused by polycystic kidney disease develops past the childhood years, as does that due to diabetes mellitus and hypertension, which are 2 major causes of ESRD worldwide[59,76] and account for 71% of new ESRD cases in United States.[61,77] The Developmental Origins of Health and Disease postulates a complex interplay of multiple factors that lead to ESRD. This begins with reduced nephron endowment in utero. Repeated insults over the lifetime, such as infections and obesity, lead to compromised renal function and, ultimately, ESRD.[78,79]

DIABETES

Rates of type 2 diabetes are disproportionately high in the indigenous populations in developed countries. This is well documented in American Indians[49,80] and Aboriginal Australians.[68] Reported incidence is 10 times higher in First Nations Canadians.[81] Some studies have suggested that the prepubertal years contribute less to the diabetic kidney disease, but this is not borne out in long-term follow-up studies.[82] The duration of diabetes, in type 1 and 2 diabetes, seems to be the major factor, with renal complications occurring, on an average, 15 years (usually 20–25 years) after the onset of diabetes.[82] Adequacy of control of hyperglycemia and hypertension are the other important factors.[82–85] However, not all renal disease in diabetes is because of classical diabetic nephropathy. In a study of First Nations Canadians with maturity-onset diabetes of the young and albuminuria who underwent a renal biopsy, not a single biopsy result showed classical diabetic pathology, whereas 9 of 10 showed immune complex disease or glomerulosclerosis.[86]

OBESITY

Obesity is increasing worldwide. It has a significant role in the current epidemic of lifestyle diseases, including type 2 diabetes.[87–89] Obesity-related glomerulopathy is a documented entity in its own right, presenting with albuminuria and characterized by focal glomerulosclerosis on renal biopsy.[87,90–93] Obesity also has a detrimental effect on nephron number.[87]

NEPHRON ENDOWMENT AND THE DEVELOPMENT ORIGINS OF KIDNEY DISEASE

The progressive deterioration of renal function results from nephron loss, which leads to compensatory glomerular hyperfiltration, which in turn causes relentless injury of the remaining nephrons.[94] The initial nephron loss could be the result of poorer nephron endowment due to prematurity or intrauterine growth restriction.[95–98] Multiple factors have been implicated in the development of ESRD in this setting of low nephron numbers and hyperfiltration. These are low birth weight (LBW), increased central fat deposition, inflammation, infection, including PSGN, diabetes, and hypertension. This scenario explains the epidemic proportions of ESRD seen in some high-risk populations, such as Aboriginal Australian, and provides an explanation for the glomerulosclerosis seen in the kidney biopsies from these populations.

Management of Risk Factors for CKD

The management of risk factors for CKD can be stratified according to the stage of CKD as shown in **Table 3**. These were developed by the KDOQI in 2002 and revised in 2005 under the auspices of KDIGO (Kidney Disease: Improving Global Outcomes).

SCREENING PROGRAMS: EARLY IDENTIFICATION OF RISK FACTORS

CKD has a long latent period and generally evolves slowly over a period of time. CKD is a silent disease and about half the patients in early-stage CKD have no discernable symptoms.[111] Early stages of CKD maybe reversible. Screening programs are based on early detection of risk factors and development of strategies that seek to modify these to delay or prevent CKD. Screening the general populations in the United States (National Health and Nutrition Examination Survey[61]), Australia (AusDiab[60]), Japan (Okinawa study[112]), Europe (Prevention of Renal and Vascular End stage Disease

Table 3
Strategies for management of CKD by stage

'Intervention'	Recommendation	Recommendation Grade	Quality of Supporting Evidence
Primary prevention	Screening and risk reduction		
Screening using albuminuria and eGFR	Target groups of high-risk populations • High-risk population: older age, ethnic minorities, decreased kidney mass, hyperfiltration • Specific renal damaging conditions: diabetes, hypertension, obesity, infections, congenital conditions, LBW, prematurity	Weak	Moderate
Secondary prevention	Prevention of progression		
Life style factors	Weight reduction	Strong	Moderate[99,100]
Glycemia	Strict control in diabetics	Strong	High[101,102]
Dyslipidemia	Statins to control lipids	Weak	High,[103,104]
Albuminuria	ACE inhibitors	Strong	Moderate[105–107]
Tertiary prevention	Improving outcomes		
Complications of ESRD	Hypertension Anemia Malnutrition Bone and mineral disorders	Strong	Moderate[108,109]
CVD risk factors	Dyslipidemia	Weak	High,[103,104]
Comorbid conditions	Diabetes Sepsis	Strong	Moderate[110]
Access to RRT	Decrease delay in referral Improve access	Strong	Low

Abbreviations: ACE, angiotensin-converting enzyme; CVD, cardiovascular disease; eGFR, estimated glomerular filtration rate.

[PREVEND][113]), Iceland,[114] Singapore,[115] and India[116] detected albuminuria in 3% to 11% of the population screened. Similar rates were found in Taiwanese[111] and Australian children, Aboriginal and non-Aboriginal.[117] Rates in high-risk groups, such as ethnic minorities like Zuni Indians[118,119] and Australian Aborigines,[46,70] show higher rates of albuminuria.

Screening of the general population for CKD is not found to be cost-effective.[120–122] Targeted screening for high-risk groups yield better results; such as in high-risk populations[119,123] or those with diabetes, hypertension, and in first-degree relatives of those with diabetes and hypertension.[124] In addition to diabetes and hypertension, other risk factors were increasing age,[125] smoking[125] and obesity.[125,126] Birth weight and prematurity are also risk factors.[46,127–129] In addition to ESRD, CKD (low GFR and albuminuria) is also a risk factor for CVD, and interventions targeting this group would reduce renal and cardiovascular disease.

Current screening methods use albuminuria with or without a measure of estimated glomerular filtration rate (eGFR) calculated from serum creatinine. Neutrophil gelatinase-associated lipocalin, a 25-kD protein initially found in activated neutrophils, is found in many cells including kidney tubules and can be measured in urine and serum.[130] Initially considered a predictor of acute kidney injury, it is emerging as a marker of CKD and of its severity.[130]

PREVENTATIVE MEASURES AND PROTECTIVE THERAPIES
Lifestyle Modification

Life style factors, such as weight reduction, diet modification, and exercise, have been found to be effective in preventing the development of diabetes in overweight individuals with impaired glucose tolerance.[99,100,131,132] Smoking and alcohol have been implicated in the development of albuminuria.[131,133] Improved living conditions and urbanization are believed to have decreased the prevalence of GAS disease and PSGN.[12]

Strict Control of Glycemia and Hypertension

A major factor in preventing diabetic nephropathy and slowing its progression is the strict control of glycemia in type 1[101,134] and type 2 diabetes.[102,135,136] Control of hypertension is equally important.[136,137]

Strict Control of Proteinuria

The severity of albuminuria predicts the severity of ESRD. Its control is important in slowing the progression of ESRD. Angiotensin-converting enzyme (ACE) inhibitors or angiotensin receptor blockers[138] are advocated in antihypertensive therapies for their effect on renal function.[139] The effect of these therapies on renal function is proportional to their protein-lowering effect. This effect has been demonstrated in different populations,[105–107,113] including high-risk groups such as Aboriginal Australians.[106]

Control of Dyslipidemia

A systematic review of trials of lipid reduction with 3-hydroxy-3-methyl-glutaryl-CoA reductase inhibitors (statins) showed that in populations with CVD, there is a modest reduction in proteinuria and a slight reduction in the rate of kidney function loss.[103] However this benefit did not extend to those with diabetes or GN.[103,104]

Multiple Therapies

Several large randomized trials have shown that lowering cholesterol with statins reduces coronary mortality and morbidity across a wide range of cholesterol levels and in patients with proteinuric disease.[104,140] It has been hypothesized that statins may directly modulate intracellular signaling systems involved in cellular proliferation and inflammatory and fibrogenic responses. Studies in animals have shown that the mevalonate pathway also may be involved in the regulation of the renin-angiotensin system, providing the rationale for the use of statins in combination with ACE inhibitors or angiotensin II receptor antagonists. Preliminary studies have shown that a multidrug approach may induce remission of proteinuria, lessen renal injury and protect from loss of function in those patients whose condition does not fully respond to a single treatment. A meta-analysis of 750 trials involving 400,000 participants showed up to 80% reduction in CVD events by a combination polypill containing an ACE inhibitor, a statin, cardioprotective agents like aspirin, and vitamins.[141] Similar trials are not yet available for the effect of the polypill on CKD. Neither the safety nor the efficacy of these treatments for children is known with certainty. As ACE inhibitors and angiotensin blockers pose a significant risk to the developing fetus, they must be used with caution, especially in young diabetic women of childbearing age.[82]

REFERENCES

1. Nordstrand A, Norgren M, Holm SE. Pathogenic mechanism of acute post-streptococcal glomerulonephritis. Scand J Infect Dis 1999;31(6):523–37.
2. Carapetis JR, Steer AC, Mulholland EK, et al. The global burden of group A streptococcal diseases. Lancet Infect Dis 2005;5(11):685–94.
3. Steer AC, Danchin MH, Carapetis JR. Group A streptococcal infections in children. J Paediatr Child Health 2007;43(4):203–13.
4. Rodriguez-Iturbe B, Musser JM. The current state of poststreptococcal glomerulonephritis. J Am Soc Nephrol 2008;19(10):1855–64.
5. Rodriguez-Iturbe B, Rubio L, Garcia R. Attack rate of poststreptococcal nephritis in families. A prospective study. Lancet 1981;1(8217):401–3.
6. Sagel I, Treser G, Ty A, et al. Occurrence and nature of glomerular lesions after group A streptococci infections in children. Ann Intern Med 1973;79(4):492–9.
7. Stetson CA, Rammelkamp CH Jr, Krause RM, et al. Epidemic acute nephritis: studies on etiology, natural history and prevention. Medicine (Baltimore) 1955; 34(4):431–50.
8. Tejani A, Ingulli E. Poststreptococcal glomerulonephritis. Current clinical and pathologic concepts. Nephron 1990;55(1):1–5.
9. Kanjanabuch T, Kittikowit W, Eiam-Ong S. An update on acute postinfectious glomerulonephritis worldwide. Nat Rev Nephrol 2009;5(5):259–69.
10. Yoshizawa N. Acute glomerulonephritis. Intern Med 2000;39(9):687–94.
11. Ilyas M, Tolaymat A. Changing epidemiology of acute post-streptococcal glomerulonephritis in Northeast Florida: a comparative study. Pediatr Nephrol 2008;23(7):1101–6.
12. Yap HK, Chia KS, Murugasu B, et al. Acute glomerulonephritis–changing patterns in Singapore children. Pediatr Nephrol 1990;4(5):482–4.
13. Markowitz M. Changing epidemiology of group A streptococcal infections. Pediatr Infect Dis J 1994;13(6):557–60.
14. White AV, Hoy WE, McCredie DA. Childhood post-streptococcal glomerulonephritis as a risk factor for chronic renal disease in later life. Med J Aust 2001; 174(10):492–6.
15. Streeton CL, Hanna JN, Messer RD, et al. An epidemic of acute post-streptococcal glomerulonephritis among aboriginal children. J Paediatr Child Health 1995;31(3):245–8.
16. Marshal C, Taylor C. Northern Territory Disease Control Bulletin. 2008;15(3):1–4.

17. Wong W, Morris MC, Zwi J. Outcome of severe acute post-streptococcal glomer-ulonephritis in New Zealand children. Pediatr Nephrol 2009;24(5):1021–6.
18. Pan CG. Evaluation of gross hematuria. Pediatr Clin North Am 2006;53(3): 401–12, vi.
19. Pan CG. Glomerulonephritis in childhood. Curr Opin Pediatr 1997;9(2):154–9.
20. El-Husseini AA, Sheashaa HA, Sabry AA, et al. Acute postinfectious crescentic glomerulonephritis: clinicopathologic presentation and risk factors. Int Urol Nephrol 2005;37(3):603–9.
21. Tasic V, Polenakovic M. Occurrence of subclinical post-streptococcal glomeru-lonephritis in family contacts. J Paediatr Child Health 2003;39(3):177–9.
22. Sorger K, Gessler U, Hubner FK, et al. Subtypes of acute postinfectious glomer-ulonephritis. Synopsis of clinical and pathological features. Clin Nephrol 1982; 17(3):114–28.
23. Seegal D, Earle DP. A consideration of certain biological differences between glomerulonephritis and rheumatic fever. Am J Med Sci 1941;201:528–39.
24. Rodriguez-Iturbe B, Batsford S. Pathogenesis of poststreptococcal glomerulo-nephritis a century after Clemens von Pirquet. Kidney Int 2007;71(11):1094–104.
25. Batsford SR, Mezzano S, Mihatsch M, et al. Is the nephritogenic antigen in post-streptococcal glomerulonephritis pyrogenic exotoxin B (SPE B) or GAPDH? Kidney Int 2005;68(3):1120–9.
26. Read SE, Reid H, Poon-King T, et al. HLA and predisposition to the nonsuppur-ative sequelae of group A streptococcal infections. Transplant Proc 1977;9(1): 543–6.
27. Layrisse Z, Rodriguez-Iturbe B, Garcia-Ramirez R, et al. Family studies of the HLA system in acute post-streptococcal glomerulonephritis. Hum Immunol 1983;7(3):177–85.
28. Bakr A, Mahmoud LA, Al-Chenawi F, et al. HLA-DRB1* alleles in Egyptian chil-dren with post-streptococcal acute glomerulonephritis. Pediatr Nephrol 2007; 22(3):376–9.
29. Dursun H, Noyan A, Matyar S, et al. Endothelial nitric oxide synthase gene intron 4 a/b VNTR polymorphism in children with APSGN. Pediatr Nephrol 2006; 21(11):1661–5.
30. Robson WL, Leung AK. Post-streptococcal glomerulonephritis with minimal abnormalities in the urinary sediment. J Singapore Paediatr Soc 1992;34(3–4): 232–4.
31. Kallen AJ, Patel PR. In search of a rational approach to chronic kidney disease detection and management. Kidney Int 2007;72(1):3–5.
32. Morsi MR, Madina EH, Anglo AA, et al. Evaluation of captopril versus reserpine and frusemide in treating hypertensive children with acute post-streptococcal glomerulonephritis. Acta Paediatr 1992;81(2):145–9.
33. Parra G, Rodriguez-Iturbe B, Colina-Chourio J, et al. Short-term treatment with captopril in hypertension due to acute glomerulonephritis. Clin Nephrol 1988; 29(2):58–62.
34. Raff A, Hebert T, Pullman J, et al. Crescentic post-streptococcal glomerulone-phritis with nephrotic syndrome in the adult: is aggressive therapy warranted? Clin Nephrol 2005;63(5):375–80.
35. Suyama K, Kawasaki Y, Suzuki H. Girl with garland-pattern poststreptococcal acute glomerulonephritis presenting with renal failure and nephrotic syndrome. Pediatr Int 2007;49(1):115–7.
36. Garin EH, Araya CE. Treatment of systemic hypertension in children and adoles-cents. Curr Opin Pediatr 2009 [Epub ahead of print].

37. Smith RJ, Alexander J, Barlow PN, et al. New approaches to the treatment of dense deposit disease. J Am Soc Nephrol 2007;18(9):2447–56.
38. Johnston F, Carapetis J, Patel MS, et al. Evaluating the use of penicillin to control outbreaks of acute poststreptococcal glomerulonephritis. Pediatr Infect Dis J 1999;18(4):327–32.
39. Bergholm AM, Holm SE. Effect of early penicillin treatment on the development of experimental poststreptococcal glomerulonephritis. Acta Pathol Microbiol Immunol Scand C 1983;91(4):271–81.
40. Buzio C, Allegri L, Mutti A, et al. Significance of albuminuria in the follow-up of acute poststreptococcal glomerulonephritis. Clin Nephrol 1994;41(5): 259–64.
41. Cleper R, Davidovitz M, Halevi R, et al. Renal functional reserve after acute post-streptococcal glomerulonephritis. Pediatr Nephrol 1997;11(4):473–6.
42. Blyth CC, Robertson PW, Rosenberg AR. Post-streptococcal glomerulonephritis in Sydney: a 16-year retrospective review. J Paediatr Child Health 2007;43(6): 446–50.
43. Sesso R, Pinto SW. Five-year follow-up of patients with epidemic glomerulone-phritis due to Streptococcus zooepidemicus. Nephrol Dial Transplant 2005; 20(9):1808–12.
44. Sesso R, Wyton S, Pinto L. Epidemic glomerulonephritis due to Streptococcus zooepidemicus in Nova Serrana, Brazil. Kidney Int Suppl 2005;97:S132–6.
45. Yamagata K, Iseki K, Nitta K, et al. Chronic kidney disease perspectives in Japan and the importance of urinalysis screening. Clin Exp Nephrol 2008; 12(1):1–8.
46. Hoy W, Kelly A, Jacups S, et al. Stemming the tide: reducing cardiovascular disease and renal failure in Australian Aborigines. Aust N Z J Med 1999;29(3): 480–3.
47. Van Buynder PG, Gaggin JA, Martin D, et al. Streptococcal infection and renal disease markers in Australian aboriginal children. Med J Aust 1992;156(8): 537–40.
48. Georgousakis MM, McMillan DJ, Batzloff MR, et al. Moving forward: a mucosal vaccine against group A streptococcus. Expert Rev Vaccines 2009;8(6):747–60.
49. Centers for Disease Control and Prevention (CDC). End-stage renal disease attributed to diabetes among American Indians/Alaska Natives with diabetes–United States, 1990–1996. MMWR Morb Mortal Wkly Rep 2000;49(42):959–62.
50. Orr NI, McDonald SP, McTaggart S, et al. Frequency, etiology and treatment of childhood end-stage kidney disease in Australia and New Zealand. Pediatr Nephrol 2009;24(9):1719–26.
51. McDonald SP, Russ GR, Kerr PG, et al. ESRD in Australia and New Zealand at the end of the millennium: a report from the ANZDATA registry. Am J Kidney Dis 2002;40(6):1122–31.
52. Ansell D, Tomson CR. Evolving trends in clinical presentation of and renal replacement therapy for chronic kidney disease. Nephron Clin Pract 2009; 111(4):c265–7.
53. Ramsay CR, Campbell MK, Cantarovich D, et al. Evaluation of clinical guidelines for the management of end-stage renal disease in europe: the EU BIOMED 1 study. Nephrol Dial Transplant 2000;15(9):1394–8.
54. Korevaar JC, Jansen MA, Dekker FW, et al. Evaluation of DOQI guidelines: early start of dialysis treatment is not associated with better health-related quality of life. National Kidney Foundation-Dialysis Outcomes Quality Initiative. Am J Kidney Dis 2002;39(1):108–15.

55. Glassock RJ. The rising tide of end-stage renal disease: what can be done? Clin Exp Nephrol 2004;8(4):291–6.

56. de Zeeuw D, Hillege HL, de Jong PE. The kidney, a cardiovascular risk marker, and a new target for therapy. Kidney Int Suppl 2005;98:S25–9.

57. Brantsma AH, Atthobari J, Bakker SJ, et al. What predicts progression and regression of urinary albumin excretion in the nondiabetic population? J Am Soc Nephrol 2007;18(2):637–45.

58. Kestenbaum B, Rudser KD, de Boer IH, et al. Differences in kidney function and incident hypertension: the multi-ethnic study of atherosclerosis. Ann Intern Med 2008;148(7):501–8.

59. Zhang QL, Rothenbacher D. Prevalence of chronic kidney disease in population-based studies: systematic review. BMC Public Health 2008;8:117.

60. Chadban SJ, Briganti EM, Kerr PG, et al. Prevalence of kidney damage in Australian adults: the AusDiab kidney study. J Am Soc Nephrol 2003;14(7 Suppl 2):S131–8.

61. Coresh J, Selvin E, Stevens LA, et al. Prevalence of chronic kidney disease in the United States. JAMA 2007;298(17):2038–47.

62. Stewart JH, McCredie MR, McDonald SP. Incidence of end-stage renal disease in overseas-born, compared with Australian-born, non-indigenous Australians. Nephrology (Carlton) 2004;9(4):247–52.

63. Tonelli M, Hemmelgarn B, Manns B, et al. Death and renal transplantation among Aboriginal people undergoing dialysis. CMAJ 2004;171(6):577–82.

64. Gilbertson D, Burrows NR, Wang J, et al. Centers for Disease Control and Prevention (CDC). Racial differences in trends of end-stage renal disease, by primary diagnosis–United States, 1994–2004. MMWR Morb Mortal Wkly Rep 2007;56(11):253–6.

65. Snyder JJ, Foley RN, Collins AJ. Prevalence of CKD in the United States: a sensitivity analysis using the National Health and Nutrition Examination Survey (NHANES) 1999–2004. Am J Kidney Dis 2009;53(2):218–28.

66. Keith DS, Nichols GA, Gullion CM, et al. Longitudinal follow-up and outcomes among a population with chronic kidney disease in a large managed care organization. Arch Intern Med 2004;164(6):659–63.

67. Scavini M, Stidley CA, Paine SS, et al. The burden of chronic kidney disease among the Zuni Indians: the Zuni Kidney Project. Clin J Am Soc Nephrol 2007;2(3):509–16.

68. White SL, Chadban SJ, Jan S, et al. How can we achieve global equity in provision of renal replacement therapy? Bull World Health Organ 2008;86(3):229–37.

69. Dirks JH, de Zeeuw D, Agarwal SK, et al. Prevention of chronic kidney and vascular disease: toward global health equity–the Bellagio 2004 Declaration. Kidney Int Suppl 2005;98:S1–6.

70. Hoy WE, Kondalsamy-Chennakesavan S, McDonald S, et al. Renal disease, the metabolic syndrome, and cardiovascular disease. Ethn Dis 2006;16(2 Suppl 2):S246–51.

71. Neild GH. What do we know about chronic renal failure in young adults? I. Primary renal disease. Pediatr Nephrol 2009;24(10):1921–8.

72. Ardissino G, Dacco V, Testa S, et al. Epidemiology of chronic renal failure in children: data from the ItalKid project. Pediatrics 2003;111(4 Pt 1):e382–7.

73. Lewis MA. Demography of renal disease in childhood. Semin Fetal Neonatal Med 2008;13(3):118–24.

74. Seikaly M, Ho PL, Emmett L, et al. The 12th annual report of the North American Pediatric Renal Transplant Cooperative Study: renal transplantation from 1987 through 1998. Pediatr Transplant 2001;5(3):215–31.

75. Barsoum RS. Chronic kidney disease in the developing world. N Engl J Med 2006;354(10):997–9.
76. Zhang R, Liao J, Morse S, et al. Kidney disease and the metabolic syndrome. Am J Med Sci 2005;330(6):319–25.
77. Castro AF, Coresh J. CKD surveillance using laboratory data from the population-based National Health and Nutrition Examination Survey (NHANES). Am J Kidney Dis 2009;53(3 Suppl 3):S46–55.
78. Mackenzie HS, Lawler EV, Brenner BM. Congenital oligonephropathy: the fetal flaw in essential hypertension? Kidney Int Suppl 1996;55:S30–4.
79. Mackenzie HS, Brenner BM. Fewer nephrons at birth: a missing link in the etiology of essential hypertension? Am J Kidney Dis 1995;26(1):91–8.
80. Shah VO, Scavini M, Stidley CA, et al. Epidemic of diabetic and nondiabetic renal disease among the Zuni Indians: the Zuni Kidney Project. J Am Soc Nephrol 2003;14(5):1320–9.
81. Young TK, Reading J, Elias B, et al. Type 2 diabetes mellitus in Canada's first nations: status of an epidemic in progress. CMAJ 2000;163(5):561–6.
82. Nelson RG. Kidney disease in childhood-onset diabetes. Am J Kidney Dis 2008; 52(3):407–11.
83. Hovind P, Tarnow L, Parving HH. Remission and regression of diabetic nephropathy. Curr Hypertens Rep 2004;6(5):377–82.
84. Sego S. Pathophysiology of diabetic nephropathy. Nephrol Nurs J 2007;34(6): 631–3.
85. Pavkov ME, Bennett PH, Knowler WC, et al. Effect of youth-onset type 2 diabetes mellitus on incidence of end-stage renal disease and mortality in young and middle-aged Pima Indians. JAMA 2006;296(4):421–6.
86. Sellers EA, Blydt-Hansen TD, Dean HJ, et al. Macroalbuminuria and renal pathology in First Nation youth with type 2 diabetes. Diabetes Care 2009; 32(5):786–90.
87. Praga M, Morales E. Obesity, proteinuria and progression of renal failure. Curr Opin Nephrol Hypertens 2006;15(5):481–6.
88. Hall JE, Henegar JR, Dwyer TM, et al. Is obesity a major cause of chronic kidney disease? Adv Ren Replace Ther 2004;11(1):41–54.
89. Knowler WC, Pettitt DJ, Saad MF, et al. Obesity in the Pima Indians: its magnitude and relationship with diabetes. Am J Clin Nutr 1991;53(Suppl 6): 1543S–51S.
90. Chen HM, Li SJ, Chen HP, et al. Obesity-related glomerulopathy in China: a case series of 90 patients. Am J Kidney Dis 2008;52(1):58–65.
91. Fowler SM, Kon V, Ma L, et al. Obesity-related focal and segmental glomerulosclerosis: normalization of proteinuria in an adolescent after bariatric surgery. Pediatr Nephrol 2009;24(4):851–5.
92. Wu Y, Liu Z, Xiang Z, et al. Obesity-related glomerulopathy: insights from gene expression profiles of the glomeruli derived from renal biopsy samples. Endocrinology 2006;147(1):44–50.
93. Kambham N, Markowitz GS, Valeri AM, et al. Obesity-related glomerulopathy: an emerging epidemic. Kidney Int 2001;59(4):1498–509.
94. Remuzzi G, Ruggenenti P, Perico N. Chronic renal diseases: renoprotective benefits of renin-angiotensin system inhibition. Ann Intern Med 2002;136(8): 604–15.
95. Kojima T, Sasai-Takedatsu M, Hirata Y, et al. Characterization of renal tubular damage in preterm infants with renal failure. Acta Paediatr Jpn 1994;36(4): 392–5.

96. Hodgin JB, Rasoulpour M, Markowitz GS, et al. Very low birth weight is a risk factor for secondary focal segmental glomerulosclerosis. Clin J Am Soc Nephrol 2009;4(1):71–6.

97. Yeung MY. Oligonephropathy, developmental programming and nutritional management of low-gestation newborns. Acta Paediatr 2006;95(3):263–7.

98. Al Salmi I, Hoy WE, Kondalsamy-Chennakes S, et al. Birth weight and stages of CKD: a case-control study in an Australian population. Am J Kidney Dis 2008; 52(6):1070–8.

99. Lindstrom J, Eriksson JG, Valle TT, et al. Prevention of diabetes mellitus in subjects with impaired glucose tolerance in the Finnish Diabetes Prevention Study: results from a randomized clinical trial. J Am Soc Nephrol 2003;14(7 Suppl 2):S108–13.

100. Lindstrom J, Peltonen M, Tuomilehto J. Lifestyle strategies for weight control: experience from the Finnish Diabetes Prevention Study. Proc Nutr Soc 2005; 64(1):81–8.

101. Type 1 diabetes: benefits of intensive insulin therapy. Patients should control blood glucose strictly. Prescrire Int 2002;11(58):61.

102. Genuth S. The UKPDS and its global impact. Diabet Med 2008;25(Suppl 2): 57–62.

103. Sandhu S, Wiebe N, Fried LF, et al. Statins for improving renal outcomes: a meta-analysis. J Am Soc Nephrol 2006;17(7):2006–16.

104. Fried LF. Effects of HMG-CoA reductase inhibitors (statins) on progression of kidney disease. Kidney Int 2008;74(5):571–6.

105. Hillege HL, Janssen WM, Bak AA, et al. Microalbuminuria is common, also in a nondiabetic, nonhypertensive population, and an independent indicator of cardiovascular risk factors and cardiovascular morbidity. J Intern Med 2001; 249(6):519–26.

106. Hoy WE, Kondalsamy-Chennakesavan S, Scheppingen J, et al. A chronic disease outreach program for Aboriginal communities. Kidney Int Suppl 2005; 98:S76–82.

107. Mann JF, Gerstein HC, Pogue J, et al. Cardiovascular risk in patients with early renal insufficiency: implications for the use of ACE inhibitors. Am J Cardiovasc Drugs 2002;2(3):157–62.

108. Groothoff JW. Long-term outcomes of children with end-stage renal disease. Pediatr Nephrol 2005;20(7):849–53.

109. Groothoff J, Gruppen M, de Groot E, et al. Cardiovascular disease as a late complication of end-stage renal disease in children. Perit Dial Int 2005;25(Suppl 3):S123–6.

110. Ishimura E, Okuno S, Taniwaki H, et al. Different risk factors for vascular calcification in end-stage renal disease between diabetics and nondiabetics: the respective importance of glycemic and phosphate control. Kidney Blood Press Res 2008;31(1):10–5.

111. Lin CY, Sheng CC, Lin CC, et al. Mass urinary screening and follow-up for school children in Taiwan Province. Acta Paediatr Taiwan 2001;42(3):134–40.

112. Iseki K. Chronic kidney disease in Japan. Intern Med 2008;47(8):681–9.

113. Hillege HL, Fidler V, Diercks GF, et al. Urinary albumin excretion predicts cardiovascular and noncardiovascular mortality in general population. Circulation 2002;106(14):1777–82.

114. Magnason RL, Indridason OS, Sigvaldason H, et al. Prevalence and progression of CRF in Iceland: a population-based study. Am J Kidney Dis 2002; 40(5):955–63.

115. Ramirez SP. A comprehensive public health approach to address the burden of renal disease in singapore. J Am Soc Nephrol 2003;14(7 Suppl 2): S122–6.
116. Mani MK. Prevention of chronic renal failure at the community level. Kidney Int Suppl 2003;83:S86–9.
117. Haysom L, Williams R, Hodson E, et al. Risk of CKD in Australian indigenous and nonindigenous children: a population-based cohort study. Am J Kidney Dis 2009;53(2):229–37.
118. Stidley CA, Shah VO, Narva AS, et al. A population-based, cross-sectional survey of the Zuni Pueblo: a collaborative approach to an epidemic of kidney disease. Am J Kidney Dis 2002;39(2):358–68.
119. Stidley CA, Shah VO, Scavini M, et al. The Zuni kidney project: a collaborative approach to an epidemic of kidney disease. J Am Soc Nephrol 2003;14(7 Suppl 2):S139–43.
120. Archibald G, Bartlett W, Brown A, et al. UK Consensus Conference on early chronic kidney disease–6 and 7 February 2007. Nephrol Dial Transplant 2007; 22(9):2455–7.
121. Powe NR, Plantinga L, Saran R. Public health surveillance of CKD: principles, steps, and challenges. Am J Kidney Dis 2009;53(3 Suppl 3):S37–45.
122. Yap HK, Quek CM, Shen Q, et al. Role of urinary screening programmes in children in the prevention of chronic kidney disease. Ann Acad Med Singap 2005; 34(1):3–7.
123. Scavini M, Shah VO, Stidley CA, et al. Kidney disease among the Zuni Indians: the Zuni Kidney Project. Kidney Int Suppl 2005;97:S126–31.
124. Vassalotti JA, Li S, Chen SC, et al. Screening populations at increased risk of CKD: the Kidney Early Evaluation Program (KEEP) and the public health problem. Am J Kidney Dis 2009;53(3 Suppl 3):S107–14.
125. Fox CS, Larson MG, Leip EP, et al. Predictors of new-onset kidney disease in a community-based population. JAMA 2004;291(7):844–50.
126. Iseki K. Screening for renal disease–what can be learned from the Okinawa experience. Nephrol Dial Transplant 2006;21(4):839–43.
127. Winberg J. Does low birthweight facilitate postinfectious focal renal scarring? Acta Paediatr 2001;90(8):835–6.
128. Vikse BE, Irgens LM, Leivestad T, et al. Low birth weight increases risk for end-stage renal disease. J Am Soc Nephrol 2008;19(1):151–7.
129. Wani M, Kalra V, Agarwal SK. Low birth weight and its implication in renal disease. J Assoc Physicians India 2004;52:649–52.
130. Bolignano D, Donato V, Coppolino G, et al. Neutrophil gelatinase-associated lipocalin (NGAL) as a marker of kidney damage. Am J Kidney Dis 2008;52(3): 595–605.
131. Lindstrom J, Ilanne-Parikka P, Peltonen M, et al. Sustained reduction in the incidence of type 2 diabetes by lifestyle intervention: follow-up of the Finnish Diabetes Prevention Study. Lancet 2006;368(9548):1673–9.
132. Molitch ME, Fujimoto W, Hamman RF, et al. The diabetes prevention program and its global implications. J Am Soc Nephrol 2003;14(7 Suppl 2):S103–7.
133. Perneger TV, Whelton PK, Puddey IB, et al. Risk of end-stage renal disease associated with alcohol consumption. Am J Epidemiol 1999;150(12):1275–81.
134. Effect of intensive therapy on the development and progression of diabetic nephropathy in the Diabetes Control and Complications Trial. The Diabetes Control and Complications (DCCT) Research Group. Kidney Int 1995;47(6): 1703–20.

135. Home PD. Impact of the UKPDS–an overview. Diabet Med 2008;25(Suppl 2):2–8.

136. Intensive blood-glucose control with sulphonylureas or insulin compared with conventional treatment and risk of complications in patients with type 2 diabetes (UKPDS 33). UK Prospective Diabetes Study (UKPDS) Group. Lancet 1998; 352(9131):837–53.

137. Tight blood pressure control and risk of macrovascular and microvascular complications in type 2 diabetes: UKPDS 38. UK Prospective Diabetes Study Group. BMJ 1998;317(7160):703–13.

138. Bomback AS, Kshirsagar AV, Amamoo MA, et al. Change in proteinuria after adding aldosterone blockers to ACE inhibitors or angiotensin receptor blockers in CKD: a systematic review. Am J Kidney Dis 2008;51(2):199–211.

139. Ruggenenti P, Perna A, Remuzzi G. ACE inhibitors to prevent end-stage renal disease: when to start and why possibly never to stop: a post hoc analysis of the REIN trial results. Ramipril efficacy in nephropathy. J Am Soc Nephrol 2001;12(12):2832–7.

140. Tonelli M, Bohm C, Pandeya S, et al. Cardiac risk factors and the use of cardioprotective medications in patients with chronic renal insufficiency. Am J Kidney Dis 2001;37(3):484–9.

141. Wald NJ, Law MR. A strategy to reduce cardiovascular disease by more than 80%. BMJ 2003;326(7404):1419.

Acute and Chronic Otitis Media

Peter S. Morris, MBBS, FRACP, PhD[a,b,c,*], Amanda J. Leach, PhD[a,b]

KEYWORDS

- Upper respiratory tract infection ● Chronic otitis media
- Randomized controlled trials ● Acute otitis media

Upper respiratory tract infections (including otitis media) are the most common illnesses affecting children.[1] The term "otitis media" (OM) covers a wide spectrum of disease, and is used to describe illnesses with predominantly middle ear symptoms (including acute otitis media, otitis media with effusion, and chronic suppurative otitis media). Children can expect to experience around 6 to 8 upper respiratory infections (URTIs) each year.[2] Nearly all children will experience at least one episode of OM during childhood. On average, they experience around one episode of acute otitis media (AOM) per year in the first 3 years of life.[3]

The initial cause of respiratory mucosal infections (including OM) is most commonly a viral infection but can be bacterial (**Table 1**).[4] Of importance is that many infections involve both viruses and bacteria.[5] Most commonly, an initial viral infection is complicated by a secondary bacterial infection. In developed countries, both viral and bacterial infections are likely to be self-limited. Persistent symptomatic disease is an indication that the child has an ongoing bacterial infection.

By understanding the evidence available from high quality studies, the clinician is in a position to advise the families on appropriate action.[6] Well designed randomized controlled trials (RCTs) provide the most reliable evidence of effect (**Table 2**).[7] The aim of this article is to support clinicians in answering the following questions:

(i) What happens to children with these conditions when no additional treatment is provided?
(ii) Which interventions have been assessed in well-designed studies?
(iii) Which interventions have been shown to improve outcomes?
(iv) If an intervention is considered appropriate, how large is the overall benefit?

a Child Health Division, Menzies School of Health Research, PO Box 41096, Casuarina, NT 0811, Australia
b Institute of Advanced Studies, Charles Darwin University, Darwin, NT 0909, Australia
c Northern Territory Clinical School, Flinders University, PO Box 41326, Darwin, NT 0811, Australia
* Corresponding author. Child Health Division, Menzies School of Health Research, PO Box 41096, Casuarina, NT 0811, Australia.
E-mail address: peterm@menzies.edu.au (P.S. Morris).

Pediatr Clin N Am 56 (2009) 1383–1399
doi:10.1016/j.pcl.2009.09.007
0031-3955/09/$ – see front matter © 2009 Published by Elsevier Inc.

Table 1
Spectrum of disease, accepted terminology, and etiology of the common upper respiratory tract infections in children

Condition	Related Diagnoses	Etiology
Otitis media	Otitis media with effusion, acute otitis media without perforation, acute otitis media with perforation, chronic suppurative otitis media	Viral: respiratory syncytial virus, influenza, adenovirus, rhinovirus, coronavirus, enterovirus, parainfluenza, metapneumovirus Bacterial: *Streptococcus pneumoniae, Haemophilus influenzae, Moraxella catarrhalis, Streptococcus pyogenes*

THE APPROACH TO EVIDENCE USED IN THIS ARTICLE

There is a long list of potential interventions for the different forms of OM. Many families have strong personal preferences about their treatment options. The challenge for the clinician is to make an accurate diagnosis and then to match the effective treatment options to the preferences of the family.

In this article, the authors have initially considered the effects of an intervention compared with no intervention. Their focus on trial evidence means that the authors may not review all the relevant information to an individual decision. The overall effects of an intervention may need to be adjusted with this in mind. It is hoped that clinicians using this article should be able to determine which interventions have been rigorously assessed and the overall findings of these assessments.

The GRADE Working Group has described the steps required to review evidence.[8–10] The GRADE Working Group proposes that a recommendation should indicate a decision that the majority of well-informed individuals would make. For self-limited conditions with low risk of complications, even well-informed individuals may reach different conclusions. Therefore, the authors have tried to provide an evidence summary that will assist discussions with families (**Table 3**). The authors' own approach (informed by the best available evidence) is described in **Box 1**.

IMPORTANT HEALTH OUTCOMES AND TREATMENT EFFECTS

The self-limiting nature of modern OM in developed countries is of the utmost importance in determining which treatments are indicated. In this article, groups of children

Table 2
Typical clinical features of the common upper respiratory infections in children that have been assessed in randomized controlled trials

Condition	Typical Clinical Features
Otitis media with effusion	Asymptomatic persistent middle ear effusion confirmed by tympanometry
Acute otitis media	Recurrent clinical diagnosis of AOM ($\geq$3 in 6 mo) with red tympanic membrane and ear pain
Recurrent acute otitis media	Clinical diagnosis of AOM with red tympanic membrane and ear pain
Chronic suppurative otitis media	Discharge through a perforated tympanic membrane for 2–6 wk

Table 3
Treatment effects of interventions for otitis media in children who have been assessed in randomized controlled trials

Intervention	Evidence	Effect (no Intervention vs Intervention)
Prevention		
Pneumococcal conjugate vaccine[11]	3 studies (39,749 participants)	Acute otitis media episodes reduced by 6% (eg, 1.0 vs 0.94 episodes per year). Insertion of tympanostomy tubes reduced (3.8% vs 2.9%)
Influenza vaccine[12,13]	11 studies (11,349 participants)	Inconsistent results. Modest protection against otitis media during influenza season in some studies
Treatment of persistent otitis media with effusion		
Antibiotics[14,15]	9 studies (1534 participants)	Persistent OME at around 4 weeks reduced (81% vs 68%)
Tympanostomy tubes[16,17]	11 studies (~1300 participants)	Modest improvement in hearing: 9dB at 6 mo and 6dB at 12 mo. No improvement in language or cognitive assessment
Antihistamines and decongestants[18]	7 studies (1177 participants)	No difference in persistent OME at 4 wk (75%)
Autoinflation[19]	6 studies (602 participants)	Inconsistent results. Modest improvement in tympanometry at 4 wk in some studies
Antibiotics plus steroids[20]	5 studies (418 participants)	Persistent OME at 2 wk reduced (75% vs 52%)
Treatment of initial acute otitis media		
Antihistamines and decongestants[21]	12 studies (2300 participants)	No significant difference in persistent AOM at 2 wk
Antibiotics[22,23]	8 studies (2287 participants) 6 studies (1643 participants)	Persistent pain on day 2–7 reduced (22% vs 16%) Persistent AOM reduced in children <2 y old with bilateral AOM (55% vs 30%) and in children with AOM with perforation (53% vs 19%)
Myringotomy[24]	3 studies (812 participants)	Early treatment failure increased (5% vs 20%).
Analgesics[25]	1 study (219 participants)	Persistent pain reduced on day 2 (25% vs 9%).
Treatment of recurrent acute otitis media		
Antibiotics[26]	16 studies (1483 participants)	Acute otitis media episodes reduced (3.0 vs 1.5 episodes per year)

(*continued on next page*)

Table 3
(continued)

Intervention	Evidence	Effect (no intervention vs Intervention)
Adenoidectomy[27–29]	6 studies (1060 participants)	No significant reduction in rates of AOM
Tympanostomy tubes[27,30]	5 studies (424 participants)	Acute otitis media episodes reduced (2.0 vs 1.0 episodes per year)
Treatment of chronic suppurative otitis media		
Topical antibiotics[31–33]	7 studies (1074 participants)	Persistent CSOM at 2–16 wk reduced (around 75% vs 20%–50%
Ear cleaning[31,34]	2 studies (658 participants)	Inconsistent results. No reduction in persistent CSOM at 12–16 wk (78%) in large African study

with low rates of suppurative complications of OM are categorized as low-risk populations. Communities where more than 4% of children experience chronic tympanic membrane perforation secondary to suppurative infection are high-risk populations.[35]

In low-risk populations, OM is generally a condition that resolves without treatment or complications. Unfortunately, tympanic membrane perforation remains a common occurrence for many Indigenous groups.

The outcomes considered important in this article are: (i) persistent disease (short term ≤14 days, medium term >2 weeks to 6 months, long term >6 months); (ii) time to cure; and (iii) complications arising from progressive disease. The authors considered interventions to have very large effects if they were associated with a relative reduction in the outcome of interest of more than 80%; large effects were associated with a reduction in outcome of at least 50%.[36] Reductions of between 20% and 50% were considered modest and reductions less than 20% were considered slight (or small). Because only a proportion of children with OM experience bad outcomes, even large relative effects may have modest absolute benefits.

SEARCH STRATEGY

The search targeted evidence-based guidelines, evidence-based summaries, systematic reviews, and RCTs of interventions for otitis media (see **Box 2**). This simple strategy identified over 1600 hits using PubMed alone. To be included as an evidence-based guideline, summary, or systematic review, one needed to provide an explicit search strategy and criteria for study inclusion. To be included as a clinical trial, randomization needed to be used. Four primary sources to identify relevant information were used: Clinical Evidence (Issue 1 2009),[36] the Cochrane Library (Issue 2 2009),[37] Evidence-Based Otitis Media[27] and Medline (last accessed via PubMed on 26 June, 2009). The evidence-based summaries in Clinical Evidence have links to major guidelines and use the GRADE Working Group approach to assess quality of evidence and strength of recommendations.[36] PubMed was also searched to identify publications specifically addressing OM in Indigenous populations.

RESULTS OF SEARCH

The search identified over 50 evidence-based guidelines, evidence summaries, and systematic reviews (and many more additional RCTs) published since 2000. In this

---

Box 1
Suggested approach when assessing and managing a child with OM

1. Take a history of the presenting complaint to elicit the primary symptoms: nasal discharge or sore throat (nonspecific URTI), ear pain, ear discharge, or hearing loss (OM). Ask about frequency and severity of previous episodes. Clarify duration of illness and presence of any associated features including cough (bronchitis), fever, respiratory distress, cyanosis, poor feeding, or lethargy. Determine the concerns, expectations, and preferences of the child and their carer. (Grade: very low; Level of evidence: cohort studies and other evidence.)

2. Examine the child to confirm whether investigation and management strategy should include OM. Assess temperature, pulse, and respiratory rate, presence and color of nasal discharge, nasal obstruction, facial tenderness, tonsillar enlargement, tonsillar exudate, cervical lymphadenopathy, presence of cough, presence of middle ear effusion (using pneumatic otoscopy or tympanometry), and position and integrity of tympanic membrane. Ensure normal hydration, perfusion, conscious state, and no meningism, periorbital swelling, proptosis, limitation of eye movements, upper airway obstruction, respiratory distress, or mastoid tenderness. (Grade: very low; Level of evidence: cohort studies and other evidence.)

3. Investigations:

   - Otitis media with effusion (OME): None required for most children. If effusions are bilateral and persistent for >3 months, then organize a hearing test. (Grade: low; Level of evidence: cohort studies.)

   - AOM: None required unless febrile and <3 months of age, or danger signs present (respiratory distress, cyanosis, poor feeding, or lethargy). (Grade: low; Level of evidence: cohort studies.)

   - Chronic suppurative otitis media (CSOM): Organize a hearing test. Imaging (computed tomography scan) is appropriate if CSOM is persistent despite treatment and the tympanic membrane cannot be visualized. (Grade: low; Level of evidence: cohort studies)

4. Management:

   - OME: No immediate treatment required. Review at 3 months is appropriate if bilateral effusions are present and child is from a high-risk population. (Grade: low; Level of evidence: cohort studies.)

   - AOM: Symptomatic pain relief if indicated, watchful waiting with advice to parents on likely course and possible complications. For low-risk populations, antibiotics are most likely to benefit those who have AOM with perforation, <2 years and bilateral AOM, already had 48 hours of watchful waiting and no improvement, or are at high risk of suppurative complications (especially perforation of the tympanic membrane). For high-risk populations, antibiotics are recommended. (Grade: high; Level of evidence: RCTs.)

   - CSOM: Cleaning ear discharge from external canal and topical antibiotics are recommended. (Grade: high; Level of evidence: RCTs.)

---

article, the authors have not considered interventions that have been assessed in non-randomized studies, interventions that have been assessed in studies with less than 200 participants (sparse data),[36] or studies of interventions that are only available experimentally. The simple search strategy for Indigenous studies identified 291 hits. Of these, 17 hits were also identified by the strategy to identify high-quality intervention studies. These hits included 1 systematic review and 5 RCTs. The systematic review described clinical research studies of OM in Australian Aboriginal children.[38] Two RCTs addressed the effect of antibiotic prophylaxis in Alaskan Inuit children and Australian Aboriginal children.[39,40] Two of the RCTs addressed the effect of topical antibiotics for CSOM in Australian Aboriginal children.[41,42] One RCT assessed

---

Box 2
A simple PubMed search strategy to identify evidence-based guidelines, evidence-based summaries, systematic reviews, and RCTs on otitis media and additional studies involving Indigenous children

1. "otitis"[MeSH Terms] AND (practice guideline[pt] OR systematic[sb] OR clinical evidence[jour] OR clinical trial[pt]) = 1625 hits

2. "otitis"[MeSH Terms] AND ("American Native Continental Ancestry Group"[MeSH Terms] OR "Oceanic Ancestry Group"[MeSH Terms] OR "ethnic groups"[MeSH Terms] OR Inuit OR "Native American" OR Indian OR "First Nation" OR Maori OR Indig* OR Aborig*) = 291 hits

3. 1 AND 2 = 17 hits

---

the impact of the conjugate pneumococcal vaccine on OM in Navajo and Apache children.[43] Although they were not identified by a search strategy, the authors were also aware of an additional systematic review and evidence-based clinical guidelines developed specifically to assist in the care of Australian Aboriginal children with OM.[44,45]

BURDEN OF OTITIS MEDIA

Otitis media (OM) is an acute upper respiratory tract infection that affects the respiratory mucosa of the middle ear cleft. OM is a common illness in young children (and occurs much less frequently in children >6 years).[24,46] In developed countries, OM is the commonest indication for antibiotic prescribing and surgery in young children. In the United States, annual costs were estimated to be $3 to $5 billion in the 1990s.[46] The costs per capita are likely to be considerably greater in high-risk populations.

COMMON TYPES OF OTITIS MEDIA

Otitis media is best regarded as a spectrum of disease. The most important conditions are OME, acute otitis media without perforation (AOMwoP), acute otitis media with perforation (AOMwiP), and CSOM. OME is usually the mildest form of the disease and CSOM the most severe. Children who end up with CSOM usually progress through the stages of OME, AOM without perforation, AOM with perforation, and finally to CSOM. Unfortunately, there is currently a lack of consistency in definitions of different forms of OM (especially AOM).[47] This can lead to confusion when you need to describe the progress of a child over time.

OME is usually defined as the presence of a middle ear effusion without symptoms or signs of an acute infection. OME is by far the most common form of OM in all populations. Brief periods of OME (often in association with upper respiratory tract infections) should be regarded as a normal phenomenon in early childhood.

AOM is usually defined as the presence of a middle ear effusion plus the presence of the symptoms (especially pain) or signs (especially bulging of the tympanic membrane or fresh discharge). The diagnostic criteria used in studies of AOM vary. Some use symptomatic criteria, some use otoscopic criteria, and some require both symptomatic and otoscopic criteria to be met.

CSOM is usually defined as discharge through a perforated tympanic membrane for greater than 2 to 6 weeks. If the duration of the discharge is uncertain, perforations that are easily visible (covering >2% of the tympanic membrane) are more likely to be associated with CSOM.

Children with immunodeficiency or craniofacial abnormalities (cleft palate, Down syndrome, and so forth) are at increased risk of OM. Other risk factors that have been identified in epidemiologic studies include recent respiratory infection, family history, siblings, child care attendance, lack of breast feeding, passive smoke exposure, and use of a pacifier.[48]

FEATURES OF OTITIS MEDIA IN INDIGENOUS POPULATIONS

High rates of severe otitis media have been described in Indigenous children for over 40 years. The first publication identified by the authors' search was published in 1960,[49] and publications have appeared regularly from 1965 on.[50] In the recent past, Indigenous children from the United States, Canada, Northern Europe, Australia, and New Zealand have all been affected.[51–60] The rates of tympanic membrane perforation in these populations remain among the highest ever described in the medical literature.[61] Many investigators have puzzled over the high rates of severe disease and wondered whether ear discharge was a new illness that occurred during the transition from a nomadic lifestyle typical of many of these Indigenous groups. The search reported here did not identify any studies that were able to answer this question.

The rates of tympanic membrane perforation vary enormously, even with Indigenous groups within the same region. Furthermore, discharging ears as described in Indigenous children ("the running ear are the heritage of the poor")[62] were common in disadvantaged children living in developed countries in the pre-antibiotic era.[63] For these reasons, the authors believe the most important underlying causes of severe ear infections are likely to be environmental. Indigenous populations at high risk of severe OM also have high rates of rhinosinusitis, bronchitis, pneumonia, invasive pneumococcal disease, and chronic suppurative lung disease (including bronchiectasis).[64–71] It is likely that the same risk factors contribute to the excessive frequency of all of these conditions.

Early exposure to otitis media pathogens has been demonstrated in Australian Aboriginal infants, and this is the most important determinant of subsequent OM (**Fig. 1**).[72–74] Of importance is that in this high-risk population, children usually have multiple pathogens (and often multiple types of each pathogen) and their total bacterial load is high. International comparisons show that a similar early onset of carriage of the pneumococcus is seen in other populations with high rates of invasive pneumococcal disease (**Fig. 2**).[75]

Although genetic factors are known to contribute to the risk of OM, their importance in high-risk populations has not been determined. Some investigators have proposed that genetic susceptibility is linked to poor Eustachian tube function.[52] However, this does not explain the associated high rates of other bacterial respiratory infection.

DIAGNOSIS OF OTITIS MEDIA

Children with OM will usually present with features related to either: (i) pain and fever (AOM); (ii) hearing loss (OME); or (iii) ear discharge (AOM with perforation or CSOM). In some children, OM will be detected as part of a routine examination. Making an accurate diagnosis is not easy. In general it requires a good view of the whole tympanic membrane, and the use of either pneumatic otoscopy or tympanometry (to confirm the presence of a middle ear effusion).[47,76] Studies of diagnostic accuracy in AOM have found ear pain to be the most useful symptom (but not very reliable on it is own). Presence of bulging, opacity, and immobility of the tympanic membrane are

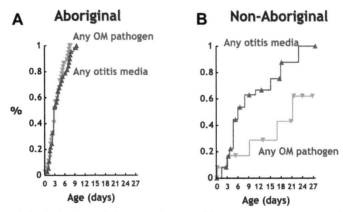

Fig. 1. Bacterial colonization of the nasopharynx with pneumococcus, nontypable *Haemophilus influenzae*, or *Moraxella catarrhalis* predicts early onset of persistent otitis media in Aboriginal infants. (*From* Leach AJ, Boswell JB, Asche V, et al. Bacterial colonization of the nasopharynx predicts very early onset and persistence of otitis media in Australian aboriginal infants. Pediatr Infect Dis J 1994;13(11):983–9; with permission.)

all highly predictive of AOM. Normal (pearly gray) color of the tympanic membrane makes AOM unlikely.[77]

OTITIS MEDIA WITH EFFUSION

The commonest form of OM is OME. The point prevalence in screening studies is around 20% in young children.[46] OME can occur spontaneously, as part of rhinosinusitis, or following an episode of AOM. The same respiratory bacterial pathogens associated with AOM have been implicated in the pathogenesis. Most children with OME will improve spontaneously within 3 months, and complications from this illness are uncommon.[46] The average hearing loss associated with OME is around 25 dB.[46] Despite large numbers of studies, a causal relationship between OME and speech and language delay has not been proven.[27,78]

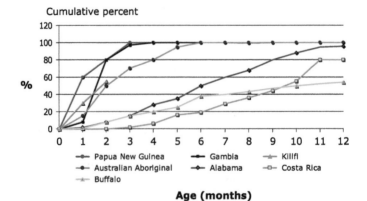

Fig. 2. Time to acquisition of pneumococcus in the nasopharynx of infants enrolled in birth cohort studies. (*Adapted from* O'Brien KL, Nohynek H. Report from a WHO Working Group: standard method for detecting upper respiratory carriage of *Streptococcus pneumoniae*. Pediatr Infect Dis J 2003;22(2):e1–11; with permission.)

ACUTE OTITIS MEDIA

Most children will experience at least one episode of AOM.[46] The peak incidence of infection occurs between 6 and 12 months. Although the pathogenesis of AOM is multifactorial, both viruses and bacteria are implicated.[46] Bacterial infection with the common respiratory pathogens (*Streptococcus pneumoniae*, *Haemophilus influenzae*, and *Moraxella catarrhalis*) is often preceded by a viral infection. Viruses (especially respiratory syncytial virus and influenza) can cause AOM without coinfection with bacteria.[46] The pain associated with AOM resolves within 24 hours in around 60% and within 3 days in around 80%.[24] Young children with AOM (<2 years) are less likely to experience spontaneous resolution.[22] Complications of AOM include CSOM, mastoiditis, labyrinthitis, facial palsy, meningitis, intracranial abscess, and lateral sinus thrombosis.[27] Mastoiditis was the most common life-threatening complication in the pre-antibiotic era. Mastoiditis occurred in 18% of children admitted to hospital with AOM in one study.[23] Mastoiditis (and all other complications) is now rare in developed countries.

CHRONIC SUPPURATIVE OTITIS MEDIA

CSOM is the most severe form of OM.[79] Although there is a lack of well-designed longitudinal studies, CSOM is the type of OM most likely to persist without treatment. In developing countries, CSOM occurs as a complication of AOM with perforation and can be a major health issue. The range of bacterial pathogens associated with CSOM is considerably broader than those seen in AOM. *Pseudomonas*, *Staphylococcus*, *Proteus*, and *Klebsiella* species are most commonly isolated, and mixed infections are common.[79] Multidrug antibiotic resistance is often seen in *Pseudomonas* infections. The associated hearing loss is usually more than that seen in OME (and CSOM represents the most important cause of moderate conductive hearing loss [>40dB] in many developing countries).[31]

  In developed countries, CSOM is now very uncommon. A recent risk factor study in the Netherlands found that most cases of CSOM are now occurring as a complication of tympanostomy tubes insertion.[80] Children with immunodeficiency and some Indigenous populations are also at greatly increased risk. In rural and remote communities in northern Australia, more than 20% of young children are affected.[71]

OPTIONS FOR INTERVENTIONS: OTITIS MEDIA WITH EFFUSION

OME affects all children but is usually asymptomatic.[46] A small proportion of children have persistent OME with associated hearing loss. There is evidence on the effects of screening to identify young children with OME (or hearing loss associated with OME), and this is not effective in developed countries.[81] There is also evidence on treatment effects of antibiotics, insertion of tympanostomy tubes, autoinflation devices, antihistamines and decongestants, and antibiotics plus steroids (see **Table 3**).[14–20,22,23,82] Of these interventions, early insertion of tympanostomy tubes (compared with watchful waiting and option of insertion later) is proven to improve hearing at 6 and 12 months, but the beneficial effect is modest.[14–16] This improvement in hearing has not been associated with improvement in language development or cognitive assessment scores.[16] Tympanostomy tubes usually last 6 to 12 months, and there is no evidence that there is any ongoing benefit after they have been extruded. Antibiotics have also been shown to be an effective treatment, but the beneficial effects are slight and do not seem to persist over the long term.[14,15,27] There seem to be additional short-term benefits when antibiotics are combined with steroids, but again the beneficial effect is modest.[14,20] There is some evidence that autoinflation devices are effective.[14,19] The benefits are modest and have only been documented to be short term. Antihistamines and decongestants provide no benefit (see **Table 3**).[14,15,18]

Given the available evidence from RCTs on OME, most well-informed individuals in low-risk populations would choose a course of watchful waiting initially. For those children with persistent OME in both ears associated with hearing loss despite watching and waiting for 6 to 12 months, a trial of antibiotics is reasonable. Insertion of tympanostomy tubes is most appropriate in children for whom the primary concern is the conductive hearing loss and communication difficulties. Children with the most severe conductive hearing loss are most likely to benefit. Families should be informed that a small proportion of children will suffer recurrent persistent OME when the tympanostomy tubes are extruded, and may need a second operation. In these children, tympanostomy tubes plus adenoidectomy is a reasonable option.[14,82]

Children who experience frequent suppurative infections (including those with immunodeficiency or persistent bacterial rhinosinusitis) are at greatest risk of developing CSOM as a complication of tympanostomy tubes. Indigenous children in high-risk populations would fall into this group.

None of the RCTs assessing interventions for OME were conducted with Indigenous children. However, one RCT of prophylactic antibiotics in Australian Aboriginal children enrolled only infants with OME. None of the children in the placebo group had resolution of their OME within 6 months. Around 10% of children in the antibiotic group had resolution of their OME.[40] This result suggests that OME is a persistent condition that does not respond well to established treatment options. Although no reliable evidence from RCTs was found, strategies that aim to improve hearing and communication in those with moderate hearing loss might provide most benefit in high-risk populations.

Although not a primary outcome measure, pneumococcal conjugate vaccine reduced the number of children who received tympanostomy tube insertion by around 20%. It is possible that some of this effect was mediated through a reduction in chronic bilateral OME with hearing loss. Consistent with this, substantial declines in this procedure have been described in the United States in recent years, but not amongst Alaskan Native children.[83]

OPTIONS FOR INTERVENTIONS: ACUTE OTITIS MEDIA

Most children with AOM will improve spontaneously within 14 days, and complications from this illness are uncommon. When considering the onset of the illness, there is evidence on the preventive effects of pneumococcal conjugate vaccine and influenza vaccine (see **Table 3**).[11–13,24] Both of these vaccines have been shown to be effective, but the beneficial effects in terms of overall rates of infection are slight. The beneficial effects of the pneumococcal conjugate vaccine are modest in terms of reductions in the insertion of tympanostomy tubes.[84] Most children in low-risk populations will not meet the criteria for tympanostomy tube insertion. There is also evidence on the treatment effects of antihistamines and decongestants, antibiotics, myringotomy, and analgesics (see **Table 3**).[21,23–25,27] Regular analgesics (paracetamol or ibuprofen) provide a benefit (assessment on day 2), and the beneficial effects were large.[24] Antibiotics are also proven to be effective.[22,23] The short-term beneficial effects are slight in most children. The beneficial effects are modest in children younger than 2 years with bilateral AOM, and large in those with AOM with perforation. Studies of initial treatment with antibiotics have not documented a long-term effect. If antibiotics are to be used, there is evidence that a longer course of treatment (≥7 days) is more effective but the beneficial effects are modest (persistent AOM reduced from 22% to 15%).[85] There is no evidence to support the belief that any one of the commonly used antibiotics is more effective than the others. The use of antihistamines and deconges-tants has not been shown to be beneficial, and myringotomy seems to be harmful compared with no treatment or antibiotics (see **Table 3**).[21,24,27]

Given the available evidence from RCTs on AOM, most well-informed individuals in low-risk populations would choose symptomatic relief with analgesics and either watchful waiting or antibiotics. Antibiotics would be most appropriate in children younger than 2 years with bilateral AOM, those with AOM with perforation, children with high risk of complications, and those who have already had 48 hours of watchful waiting.

If the child is not in a high-risk group but the family prefers antibiotic treatment, the clinician should discuss "wait and see prescribing." Provision of a script for antibiotic along with advice only to use it if the pain persists 48 hours will reduce antibiotic use by two-thirds (with no negative impact on family satisfaction).[86–88]

A small proportion of children with AOM will experience recurrent AOM (3 episodes in 6 months or 4 episodes within 12 months).[46] There is evidence on the treatment effects of prophylactic antibiotics, adenoidectomy, and tympanostomy tube inser-tion.[24,26–30] Antibiotics are proven to be effective but the beneficial effects are modest. The rates of AOM also reduce spontaneously without treatment so that absolute bene-fits are less impressive than anticipated. Two of the RCTs assessing prophylactic anti-biotics have been conducted in Indigenous children.[39,40] These studies demonstrate that prophylactic antibiotics will prevent perforation of the tympanic membrane. The size of the benefit is similar to prevention of any AOM. Insertion of tympanostomy tubes also seems to reduce rates of AOM, and the effect is similar to antibiotics. Either of these options could be considered in those children from low-risk populations with very frequent infections (especially if occurring before the peak of respiratory illness in winter). However, children with tympanostomy tubes may develop a discharging ear, so this is not a good option in children at increased risk of suppurative infections (including those with immunodeficiency or persistent bacterial rhinosinusitis). For Indigenous children in high-risk populations, prophylactic antibiotics or prompt antibi-otic treatment of infections are probably the more appropriate treatment options. Adenoidectomy does not seem to be an effective treatment.[27–29]

Because Indigenous children in high-risk populations are known to have high rates of pneumococcal diseases, there was hope that introduction of the pneumococcal conjugate vaccine would have a greater impact on OM in these populations. One RCT in Navajo and Apache children assessed the impact on OM and could not demonstrate substantially improved outcomes.[43] Of note, comparison of longitudinal cohorts before and after the introduction of the pneumococcal conjugate vaccine found a reduction in OM visits for American Indian children but not for Alaskan Native children.[83] In Australia, comparison of longitudinal cohorts of Aboriginal infants before and after the introduction of the vaccine did not document substantial reductions in severe OM.[43,89]

OPTIONS FOR INTERVENTIONS: CHRONIC SUPPURATIVE OTITIS MEDIA

A small proportion of children with AOM with perforation go on to develop CSOM. In developed countries, CSOM most commonly occurs as a complication of tympanos-tomy tube placement. There is evidence on the treatment effects of topical antibiotics, topical antiseptics, systemic antibiotics, and ear cleaning.[31–34,79] Interpretation of a large number of small studies is challenging, but topical antibiotics are proven to be effective and the beneficial effects vary from large to modest. Most studies have not documented a long-term effect. Topical antibiotics also seem to be more effective than antiseptics and systemic antibiotics.[31] The role of topical antibiotics plus systematic antibiotics is unclear.[90] Cleaning the middle ear discharge has not been proven to be effective in RCTs but is generally regarded as necessary before insertion of topical antibiotics (at least in children with profuse discharge). Although not seen in RCTs, there is also a very small risk of ototoxicity associated with most topical antibiotics (except topical quinolones) and topical antiseptics.[27] For children who fail to respond to prolonged courses of topical antibiotics, 2 small studies (85 participants) have documented high cure rates and large beneficial effects associated with 2 to 3 weeks of intravenous antipseudomonal antibiotics (such as ceftazidime).[91,92]

Given the available evidence from RCTs on CSOM, most well-informed individuals would choose topical antibiotic treatment. However, even though this is an effective treatment, prolonged or repeated courses of treatment are often required. If this is the case, topical quinolones will provide a slight benefit in terms of risk of ototoxicity. Even in high-risk Indigenous populations there is a considerable difference in the likely response to treatment. Two RCTs comparing ciprofloxacin drops with framycetin-gramycidin-dexamethasone drops in Australian Aboriginal children with CSOM have been conducted. One trial found most children could be effectively treated within 9 days, whereas the other reported most children with persistent CSOM despite 6 weeks of treatment.[41,42]

Although not the subject of RCTs, the outcomes of tympanoplasty in Indigenous children and adults have been described. These studies usually report effective surgical repair of the tympanic membrane in around 50% to 70% and a modest improvement in hearing.[57,93,94] These results are not as good as those seen in other populations, where effective repair is usually achieved in 80% to 90%. This operation is probably most appropriate for Indigenous children with bilateral large, dry tympanic membrane perforations associated with a moderate hearing loss or frequent episodes of discharge.

SUMMARY

OM is one of the most common illnesses affecting children. In low-risk populations, most illnesses are mild and will resolve completely without specific treatment. Unfortunately, this is not always the case for Indigenous children in high-risk populations. Multiple interventions have been assessed in the treatment of OM. None of the interventions have had substantial absolute benefits for the populations studied. Therefore, for low-risk children symptomatic relief and watchful waiting (including education of the parents about important danger signs) is the most appropriate treatment option. Antibiotics have a role in children with persistent bacterial infection, or those at risk of complications. Even today, many Indigenous children will often fall into these high-risk groups.

REFERENCES

1. Monto AS. Epidemiology of viral respiratory infections. Am J Med 2002;112(Suppl 6A):4S–12S.
2. Heikkinen T, Jarvinen A. The common cold. Lancet 2003;361(9351):51–9.
3. Bluestone CD, Klein JO. Otitis media in infants and children. 4th edition. Philadelphia: W.B. Saunders Company; 2007.
4. Nelson WE. In: Nelson WE, Behman RE, Kliegman RM, et al, editors. Textbook of pediatrics. 15th edition. Philadelphia: W.B. Saunders Company; 1996.

5. Revai K, Dobbs LA, Nair S, et al. Incidence of acute otitis media and sinusitis complicating upper respiratory tract infection: the effect of age. Pediatrics 2007;119(6):e1408–12.
6. Irwig L, Irwig J, Sweet M, et al. Smart health choices: making sense of health advice. Sydney: Hammersmith Press; 2007.
7. Altman DG, Bland JM. Statistics notes. Treatment allocation in controlled trials: why randomise? BMJ 1999;318(7192):1209.
8. Atkins D, Best D, Briss PA, et al. Grading quality of evidence and strength of recommendations. BMJ 2004;328(7454):1490.
9. Guyatt GH, Oxman AD, Vist GE, et al. GRADE: an emerging consensus on rating quality of evidence and strength of recommendations. BMJ 2008;336(7650):924–6.
10. Atkins D, Briss PA, Eccles M, et al. Systems for grading the quality of evidence and the strength of recommendations II: pilot study of a new system. BMC Health Serv Res 2005;51:25.
11. Straetemans M, Sanders EA, Veenhoven RH, et al. Pneumococcal vaccines for preventing otitis media. Cochrane Database Syst Rev 2004;(1):CD001480.
12. Jefferson T, Rivetti A, Harnden A, et al. Vaccines for preventing influenza in healthy children. Cochrane Database Syst Rev 2008;(2):CD004879.
13. Manzoli L, Schioppa F, Boccia A, et al. The efficacy of influenza vaccine for healthy children: a meta-analysis evaluating potential sources of variation in efficacy estimates including study quality. Pediatr Infect Dis J 2007;26(2):97–106.
14. Williamson I. Otitis media with effusion. Clin Evid 2006;15:814–21.
15. American Academy of Family Physicians, American Academy of Otolaryngology-Head and Neck Surgery, American Academy of Pediatrics Subcommittee on Otitis Media With Effusion. Otitis media with effusion. Pediatrics 2004;113(5):1412–29.
16. Lous J, Burton MJ, Felding JU, et al. Grommets (ventilation tubes) for hearing loss associated with otitis media with effusion in children. Cochrane Database Syst Rev 2005;(1):CD001801.
17. Rovers MM, Black N, Browning GG, et al. Grommets in otitis media with effusion: an individual patient data meta-analysis. Arch Dis Child 2005;90(5):480–5.
18. Griffin GH, Flynn C, Bailey RE, et al. Antihistamines and/or decongestants for otitis media with effusion (OME) in children. Cochrane Database Syst Rev 2006;(4):CD003423.
19. Perera R, Haynes J, Glasziou P, et al. Autoinflation for hearing loss associated with otitis media with effusion. Cochrane Database Syst Rev 2006;(4):CD006285.
20. Thomas CL, Simpson S, Butler CC, et al. Oral or topical nasal steroids for hearing loss associated with otitis media with effusion in children. Cochrane Database Syst Rev 2006;(3):CD001935.
21. Flynn CA, Griffin GH, Schultz JK. Decongestants and antihistamines for acute otitis media in children. Cochrane Database Syst Rev 2004;(3):CD001727.
22. Rovers MM, Glasziou P, Appelman CL, et al. Antibiotics for acute otitis media: a meta-analysis with individual patient data. Lancet 2006;368(9545):1429–35.
23. Glasziou PP, Del Mar CB, Sanders SL, et al. Antibiotics for acute otitis media in children. Cochrane Database Syst Rev 2004;(1):CD000219.
24. O'Neill P, Roberts T, Bradley SC. Otitis media in children (acute). Clin Evid 2006;15:500–10.
25. Bertin L, Pons G, d'Athis P, et al. A randomized, double-blind, multicentre controlled trial of ibuprofen versus acetaminophen and placebo for symptoms of acute otitis media in children. Fundam Clin Pharmacol 1996;10(4):387–92.

26. Leach AJ, Morris PS. Antibiotics for the prevention of acute and chronic suppurative otitis media in children. Cochrane Database Syst Rev 2006;(4):CD004401.
27. Rosenfeld RM, Bluestone CD. Evidence-based otitis media. Hamilton: B.C. Decker Inc; 2003.
28. Mattila PS, Joki-Erkkila VP, Kilpi T, et al. Prevention of otitis media by adenoidectomy in children younger than 2 years. Arch Otolaryngol Head Neck Surg 2003; 129(2):163–8.
29. Hammaren-Malmi S, Saxen H, Tarkkanen J, et al. Adenoidectomy does not significantly reduce the incidence of otitis media in conjunction with the insertion of tympanostomy tubes in children who are younger than 4 years: a randomized trial. Pediatrics 2005;116(1):185–9.
30. McDonald S, Langton Hewer CD, Nunez DA. Grommets (ventilation tubes) for recurrent acute otitis media in children. Cochrane Database Syst Rev 2008;(4):CD004741.
31. Acuin J. Chronic suppurative otitis media. Clin Evid 2006;15:772–87.
32. Macfadyen CA, Acuin JM, Gamble C. Topical antibiotics without steroids for chronically discharging ears with underlying eardrum perforations. Cochrane Database Syst Rev 2005;(4):CD004618.
33. Macfadyen CA, Acuin JM, Gamble C. Systemic antibiotics versus topical treatments for chronically discharging ears with underlying eardrum perforations. Cochrane Database Syst Rev 2006;(1):CD005608.
34. Acuin J, Smith A, Mackenzie I. Interventions for chronic suppurative otitis media. Cochrane Database Syst Rev 2000;(2):CD000473.
35. Report of a WHO/CIBA Foundation Workshop. Prevention of hearing impairment from chronic otitis media. Geneva: World Health Organisation; 1996.
36. Clinical evidence. Issue 1. London: BMJ Publishing Group; 2009.
37. The Cochrane Library. Oxford: Wiley interScience; 2009.
38. Morris PS. A systematic review of clinical research addressing the prevalence, aetiology, diagnosis, prognosis and therapy of otitis media in Australian Aboriginal children. J Paediatr Child Health 1998;34(6):487–97.
39. Maynard JE, Fleshman JK, Tschopp CF. Otitis media in Alaskan Eskimo children. Prospective evaluation of chemoprophylaxis. JAMA 1972;219(5):597–9.
40. Leach AJ, Morris PS, Mathews JD. Compared to placebo, long-term antibiotics resolve otitis media with effusion (OME) and prevent acute otitis media with perforation (AOMwiP) in a high-risk population: a randomized controlled trial. BMC Pediatr 2008;8(1):23.
41. Couzos S, Lea T, Mueller R, et al. Effectiveness of ototopical antibiotics for chronic suppurative otitis media in Aboriginal children: a community-based, multicentre, double-blind randomised controlled trial. Med J Aust 2003;179(4): 185–90.
42. Leach A, Wood Y, Gadil E, et al. Topical ciprofloxin versus topical framycetin-gramicidin-dexamethasone in Australian aboriginal children with recently treated chronic suppurative otitis media: a randomized controlled trial. Pediatr Infect Dis J 2008;27(8):692–8.
43. O'Brien KL, David AB, Chandran A, et al. Randomized, controlled trial efficacy of pneumococcal conjugate vaccine against otitis media among Navajo and White Mountain Apache infants. Pediatr Infect Dis J 2008;27(1):71–3.
44. Couzos S, Metcalf S, Murray R. Systematic review of existing evidence and primary care guidelines on the management of otitis media in Aboriginal and Torres Strait Islander populations. Canberra: Office of Aboriginal and Torres Strait Islander Health; 2001.

45. Morris P, Ballinger D, Leach A, et al. Recommendations for clinical care guidelines on the management of otitis media in Aboriginal and Torres Strait Islander populations. Canberra: Office of Aboriginal and Torres Strait Islander Health; 2001.
46. Rovers MM, Schilder AG, Zielhuis GA, et al. Otitis media. Lancet 2004;363(9407): 465–73.
47. American Academy of Pediatrics Subcommittee on Management of Acute Otitis Media. Diagnosis and management of acute otitis media. Pediatrics 2004;113(5): 1451–65.
48. Uhari M, Mantysaari K, Niemela M. A meta-analytic review of the risk factors for acute otitis media [see comments]. Clin Infect Dis 1996;22(6):1079–83.
49. Ensign PR, Urbanich EM, Moran M. Prophylaxis for otitis media in an Indian population. Am J Public Health Nations Health 1960;50:195–9.
50. Brody A. Draining ears and deafness among Alaskan Eskimos. Arch Otorhinolaryngol 1965;81:29–33.
51. Wiet RJ. Patterns of ear disease in the southwestern American Indian. Arch Otolaryngol 1979;105(7):381–5.
52. Beery QC, Doyle WJ, Cantekin EI, et al. Eustachian tube function in an American Indian population. Ann Otol Rhinol Laryngol Suppl 1980;89(3 Pt 2):28–33.
53. Daly KA, Pirie PL, Rhodes KL, et al. Early otitis media among Minnesota American Indians: the little ears study. Am J Public Health 2007;97(2):317–22.
54. Baxter JD. An overview of twenty years of observation concerning etiology, prevalence, and evolution of otitis media and hearing loss among the Inuit in the eastern Canadian Arctic. Arctic Med Res 1991;(Suppl):616–9.
55. Homoe P, Prag J, Farholt S, et al. High rate of nasopharyngeal carriage of potential pathogens among children in Greenland: results of a clinical survey of middle-ear disease. Clin Infect Dis 1996;23(5):1081–90.
56. Homoe P, Christensen RB, Bretlau P. Prevalence of otitis media in a survey of 591 unselected Greenlandic children. Int J Pediatr Otorhinolaryngol 1996;36(3): 215–30.
57. Homoe P, Siim C, Bretlau P. Outcome of mobile ear surgery for chronic otitis media in remote areas. Otolaryngol Head Neck Surg 2008;139(1):55–61.
58. Leach AJ. Otitis media in Australian Aboriginal children: an overview. Int J Pediatr Otorhinolaryngol 1999;49(Suppl 1):S173–8.
59. Giles M, O'Brien P. The prevalence of hearing impairment amongst Maori schoolchildren. Clin Otolaryngol 1991;16(2):174–8.
60. Giles M, Asher I. Prevalence and natural history of otitis media with perforation in Maori school children. J Laryngol Otol 1991;105(4):257–60.
61. Bluestone CD. Epidemiology and pathogenesis of chronic suppurative otitis media: implications for prevention and treatment. Int J Pediatr Otorhinolaryngol 1998;42(3):207–23.
62. Cambon K, Galbraith JD, Kong G. Middle-ear disease in Indians of the Mount Currie Reservation, British Columbia. Can Med Assoc J 1965;93(25):1301–5.
63. Miller FJ. Childhood morbidity and mortality in Newcastle-Upon-Tyne. Further report on the thousand family study. N Engl J Med 1966;275(13):683–90.
64. Fleshman JK, Wilson JF, Cohen JJ. Bronchiectasis in Alaska Native children. Arch Environ Health 1968;17(4):517–23.
65. Baxter JD. Otitis media in Inuit children in the Eastern Canadian Arctic—an overview 1968 to date. Int J Pediatr Otorhinolaryngol 1999;49(Suppl 1):S165–8.
66. Singleton R, Morris A, Redding G, et al. Bronchiectasis in Alaska Native children: causes and clinical courses. Pediatr Pulmonol 2000;29(3):182–7.

67. Peck AJ, Holman RC, Curns AT, et al. Lower respiratory tract infections among American Indian and Alaska Native children and the general population of U.S. children. Pediatr Infect Dis J 2005;24(4):342–51.

68. Singleton RJ, Hennessy TW, Bulkow LR, et al. Invasive pneumococcal disease caused by nonvaccine serotypes among Alaska native children with high levels of 7-valent pneumococcal conjugate vaccine coverage. JAMA 2007;297(16):1784–92.

69. Torzillo PJ, Hanna JN, Morey F, et al. Invasive pneumococcal disease in central Australia [see comments]. Med J Aust 1995;162(4):182–6.

70. Chang AB, Grimwood K, Mulholland EK, et al. Bronchiectasis in indigenous children in remote Australian communities. Med J Aust 2002;177(4):200–4.

71. Leach AJ, Morris PS. The burden and outcome of respiratory tract infection in Australian and aboriginal children. Pediatr Infect Dis J 2007;26(10 suppl):S4–7.

72. Leach AJ, Boswell JB, Asche V, et al. Bacterial colonization of the nasopharynx predicts very early onset and persistence of otitis media in Australian aboriginal infants. Pediatr Infect Dis J 1994;13(11):983–9.

73. Smith-Vaughan HC, Leach AJ, Shelby JT, et al. Carriage of multiple ribotypes of nonencapsulated *Haemophilus influenzae* in aboriginal infants with otitis media. Epidemiol Infect 1996;116(2):177–83.

74. Smith-Vaughan H, Byun R, Nadkarni M, et al. Measuring nasal bacterial load and its association with otitis media. BMC Ear Nose Throat Disord 2006;6:10.

75. O'Brien KL, Nohynek H. Report from a WHO working group: standard method for detecting upper respiratory carriage of *Streptococcus pneumoniae*. Pediatr Infect Dis J 2003;22(2):e1–e11.

76. Takata GS, Chan LS, Morphew T, et al. Evidence assessment of the accuracy of methods of diagnosing middle ear effusion in children with otitis media with effusion. Pediatrics 2003;112(6 Pt 1):1379–87.

77. Rothman R, Owens T, Simel DL. Does this child have acute otitis media? JAMA 2003;290(12):1633–40.

78. Roberts JE, Rosenfeld RM, Zeisel SA. Otitis media and speech and language: a meta-analysis of prospective studies. Pediatrics 2004;113(3 Pt 1):e238–48.

79. Verhoeff M, van der Veen EL, Rovers MM, et al. Chronic suppurative otitis media: a review. Int J Pediatr Otorhinolaryngol 2006;70(1):1–12.

80. van der Veen EL, Schilder AG, van Heerbeek N, et al. Predictors of chronic suppurative otitis media in children. Arch Otolaryngol Head Neck Surg 2006; 132(10):1115–8.

81. Simpson SA, Thomas CL, van der Linden MK, et al. Identification of children in the first four years of life for early treatment for otitis media with effusion. Cochrane Database Syst Rev 2007;(1):CD004163.

82. Rosenfeld RM. Surgical prevention of otitis media. Vaccine 2000;19(Suppl 1): S134–9.

83. Singleton RJ, Holman RC, Plant R, et al. Trends in otitis media and myringtomy with tube placement among American Indian/Alaska native children and the US general population of children. Pediatr Infect Dis J 2009;28(2):102–7.

84. Fireman B, Black SB, Shinefield HR, et al. Impact of the pneumococcal conjugate vaccine on otitis media. Pediatr Infect Dis J 2003;22(1):10–6.

85. Kozyrskyj AL, Hildes-Ripstein GE, Longstaffe SE, et al. Short course antibiotics for acute otitis media. Cochrane Database Syst Rev 2000;(2):CD001095.

86. Spurling GK, Del Mar CB, Dooley L, et al. Delayed antibiotics for respiratory infections. Cochrane Database Syst Rev 2007;(3):CD004417.

87. Spiro DM, Tay KY, Arnold DH, et al. Wait-and-see prescription for the treatment of acute otitis media: a randomized controlled trial. JAMA 2006;296(10):1235–41.

88. Little P, Gould C, Williamson I, et al. Pragmatic randomised controlled trial of two prescribing strategies for childhood acute otitis media. BMJ 2001;322(7282): 336–42.
89. Mackenzie GA, Carapetis JR, Leach AJ, et al. Pneumococcal vaccination and otitis media in Australian Aboriginal infants: comparison of two birth cohorts before and after introduction of vaccination. BMC Pediatr 2009;9:14.
90. van der Veen EL, Rovers MM, Albers FW, et al. Effectiveness of trimethoprim/sulfamethoxazole for children with chronic active otitis media: a randomized, placebo-controlled trial. Pediatrics 2007;119(5):897–904.
91. Leiberman A, Fliss DM, Dagan R. Medical treatment of chronic suppurative otitis media without cholesteatoma in children—a two-year follow-up. Int J Pediatr Otorhinolaryngol 1992;24(1):25–33.
92. Dagan R, Fliss DM, Einhorn M, et al. Outpatient management of chronic suppurative otitis media without cholesteatoma in children. Pediatr Infect Dis J 1992; 11(7):542–6.
93. Mak D, MacKendrick A, Bulsara M, et al. Outcomes of myringoplasty in Australian Aboriginal children and factors associated with success: a prospective case series. Clin Otolaryngol Allied Sci 2004;29(6):606–11.
94. Guerin N, McConnell F. Myringoplasty: a post-operative survey of 90 aborigine patients. Rev Laryngol Otol Rhinol (Bord) 1988;109(2):123–7.

Acute Rheumatic Fever and Rheumatic Heart Disease in Indigenous Populations

Andrew C. Steer, MBBS, BMedSc, FRACP[a,b,*],
Jonathan R. Carapetis, MBBS, BMedSc, PhD, FRACP, FAFPHM[c]

KEYWORDS

- Acute rheumatic fever • Rheumatic heart disease
- *Streptococcus pyogenes*

Acute rheumatic fever (ARF) is an autoimmune disease characterized by inflammation of several tissues that gives rise to typical clinical characteristics including carditis/valvulitis, arthritis, chorea, erythema marginatum, and subcutaneous nodules. Long-term effects for all tissues are minimal, except for cardiac valves, in which fibrosis and scarring may lead to chronic rheumatic heart disease (RHD). Carditis occurs in 30% to 80% of all patients with ARF, being more common in younger patients (90%) than in adolescents and young adults. At least 60% of ARF patients develop RHD.[1–3]

ARF and RHD have been described as "classic diseases of social injustice."[4] More than 80% of the world's cases of ARF and RHD occur in people living in developing countries.[5] Rheumatic fever and RHD have all but disappeared in industrialized countries, and the cases that do occur seem to occur at disproportionately high rates among indigenous peoples in these countries. It is widely believed that the dramatic reduction in ARF and RHD witnessed in the industrialized world in the last century was the result of improvements in socioeconomic conditions, hygiene and access to medical care, and reductions in household crowding.[6] The corollary, therefore, is

[a] Department of Paediatrics, Centre for International Child Health, University of Melbourne, Flemington Road, Parkville, 3052, Melbourne, Victoria, Australia
[b] Division of Infectious and Immunologic Diseases, Department of Pediatrics, University of British Columbia, 4480 Oak Street, Vancouver, V6H 3V4, Canada
[c] Menzies School of Health Research, Charles Darwin University, Darwin, PO Box 41096, Casuarina, NT 0811, Australia
* Corresponding author. Division of Infectious and Immunologic Diseases, Department of Pediatrics, University of British Columbia, 4480 Oak Street, Vancouver, V6H 3V4, Canada.
E-mail address: andrew.steer@rch.org.au (A.C. Steer).

Pediatr Clin N Am 56 (2009) 1401–1419
doi:10.1016/j.pcl.2009.09.011   **pediatric.theclinics.com**

that these improvements have not been afforded to people in developing countries or indigenous people in wealthy countries.

This review summarizes the epidemiology and pathogenesis of ARF and RHD, and discusses current practice in the diagnosis and management of ARF and RHD, with an emphasis on issues that are relevant to indigenous populations living in affluent countries. There are many indigenous people living in low- and middle-income countries around the world, but there are few data relating to ARF and RHD in these groups, so they are not specifically addressed here.

EPIDEMIOLOGY OF ARF AND RHD IN INDIGENOUS POPULATIONS

A review of the global burden of ARF and RHD published in 2005 estimated that, worldwide, there is a minimum of 15·6 million prevalent cases of RHD, with 280,000 new cases and 230,000 deaths due to RHD each year.[5] An update of population-based RHD prevalence data for Asia in 2008 suggested that, as more data emerge from high-prevalence regions, the true figures will be substantially higher than this; using data published to 2007, the estimated number of RHD cases in school-aged children in Asia doubled from the original estimate, which was based on data published to 2002.[7] There is regional variation in the epidemiology, with the highest prevalences of RHD found in Africa (5.7 cases per 1000 school-aged children), the Pacific (3.5 cases per 1000), and Asia (3.0 per 1000).[3,7–11] ARF and RHD are particularly common in indigenous populations (**Table 1**). The best quality and greatest volume of data come from studies conducted among Aboriginal Australians in the Northern Territory of Australia and from Maori people in New Zealand; these data suggest that the highest incidence of ARF, and among the greatest prevalences of RHD, in the world are found in these populations.[12,13] However, for most indigenous populations, there are few or no data available regarding ARF and RHD disease burden.

The explanation for the stark disparity in rates of ARF and RHD among indigenous peoples is likely to be multifactorial and include environmental (particularly social) factors and host factors. Important environmental factors include access to medical care, in particular access to secondary prophylaxis (discussed further in the section on Prevention), persistent exposure to group A streptococcal (GAS) infection via skin infection (discussed in the section on Pathogenesis), and overcrowding.[14] Overcrowding has for decades been known to be an important factor in ARF epidemiology.[15] The classic studies during the 1950s in US Air Force base barracks found that rates of acquisition of streptococcal infections increased when beds were moved closer together, providing a biologic basis for a relationship between overcrowding and the incidence of ARF.[16] Data from developing countries also support overcrowding as a risk factor. In Kinshasa in the Democratic Republic of Congo, children living in households with more than 8 people were found to have 4 times the prevalence of RHD.[17] In the Northern Territory of Australia, overcrowding is a perennial problem, with a median number of people per household of 14 to 17 in 2 communities in 1 study, and is considered to be a contributing factor to high rates of ARF and RHD.[4,18]

PATHOGENESIS OF ARF AND RHD

ARF is an immune-mediated multisystem inflammatory disease that follows infection by GAS. The pathogenic mechanism of ARF and RHD has not been clearly elucidated, but it seems that an interaction between a GAS strain that is "rheumatogenic" and a host with inherited susceptibility leads to an abnormal immune response with the development of autoimmunity (**Fig. 1**).[19]

Table 1
Selected studies supporting the notion that ARF and RHD are more common in indigenous populations

Indigenous Population	Study Period	Comments
Alaskan Natives in Alaska[100]	1979–1988	Alaskan natives had an annual cardiac mortality rate due to RHD 2 times that of Alaskan whites (mortality rate 8.5 per 100,000 vs 4.2 per 100,000)
Native American Indians in the United States[101]	1989–1992	The prevalence of RHD based on echocardiographic screening in 45–74-year-old Native American Indians was 4.6 per 1000 (the overall prevalence of RHD in established market economy countries is estimated to be 0.3 per 1000)
First Nations peoples in Canada[102]	1970–1979	The incidence of ARF in native children in Manitoba was 3.5 times that of non–native children (rate 126 per 100,000 vs 29 per 100,000)
Indigenous Fijians in Fiji[3,103]	2005–2007	The incidence of ARF in indigenous Fijians was 2.2 times (95% CI 0.9–6.1) that of the nonindigenous population (rate 6.4 per 100,000 vs 2.5 per 100,000); the prevalence of RHD in indigenous children aged 5–15 years was 2 times (95% CI 0.8–5.1) that of nonindigenous children (prevalence 10.3 per 1000 vs 4.4 per 1000)
Indigenous Hawaiians in Hawaii[104]	1980–1984	The incidence of ARF in Hawaiian and part-Hawaiian people was nearly 8 times that of the white population (rate 18.0 per 100,000 vs 2.3 per 100,000)
New Zealand Maori in New Zealand[11]	1996–2005	The incidence of ARF in New Zealand Maori people was 10 times (95% CI 1.7–58.3) that of people of European descent (rate 8 per 100,000 vs 0.8 per 100,000)
Indigenous Australians in Australia[10]	1989–1993	The annual incidence of confirmed ARF in Aboriginal people aged 5–14 years in the Top End of the Northern Territory was 254 per 100,000, higher than anywhere else reported in the world

The large burden of ARF and RHD in indigenous populations has led researchers to consider several factors that may contribute to susceptibility to disease, including genetic susceptibility and the potential role of GAS impetigo in the pathogenesis of ARF.

The question of why only a small percentage (approximately 3%–5%) of people infected with rheumatogenic GAS develop ARF remains unanswered.[20] The answer most likely lies in a genetic susceptibility to disease, although the nature of this susceptibility is not clear.[21] There is epidemiologic evidence that the proportion of Aboriginal Australians living in the Northern Territory who are susceptible to developing ARF is similar to the proportion of North American military recruits who developed ARF following outbreaks of GAS pharyngitis in military camps in the 1950s[22]; this suggests that susceptibility may not vary dramatically between different populations.[20] Further evidence supporting this contention comes from a study in Melbourne's predominantly white population between 1938 and 1948, which found an annual ARF incidence of 242 per 100,000 in lower socioeconomic groups, similar to the incidence in Aboriginal people in northern and central Australia today.[23]

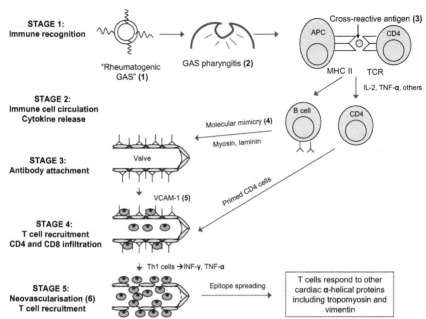

Fig. 1. Immunopathogenesis of ARF and RHD. (1) Classic rheumatogenic streptococci seem not to exist in some indigenous populations. (2) GAS impetigo may play a role as the initiating infection in indigenous populations in which impetigo is endemic. (3) The cross-reactive antigen on group A streptococci has not been identified: putative cross-reactive epitopes include the M-protein and N-acetyl glucosamine. (4) Molecular mimicry between GAS antigens and human host tissue is believed to be the basis of pathogen-host cross-reactivity, best documented with α-helical cardiac proteins such as myosin, laminin, and vimentin. (5) Vascular cell adhesion molecule 1 (VCAM-1) is upregulated at the valve and aids in recruitment and infiltration of T cells. (6) Inflammation leads to neovascularization, which allows further recruitment of T cells, leading to granulomatous inflammation and the establishment of chronic RHD. (*Adapted from* Guilherme L, Kalil J, Cunningham MW. Molecular mimicry in the autoimmune pathogenesis of rheumatic heart disease. Autoimmunity 2006;39:35; with permission.)

Multiple studies seeking the nature of genetic susceptibility to ARF and RHD have been undertaken, including studies of human leukocyte antigens, B-cell alloantigens, and immune gene polymorphisms (particularly tumor necrosis factor-α). As yet, there have been no convincing data. One promising marker, a B-cell alloantigen known as D8/17, has been studied in the Aboriginal Australian population.[24] This study found that 95% of patients with a past history of ARF tested positive for D8/17 antigen, compared with 50% of first-degree relatives and 4% of controls. Although this marker has been shown to be highly associated with ARF/RHD in several populations, including Israel and the United States,[25,26] the marker is not universal, with considerably lower correlation in studies conducted in India.[27,28] The role of D8/17 antigen in the pathogenesis of ARF remains uncertain.

Traditional teaching states that ARF follows GAS pharyngitis but not GAS impetigo.[29] However, there is some epidemiologic evidence, predominantly from Australia, to suggest that skin strains of GAS may play a role in the pathogenesis of ARF. In Aboriginal populations in Australia in which there is a high incidence of ARF, there is also a low incidence of GAS pharyngitis (one study found no episodes of symptomatic GAS pharyngitis in more than 1000 people followed prospectively for 23 months),[18] low rates of GAS carriage in the upper respiratory tract, and a high incidence of pyoderma (in the same study 40% of children experienced at least 1 episode of impetigo during the study).[18,30] In addition, in the Northern Territory and some other high-incidence ARF populations, including Maori people in New Zealand, there is an absence of the classic rheumatogenic M-serotypes of GAS (ie, serotypes associated with GAS pharyngitis), suggesting that other serotypes, possibly associated with GAS impetigo, may play a role.[31–34] The role of impetigo in the pathogenesis of ARF is the subject of speculation, but may involve direct causation of ARF after skin infection, an immune priming mechanism, or movement of strains from skin to throat where they cause ARF.[35] Confirmation of this impetigo-ARF hypothesis would necessitate reconsideration of primary prevention strategies, because primary prevention currently focuses only on treatment of GAS pharyngitis, not impetigo. In tropical settings, impetigo is often due to secondary infection of scabies infestation,[36,37] and so a further implication would potentially be the need to control endemic scabies infection to effect control of ARF.

DIAGNOSIS OF ARF AND RHD

Faced with a patient with the potential diagnosis of ARF, the clinician must take a careful history, conduct a thorough clinical examination, and order several key investigations. Because of the high rates of ARF in indigenous populations, a high index of suspicion is necessary in these populations, particularly in children who present with fever and polyarthritis. There is no single diagnostic investigation for ARF, and the diagnosis is based on clinical criteria known as the Jones Criteria. The criteria are divided into major and minor manifestations, depending on the diagnostic importance of a particular finding, and in most cases the diagnosis requires evidence of a preceding GAS infection (**Table 2**).[38] The Jones Criteria were first published in 1944 and were intended as a guide to the diagnosis of ARF.[39] With subsequent reduction in incidence of ARF in industrialized nations, the Jones Criteria have been revised several times to increase specificity and reduce sensitivity of the criteria.[38,40–42] Epidemiologists and clinicians in developing countries, and those working among indigenous populations in industrialized countries, have noted that strict application of the updated Jones Criteria may result in underdiagnosis of ARF in high-incidence populations.[43] As a result, several investigators have suggested

Table 2
1992 Updated Jones Criteria for the diagnosis of a first episode of ARF (diagnosis requires evidence of preceding GAS infection plus either (1) 2 major manifestations, or (2) 1 major manifestation and 2 minor manifestations)[38]

Major Manifestations	Minor Manifestations	Supporting Evidence of Streptococcal Infection
1. Carditis[a] 2. Polyarthritis 3. Chorea[a] 4. Erythema marginatum 5. Subcutaneous nodules	CLINICAL: 1. Arthralgia 2. Fever $\geq 39°C$ LABORATORY: 1. Elevated acute phase reactants: erythrocyte sedimentation rate, C-reactive protein 2. Prolonged P-R interval on electrocardiogram	1. Elevated or rising streptococcal antibody titer 2. Positive GAS throat culture or rapid streptococcal antigen test

[a] Chorea and insidious onset carditis do not require evidence of preceding streptococcal infection.

that the Jones Criteria be modified for these populations to increase the sensitivity of the criteria.[44–46] The major features that are the subject of debate are joint manifestations, the diagnosis of carditis, and the definition of recurrent ARF.

Joint Manifestations

In indigenous populations (and probably in many developing countries), ARF may present in an apparently subtle manner, without the typical finding of polyarthritis.[3,46,47] In a study of the clinical features of ARF in the Northern Territory of Australia, monoarthritis was a common presentation of ARF, occurring in 17% of confirmed cases and 35% of suspected but unconfirmed cases.[46] The investigators concluded that, in populations with high rates of ARF, in which the consequences of missed diagnosis may outweigh those of overdiagnosis, the inclusion of monoarthritis as a major manifestation is acceptable. Monoarthritis has been found to be a presenting feature of ARF in other settings.[47,48] A study in New Zealand suggested that these cases may be the result of early administration of antiinflammatory medication, truncating the evolution of typical rheumatic polyarthritis.[49] The investigators of the Australian study came to a similar conclusion about fever, allowing a temperature of 37.5°C or higher as acceptable evidence of fever (minor manifestation).[46] Another situation in which a high index of suspicion for the potential diagnosis of ARF is required is when a patient from an ARF high-risk population presents with a clinical picture consistent with septic arthritis, but in whom the joint fluid proves to be sterile; these patients should be considered to have ARF until proven otherwise, and appropriate investigations should be undertaken to rule out ARF.[47,48]

Carditis

Echocardiography is useful in the diagnosis and the management of ARF, as it can confirm auscultatory findings and permit the assessment of the severity of carditis. Echocardiography can also detect subclinical cases of carditis (ie, those without evidence of a clinically significant heart murmur); that is, echocardiography has greater sensitivity than auscultation for the assessment of carditis.[50,51] Expert opinion is divided as to whether the finding of subclinical carditis on echocardiography is sufficient evidence of true carditis and can be considered as a major manifestation.[52–54] Echocardiography is increasingly being used in many developing countries and in indigenous populations where clinicians are becoming expert in interpreting echocardiographic evidence of carditis.[55,56] In Australia and New Zealand, echocardiography is recommended for all patients with suspected ARF, and subclinical carditis is considered a major manifestation.[12,13] In contrast, in India, echocardiography is not considered a mandatory investigation, and subclinical carditis is not considered a major criterion.[57] The role of echocardiography in the evaluation of acute rheumatic carditis is currently being investigated through several studies conducted in settings in which acute ARF is common (including in indigenous populations).

Diagnosis of Recurrent Episodes of ARF

The Jones Criteria are applicable only to initial attacks of ARF. A World Health Organization (WHO) expert committee has proposed guidelines for how the Jones Criteria can be modified for recurrences, such that an ARF recurrence can be diagnosed on the basis of minor manifestations only (together with evidence of recent GAS infection) in a patient with preexisting RHD, because patients with RHD have a high risk of carditis in recurrent attacks of ARF.[58]

Modifications of the Jones Criteria

As a result of the considerations discussed earlier, 3 recent guidelines have been published suggesting how the 1992 Updated Jones Criteria may be modified for use in particular circumstances or populations (**Table 3**). The new guidelines are a new development internationally; until now, the Jones Criteria have been the accepted gold standard for diagnosis in all populations. These new guidelines highlight the need for clinicians working in populations with high rates of ARF and RHD, including some indigenous populations, to adapt the Jones Criteria to their local circumstances, or to interpret them in light of local experience and needs.

Table 3
Recent modifications to guidelines for the diagnosis of ARF

	2002–3 WHO Criteria[58]	2005 Australian Guidelines[12]	2006 New Zealand Guidelines[13]
Diagnosis of recurrent ARF based on minor manifestations	Yes, but only in patient with preexisting RHD	Yes, in anyone with RHD or past history of ARF	Yes, but only in patient with preexisting RHD
Different guidelines for different subgroups	No	Yes, changes to clinical features are for high-risk groups only.[a] For other groups, as per Jones and WHO criteria	No
Carditis	As per Jones Criteria	Subclinical carditis accepted as major manifestation	Subclinical carditis accepted as major manifestation
Joint manifestations	As per Jones Criteria	Aseptic monoarthritis and polyarthralgia accepted as major manifestation (if other causes excluded)	Aseptic monarthritis if history of prior NSAID, use accepted as major manifestation
Fever	Not defined	Defined as temperature $\geq 38°C$	Defined as temp $\geq 38°C$
Acute phase reactants	Elevated ESR or WCC, but not CRP. Not further defined	ESR ≥ 30 mm/h or CRP ≥ 30 mg/L	ESR ≥ 50 mm/h or CRP ≥ 30 mg/L
Evidence of GAS infection	As per Jones Criteria with addition of recent scarlet fever. Not further defined	As per Jones Criteria, but normal ranges provided for serology titers	As per Jones Criteria, but normal ranges provided for serology titers

Abbreviations: CRP, C-reactive protein; ESR, erythrocyte sedimentation rate; NSAID, nonsteroidal antiinflammatory medication; WCC, peripheral white blood cell count.
[a] High-risk groups defined as those living in communities with high rates of ARF (incidence>30 per 100,000 per year in 5–14-year-olds) or RHD (all-age prevalence>2 per 1,000).

Differential Diagnoses of ARF

The list of differential diagnoses for many of the clinical manifestations of ARF seen in isolation is long, particularly for polyarthritis. The exception to this is chorea, which is almost always due to ARF in high-incidence populations. Erythema marginatum and subcutaneous nodules are also specific for ARF, but both are rare. One differential diagnosis of polyarthritis worthy of mention is a syndrome known as poststreptococcal reactive arthritis (PSRA). The clinical characteristics of the arthritis in PSRA differ from those of ARF in several ways. There may be protracted joint involvement (up to 8 months) that is nonmigratory and symmetric, and that is poorly responsive to nonsteroidal antiinflammatory drugs, including aspirin. Although the diagnosis of PSRA may be entertained in populations in which ARF is rare, the diagnosis should generally not be considered in high-incidence settings, in which ARF is more likely to be the diagnosis.[12] The current recommendation for the management of PSRA from the American Heart Association is to commence penicillin prophylaxis for a period of 1 year, with a view to ceasing prophylaxis if an echocardiogram at 1 year shows no evidence of cardiac involvement. The authors recommend against this practice in indigenous populations in which ARF is common, and suggest that these patients require a longer period of prophylaxis and be managed in the same way as outlined for patients with ARF but no carditis (see section on Management). This is consistent with the Australian and New Zealand guidelines.[12,13]

MANAGEMENT OF ARF

Although treatment can shorten the acute inflammation of ARF, all of the various manifestations of ARF will resolve spontaneously, except for carditis, which may leave long-lasting valve damage or persist with ongoing inflammation to valvular tissue. No treatments during the acute phase of ARF have been clearly shown to affect the outcome of carditis. However, good compliance with secondary prophylaxis can positively alter the progression of RHD. The initial aim of management should be to confirm the diagnosis of ARF and to assess the severity of the attack. Severe carditis requires urgent treatment. Antiinflammatory medication can shorten the acute inflammatory phase of ARF and improve symptoms, particularly those of arthritis. A key facet of the management of ARF is patient and family education, with a particular emphasis on the importance of good adherence to secondary prophylaxis. **Table 4** summarizes treatment modalities for ARF and RHD and the evidence for their use.

Confirmation of the Diagnosis of ARF

Most patients with suspected ARF should be admitted to hospital. Hospitalization allows assessment of the severity of the attack, particularly the severity of carditis, and assessment of response to therapy. Hospitalization also allows time for health education and preparation for secondary prophylaxis. Admission to hospital is also helpful in patients who present with monoarthritis or arthralgia; in these patients, septic arthritis and other possible causes can be excluded, and salicylate therapy may be withheld initially (with pain relief provided using codeine or acetaminophen/paracetamol) and the patient observed for the development of polyarthritis, so that the diagnosis of ARF can be made with more certainty.[12]

Treatment of Arthritis

Antiinflammatory treatment is the mainstay of the treatment of the arthritis of ARF. Salicylate therapy is effective in the treatment of ARF arthritis (although simple analgesics are appropriate if there is only mild arthritis or arthralgia). If there is little

Table 4
Evidence for the various therapies used in the treatment of ARF and RHD

	Medication or Intervention	Recommendation	Grading	Quality of Supporting Evidence
Prevention	Primary prevention: oral phenoxymethyl penicillin (penicillin V) for 10 d, or intramuscular benzathine penicillin G as a single dose	Recommended for the treatment of streptococcal pharyngitis in indigenous populations (alternate regimens exist for penicillin-allergic patients)	Strong	High[77,78,105]
	Secondary prevention: intramuscular benzathine penicillin G administered 3- to 4-weekly	Recommended for the prevention of recurrent rheumatic fever in indigenous populations (alternate regimens exist for penicillin-allergic patients)	Strong	High[85,106]
Arthritis	Aspirin	Recommended as first-line treatment of the symptomatic treatment of arthritis	Strong	High[67]
	Naproxen	Recommended as second-line symptomatic treatment of arthritis for patients who are intolerant of aspirin	Weak	Low[59]
Carditis	Aspirin	Not recommended for the treatment of arthritis because there is no effect on long-term cardiac outcome	Strong	High[67]
	Glucocorticoids	Recommended for the treatment of severe carditis	Weak	Moderate[67]
	Intravenous immunoglobulin	Not recommended for the treatment of carditis	Strong	Moderate[67]
Chorea	Anticonvulsants (sodium valproate or carbamazepine)	Recommended for treatment of severe chorea only	Weak	Low[73]
	Intravenous immunoglobulin	Not recommended	Weak	Moderate[74]

or no response to salicylate treatment in the first few days of therapy, then the diagnosis of ARF should be questioned. Naproxen can be used in patients who are intolerant of aspirin.[59] Aspirin should be commenced at reasonably high doses (80–100mg/kg/d divided 4 times per day, maximum dose 4–8 g/d).[12] Some patients only require treatment for 2 weeks, after which time aspirin can be weaned or stopped, although "rebound" of symptoms should be monitored for in the 2 weeks following cessation of treatment.[60,61] For more severe episodes, a total course of 6 weeks is often required. For a 6-week course, the dose of aspirin can be reduced in a stepwise fashion after the first 2 weeks of high-dose therapy (eg, the dose can be reduced to two-thirds for the middle 2 weeks and then one-half for the last 2 weeks). If a rebound episode occurs this should not be considered as a recurrent episode, and another short course of aspirin is appropriate.

Management of Carditis

If available, all patients with suspected or confirmed ARF should undergo echocardiography to confirm the clinical diagnosis, to detect clinically silent lesions, and to assess severity of carditis.[12,13] Echocardiography may detect a lesion that requires urgent surgery, such as chordae tendinae rupture, although this is rare.

There is no evidence that antiinflammatory agents affect the outcome of carditis, and it seems that severity of residual RHD is directly related to the severity of carditis in the initial attack of ARF and the number of recurrent episodes.[62,63] Although salicylate therapy is effective in limiting the symptoms of the arthritis of ARF, salicylates should not be used specifically to treat carditis as there is no evidence that salicylates alter the rate of progression to chronic RHD.[64–67] The role of corticosteroids has been investigated in the treatment of patients with carditis.[67–69] There is little or no benefit from the use of corticosteroids in the treatment of mild to moderate carditis, and so corticosteroids are not indicated in this scenario.[67,69] However, some experts recommend the use of corticosteroids in the treatment of severe carditis (ie, carditis with associated cardiac failure) because of their more potent antiinflammatory effect and, therefore, potentially more rapid resolution of cardiac failure. It is recognized that this recommendation is not based on evidence that corticosteroids reduce the risk of developing valvular lesions in severe carditis, but it should also be noted that the existing evidence for or against such an effect is not based on studies in the post-echocardiography era or using modern corticosteroids.[67] The potential side effects of corticosteroids need to be considered, including the risk of gastrointestinal bleeding (gastric acid suppression should be instituted), the risk of fluid overload (concomitant administration of diuretics is often needed), and the risk of strongyloidiasis in endemic areas (concomitant administration of agents such as ivermectin may be necessary).[70] During corticosteroid treatment, aspirin can be discontinued, because corticosteroids will control joint pain and fever. There is a risk of rebound after steroids are discontinued, and so aspirin usually needs to be recommenced for a further 2 weeks to avoid rebound.[60,61]

Management of Chorea

Chorea is a self-limited phenomenon.[71,72] Treatment with antiinflammatory therapy does not alter the clinical course of chorea, and symptomatic treatment should only be instituted if the movement disorder becomes severe and distressing. Maintenance of a calm environment may be helpful to avoid overstimulation, which can worsen chorea. A small prospective comparison of carbamazepine, valproic acid, and haloperidol in the treatment of chorea suggested that valproic acid was the most effective agent for suppressing choreiform movements[73]; however, valproic acid may cause liver toxicity. Therefore, if treatment is considered necessary, carbamazepine may be considered as first line, with valproic acid considered as second line for refractory cases. Intravenous immunoglobulin cannot be recommended on the basis of available evidence; a small study of intravenous immunoglobulin suggested more rapid recovery from chorea, but did not affect cardiac outcome.[74] Chorea is strongly associated with carditis, and therefore all patients with chorea should undergo an echocardiogram.[12,75] The opinion of some clinicians working in high-incidence settings is that the behavioral disturbances often associated with Sydenham chorea may be long-lived, persisting long after the movement disorder has subsided. This has yet to be confirmed.

Antibiotic Treatment

Although most patients with ARF no longer have active GAS infection by the time of presentation, most experts recommend antibiotic therapy to eradicate any residual GAS infection in the pharynx, even if throat cultures are negative.[12,13,76] The sensible approach is to use a single intramuscular injection of benzathine penicillin G, as treatment of pharyngitis and as the first dose in the secondary prophylaxis regimen (see section on Secondary Prophylaxis).

MANAGEMENT OF RHD

Medical and surgical management of RHD is complex, and highly dependent on the availability of anti–heart failure medication, anticoagulant medication and monitoring tests, cardiothoracic surgery and cardiological intervention facilities (and highly trained surgeons and cardiologists), comprehensive primary health care systems, and local RHD registers and control programs. Recent evidence-based reviews provide more guidance.[12,13]

PREVENTION OF ARF AND RHD

There are 2 well-recognized methods of control of ARF and RHD: primary and secondary prophylaxis. Primary prophylaxis refers to the timely and appropriate treatment of GAS pharyngitis, which has clearly been shown to be effective in preventing ARF.[77–79] Secondary prophylaxis involves regular administration of antibiotics (usually 3- or 4-weekly benzathine penicillin G) for a sustained period of time, to prevent recurrent ARF. This strategy has been demonstrated to lead to regression of existing heart valve lesions and reduce RHD mortality.[80,81]

Primary Prevention

Primary prophylaxis has the important advantage, compared with secondary prophylaxis, of preventing cardiac damage that would otherwise occur. For the individual patient, primary prophylaxis is effective.[77–79] However, at a public health level, primary prevention programs are expensive,[82] and there are major logistical barriers that these programs need to overcome to be successful. An effective primary prophylaxis strategy relies on 3 assumptions: (1) that patients with sore throat will attend for care, (2) that clinics at which these patients attend have the ability to accurately diagnose GAS pharyngitis, and (3) that, once diagnosed, patients will be treated adequately and will adhere to the treatment regimen. All of these requirements may be difficult to achieve in indigenous populations, particularly those living in developing countries. Nonetheless, there are reasons to continue to promote investigation and treatment of sore throat in settings in which this is feasible.

Secondary Prevention

The current focus of global efforts to combat RHD is on strengthening secondary prophylaxis programs, because these programs are feasible and cost-effective.[83,84] However, there is considerable variation in practice regarding the route, dosage, frequency, and duration of penicillin as secondary prophylaxis.[12,57,58,76] Injections of benzathine penicillin G every 2 to 4 weeks are superior to daily oral penicillin.[85] Three-weekly, rather than 4-weekly, benzathine penicillin G reduced the number of recurrences of ARF in studies in Taiwan.[86,87] However, in many populations, adherence to such frequent dosing is poor. Data from New Zealand demonstrate low recurrence rates in a high-incidence population with good adherence to 4-weekly dosing, so the United States, New Zealand, and Australian guidelines recommend 4-weekly injectable benzathine penicillin G as initial standard of care, with the use of 3-weekly injections reserved for patients who have a recurrent episode of ARF despite good compliance with the 4-weekly regimen.[12,13,76]

The duration of prophylaxis depends on the severity of the lesion and the age of the patient. The minimal period of prophylaxis recommended by most guidelines for patients with a history of ARF, but without carditis, is at least 5 years, but recent guidelines suggest a minimum of 10 years, or until age 21 years, whichever is longer, with even longer duration for more severe valvular disease.[12,57,58,76] **Table 5** presents the duration of secondary prophylaxis as recommended by 4 current guidelines: Australia, New Zealand, United States, and the WHO.

From a public health perspective, it is clear that successful delivery of secondary prophylaxis to multiple patients requires effective coordination. Centralized register-based secondary prevention programs have been shown to encourage effective coordination of secondary prophylaxis.[88] Other key components of successful secondary prevention programs include strategies to increase adherence to secondary prophylaxis, programs to enable early recognition of ARF and RHD (including RHD screening programs), and health education and health promotion programs for health care workers, patients, and their families.[89]

Table 5
Duration of secondary prophylaxis for rheumatic fever and RHD according to different guidelines

Guideline	Duration
Australia[12]	No carditis: 10 y or 21 y of age (whichever is longer) Resolved ARF carditis: 10 y or 21 y of age (whichever is longer) Moderate RHD: 35 y of age Severe RHD: 40 y of age (or longer)
New Zealand[13]	No carditis: 10 y or 21 y of age (whichever is longer) Moderate carditis: 10 y or 30 y of age (whichever is longer) Severe carditis: 10 y or 30 y of age (whichever is longer), then specialist review to consider further or even lifelong
United States[76]	No carditis: 5 y or 21 y of age (whichever is longer) ARF with initial carditis but no residual RHD: 10 y or 21 y of age (whichever is longer) ARF with carditis and persistent valvular disease: 10 y or 40 y of age (whichever is longer), sometimes lifelong
WHO[58]	No carditis: 5 y or 18 y of age (whichever is longer) ARF with carditis, healed or mild mitral regurgitation: 10 y or 25 y of age (whichever is longer) More severe RHD or valve surgery: lifelong

Screening for RHD

The WHO recommends school-based screening for RHD to identify previously undiagnosed patients in high-prevalence regions and populations.[58] The rationale for screening is that early recognition of mild disease that is most amendable to secondary prophylaxis is a cost-effective strategy. There is some debate about the best method for screening. Recent advances in technology have allowed the development of small, easily portable, high-quality echocardiogram machines, which has meant that screening with echocardiography is increasingly being performed in the field. Studies in 3 countries (Mozambique, Cambodia, and Tonga) have shown that echocardiography, as a primary screening tool for RHD, is extremely sensitive.[55,56] Indeed, the prevalence of RHD detected by echocardiographic screening in the study in Mozambique was 13 times greater than that detected by auscultatory screening (prevalence by echocardiography 30.4 cases per 1000 children screened). There is a clear need to determine and standardize the best method for screening for RHD, and to establish accepted and validated criteria for diagnosis of RHD on echocardiogram (to avoid the potential for overdiagnosis); studies are currently underway to determine the sensitivity and specificity of echocardiography as a screening tool.[83,90]

PROSPECTS FOR A RHEUMATIC FEVER VACCINE

A GAS vaccine would prevent ARF and RHD by preventing the antecedent GAS infection. However, an effective GAS vaccine that is widely available remains several years away.[91,92] A multivalent M type specific vaccine has completed phase 2 trials in adults, with evidence of safety and immunogenicity.[93] However, the formulation of this vaccine may mean that it has limited effectiveness in some indigenous populations because of differing profiles of M types in these populations.[32,94,95] A vaccine that uses an antigen that is highly conserved among all GAS may be a more promising strategy for some indigenous populations, although none of these vaccines has yet reached clinical trials.[96–99] For a vaccine to be developed specifically against ARF and RHD it will be crucial that vaccine trials be performed in populations in which ARF and RHD are common, including indigenous populations.[91,92]

SUMMARY AND CONCLUSIONS

ARF and RHD are diseases of socioeconomic disadvantage, and are common in indigenous populations. The reasons for high rates in indigenous populations are not clear, but may include a potential role of GAS impetigo in the pathogenesis of ARF, and the possibility of a genetic susceptibility. The diagnosis of ARF is based on several clinical criteria, and clinicians must have a high index of suspicion for the potential diagnosis of ARF. The treatment of ARF has changed little in the last 50 years, with simple antiinflammatory drugs such as aspirin remaining the mainstay of symptomatic treatment of ARF. None of the therapies used in the acute treatment of ARF have an effect on long-term cardiac outcome, and there is a need for further research in this area. An effective and widely available GAS vaccine remains at least several years away. Secondary prevention is currently the most effective measure in controlling ARF and RHD. There is no clearly proven, cost-effective approach to primary prevention on a population-wide basis, and, although an important strategy, it should only be a major public health focus once secondary prophylaxis and a register-based control program has been established.

REFERENCES

1. Sanyal SK, Berry AM, Duggal S, et al. Sequelae of the initial attack of acute rheumatic fever in children from north India. A prospective 5-year follow-up study. Circulation 1982;65:375–9.
2. Sanyal SK, Thapar MK, Ahmed SH, et al. The initial attack of acute rheumatic fever during childhood in north India; a prospective study of the clinical profile. Circulation 1974;49:7–12.
3. Steer AC, Kado J, Jenney AW, et al. Acute rheumatic fever and rheumatic heart disease in Fiji: prospective surveillance, 2005–2007. Med J Aust 2009;190:133–5.
4. Brown A, McDonald MI, Calma T. Rheumatic fever and social justice. Med J Aust 2007;186:557–8.
5. Carapetis JR, Steer AC, Mulholland EK, et al. The global burden of group A streptococcal diseases. Lancet Infect Dis 2005;5:685–94.
6. Quinn RW. Comprehensive review of morbidity and mortality trends for rheumatic fever, streptococcal disease, and scarlet fever: the decline of rheumatic fever. Rev Infect Dis 1989;11:928–53.
7. Carapetis JR. Rheumatic heart disease in Asia. Circulation 2008;118:2748–53.
8. Neutze JM. Rheumatic fever and rheumatic heart disease in the western Pacific region. N Z Med J 1988;101:404–6.
9. Chun LT, Reddy DV, Yim GK, et al. Acute rheumatic fever in Hawaii: 1966 to 1988. Hawaii Med J 1992;51:206–11.
10. Carapetis JR, Wolff DR, Currie BJ. Acute rheumatic fever and rheumatic heart disease in the top end of Australia's Northern Territory. Med J Aust 1996;164:146–9.
11. Jaine R, Baker M, Venugopal K. Epidemiology of acute rheumatic fever in New Zealand 1996–2005. J Paediatr Child Health 2008;44:564–71.
12. National Heart Foundation of Australia (RF/RHD guideline development working group), the Cardiac Society of Australia and New Zealand. Diagnosis and management of acute rheumatic fever and rheumatic heart disease in Australia – an evidence-based review. Canberra: National Heart Foundation of Australia; 2006.
13. National Heart Foundation of New Zealand, Cardiac Society of Australia and New Zealand. Evidence-based, best practice New Zealand guidelines for rheumatic fever 1. Diagnosis, management and secondary prevention. Auckland: National Heart Foundation of New Zealand; 2006.
14. Steer AC, Carapetis JR, Nolan TM, et al. Systematic review of rheumatic heart disease prevalence in children in developing countries: the role of environmental factors. J Paediatr Child Health 2002;38:229–34.
15. Gordis L, Lilienfeld A, Rodriguez R. Studies in the epidemiology and preventability of rheumatic fever. II. Socio-economic factors and the incidence of acute attacks. J Chronic Dis 1969;21:655–66.
16. Wannamaker LW. The epidemiology of streptococcal infections. In: McCarty M, editor. Streptococcal infections. New York: Columbia University Press; 1954.
17. Longo-Mbenza B, Bayekula M, Ngiyulu R, et al. Survey of rheumatic heart disease in school children of Kinshasa town. Int J Cardiol 1998;63:287–94.
18. McDonald MI, Towers RJ, Andrews RM, et al. Low rates of streptococcal pharyngitis and high rates of pyoderma in Australian Aboriginal communities where acute rheumatic fever is hyperendemic. Clin Infect Dis 2006;43:683–9.
19. Carapetis JR, Currie BJ, Good MF. Towards understanding the pathogenesis of rheumatic fever. Scand J Rheumatol 1996;25:127–31.

20. Carapetis JR, Currie BJ, Mathews JD. Cumulative incidence of rheumatic fever in an endemic region: a guide to the susceptibility of the population? Epidemiol Infect 2000;124:239–44.
21. Bryant PA, Robbins-Browne R, Carapetis JR, et al. Some of the people, some of the time. Susceptibility to acute rheumatic fever. Circulation 2009;119:742–53.
22. Rammelkamp CH, Wannamaker LW, Denny FW. The epidemiology and prevention of rheumatic fever. 1952. Bull N Y Acad Med 1997;74:119–33.
23. Holmes MC, Rubbo SD. A study of rheumatic fever and streptococcal infection in different social groups in Melbourne. J Hyg (Lond) 1953;51:450–7.
24. Harrington Z, Visvanathan K, Skinner NA, et al. B-cell antigen D8/17 is a marker of rheumatic fever susceptibility in Aboriginal Australians and can be tested in remote settings. Med J Aust 2006;184:507–10.
25. Khanna AK, Buskirk DR, Williams RC Jr, et al. Presence of a non-HLA B cell antigen in rheumatic fever patients and their families as defined by a monoclonal antibody. J Clin Invest 1989;83:1710–6.
26. Harel L, Zeharia A, Kodman Y, et al. Presence of the d8/17 B-cell marker in children with rheumatic fever in Israel. Clin Genet 2002;61:293–8.
27. Kaur S, Kumar D, Grover A, et al. Ethnic differences in expression of susceptibility marker(s) in rheumatic fever/rheumatic heart disease patients. Int J Cardiol 1998;64:9–14.
28. Taneja V, Mehra NK, Reddy KS, et al. HLA-DR/DQ antigens and reactivity to B cell alloantigen D8/17 in Indian patients with rheumatic heart disease. Circulation 1989;80:335–40.
29. Bisno AL, Pearce IA, Wall HP, et al. Contrasting epidemiology of acute rheumatic fever and acute glomerulonephritis. N Engl J Med 1970;283:561–5.
30. Carapetis JR, Currie BJ. Group A streptococcus, pyoderma, and rheumatic fever. Lancet 1996;347:1271–2.
31. Martin DR. Rheumatogenic and nephritogenic group A streptococci. Myth or reality? An opening lecture. Adv Exp Med Biol 1997;418:21–7.
32. Bessen DE, Carapetis JR, Beall B, et al. Contrasting molecular epidemiology of group A streptococci causing tropical and nontropical infections of the skin and throat. J Infect Dis 2000;182:1109–16.
33. Steer AC, Magor G, Jenney AW, et al. emm and C-repeat region molecular typing of beta-hemolytic streptococci in a tropical country: implications for vaccine development. J Clin Microbiol 2009;47(8):2502–9.
34. Martin DR, Voss LM, Walker SJ, et al. Acute rheumatic fever in Auckland, New Zealand: spectrum of associated group A streptococci different from expected. Pediatr Infect Dis J 1994;13:264–9.
35. McDonald M, Currie BJ, Carapetis JR. Acute rheumatic fever: a chink in the chain that links the heart to the throat? Lancet Infect Dis 2004;4:240–5.
36. Steer AC, Tikoduadua LV, Manalac EM, et al. Validation of an Integrated Management of Childhood Illness algorithm for the management of common skin conditions in Fiji. Bull World Health Organ 2009;87:173–9.
37. Lawrence GW, Leafasia J, Sheridan J, et al. Control of scabies, skin sores and haematuria in children in the Solomon Islands: another role for ivermectin. Bull World Health Organ 2005;83:34–42.
38. Guidelines for the diagnosis of rheumatic fever. Jones Criteria, 1992 update. Special Writing Group of the Committee on Rheumatic Fever, Endocarditis, and Kawasaki Disease of the Council on Cardiovascular Disease in the Young of the American Heart Association. JAMA 1992;268:2069–73.
39. Jones TD. The diagnosis of rheumatic fever. JAMA 1944;126:481–4.

40. Rutstein DD, Bauer W, Dorfman A, et al. Jones Criteria (modified) for guidance in the diagnosis of rheumatic fever; report of the Committee on Standards and Criteria for programs of care. Circulation 1956;13:617–20.

41. Committee of Rheumatic Fever and Bacterial Endocarditis of the American Heart Association: Jones Criteria (revised) for guidance in the diagnosis of rheumatic fever. Circulation 1984;69:204A–8A.

42. Stollerman GH, Markowitz M, Taranta A, et al. Committee report: Jones Criteria (revised) for guidance in the diagnosis of rheumatic fever. Circulation 1965;32: 664–8.

43. Pereira BAF, da Silva NA, Andrade LEC, et al. Jones Criteria and underdiagnosis of rheumatic fever. Indian J Pediatr 2007;74:117–21.

44. Cherian G. Acute rheumatic fever–the Jones Criteria: a review and a case for polyarthralgia. J Assoc Physicians India 1979;27:453–7.

45. Padmavati S, Gupta V. Reappraisal of the Jones Criteria: the Indian experience. N Z Med J 1988;101:391–2.

46. Carapetis JR, Currie BJ. Rheumatic fever in a high incidence population: the importance of monoarthritis and low grade fever. Arch Dis Child 2001;85:223–7.

47. Mataika R, Carapetis JR, Kado J, et al. Acute rheumatic fever: an important differential diagnosis of septic arthritis. J Trop Pediatr 2008;54:205–7.

48. Harlan GA, Tani LY, Byington CL. Rheumatic fever presenting as monoarticular arthritis. Pediatr Infect Dis J 2006;25:743–6.

49. Wilson E, Wilson N, Voss L, et al. Monoarthritis in rheumatic fever? Pediatr Infect Dis J 2007;26:369–70.

50. Vasan RS, Shrivastava S, Vijayakumar M, et al. Echocardiographic evaluation of patients with acute rheumatic fever and rheumatic carditis. Circulation 1996;94: 73–82.

51. Tubridy-Clark M, Carapetis JR. Subclinical carditis in rheumatic fever: a systematic review. Int J Cardiol 2007;119:54–8.

52. Narula J, Kaplan EL. Echocardiographic diagnosis of rheumatic fever. Lancet 2000;2001:358.

53. Wilson NJ, Neutze JM. Echocardiographic diagnosis of subclinical carditis in acute rheumatic fever. Int J Cardiol 1995;50:1–6.

54. Veasy LG. Time to take soundings in acute rheumatic fever. Lancet 2001;357: 1994–5.

55. Marijon E, Ou P, Celermajer DS, et al. Prevalence of rheumatic heart disease detected by echocardiographic screening. N Engl J Med 2007;357:470–6.

56. Carapetis JR, Hardy M, Fakakovikaetau T, et al. High prevalence of rheumatic heart disease in Tongan school children, and evaluation of a screening protocol using portable echocardiography. Nat Clin Pract Cardiovasc Med 2008;5:411–7.

57. Working Group on Pediatric Acute Rheumatic Fever and Cardiology Chapter of Indian Academy of Pediatrics. Consensus guidelines on pediatric acute rheumatic fever and rheumatic heart disease. Indian Pediatr 2008;45:565–73.

58. Rheumatic fever and rheumatic heart disease: report of a WHO Expert Consultation Geneva. Geneva: World Health Organization; 2004.

59. Hashkes PJ, Tauber T, Somekh E, et al. Naproxen as an alternative to aspirin for the treatment of arthritis of rheumatic fever: a randomized trial. J Pediatr 2003; 143:399–401.

60. Feinstein AR, Spagnuolo M, Gill FA. The rebound phenomenon in acute rheumatic fever. I. Incidence and significance. Yale J Biol Med 1961;33:259–78.

61. Holt KS. The rebound phenomenon in acute rheumatic fever. Arch Dis Child 1956;31:444–51.

62. Carapetis JR, Kilburn CJ, MacDonald KT, et al. Ten-year follow up of a cohort with rheumatic heart disease (RHD). Aust N Z J Med 1997;27:691–7.

63. Rheumatic Fever Working Party. The natural history of rheumatic fever and rheumatic heart disease: ten-year report of a cooperative clinical trial of ACTH, cortisone, and aspirin. Circulation 1965;32:457–76.

64. Bywaters EGL, Thomas GT. Bed rest, salicylates and steroid in rheumatic fever. BMJ 1961;1:1628–34.

65. Dorfman A, Gross JI, Lorincz AE. The treatment of acute rheumatic fever. Pediatrics 1961;27:692–706.

66. Illingworth RS, Lorber J, Holt KS. Acute rheumatic fever in children: a comparison of six forms of treatment in 200 cases. Lancet 1957;273:653–9.

67. Cilliers AM, Manyemba J, Saloojee H. Anti-inflammatory treatment for carditis in acute rheumatic fever. Cochrane Database Syst Rev 2003;(2):CD003176.

68. Czoniczer G, Amezcua F, Pelargonio S, et al. Therapy of severe rheumatic carditis. Comparison of adrenocortical steroids and aspirin. Circulation 1964;29: 813–9.

69. Albert DA, Harel L, Karrison T. The treatment of rheumatic carditis: a review and meta-analysis. Medicine (Baltimore) 1995;74:1–12.

70. Thatai D, Turi ZG. Current guidelines for the treatment of patients with rheumatic fever. Drugs 1999;57:545–55.

71. Lessof MH, Bywaters EG. The duration of chorea. Br Med J 1956;1:1520–3.

72. Carapetis JR, Currie BJ. Rheumatic chorea in northern Australia: a clinical and epidemiological study. Arch Dis Child 1999;80:353–8.

73. Pena J, Mora E, Cardozo J, et al. Comparison of the efficacy of carbamazepine, haloperidol and valproic acid in the treatment of children with Sydenham's chorea: clinical follow-up of 18 patients. Arq Neuropsiquiatr 2002;60:374–7.

74. Voss LM, Wilson NJ, Neutze JM, et al. Intravenous immunoglobulin in acute rheumatic fever: a randomized controlled trial. Circulation 2001;103:401–6.

75. Veasy LG, Wiedmeier SE, Orsmond GS, et al. Resurgence of acute rheumatic fever in the intermountain area of the United States. N Engl J Med 1987;316: 421–7.

76. Gerber MA, Baltimore RS, Eaton CB, et al. Prevention of rheumatic fever and diagnosis and treatment of acute streptococcal pharyngitis: a scientific statement from the American Heart Association Rheumatic Fever, Endocarditis, and Kawasaki Disease Committee of the Council on Cardiovascular Disease in the Young, the Interdisciplinary Council on Functional Genomics and Translational Biology, and the Interdisciplinary Council on Quality of Care and Outcomes Research: endorsed by the American Academy of Pediatrics. Circulation 2009;119:1541–51.

77. Del Mar CB, Glasziou PP, Spinks AB. Antibiotics for sore throat. Cochrane Database Syst Rev 2000;(4):CD000023.

78. Denny F, Wannamaker L, Brink W, et al. Prevention of rheumatic fever; treatment of preceding streptococci infection. JAMA 1950;143:151–3.

79. Robertson KA, Volmink JA, Mayosi BM. Antibiotics for the primary prevention of acute rheumatic fever: a meta-analysis. BMC Cardiovasc Disord 2005;31:11.

80. Stollerman GH, Rusoff JH, Hirschfeld I. Prophylaxis against group A streptococci in rheumatic fever; the use of single monthly injections of benzathine penicillin G. N Engl J Med 1955;252:787–92.

81. Tompkins DG, Boxerbaum B, Liebman J. Long-term prognosis of rheumatic fever patients receiving regular intramuscular benzathine penicillin. Circulation 1972;45:543–51.

82. Michaud C, Rammohan R, Narula J. Cost-effectiveness analysis of intervention strategies for reduction of the burden of rheumatic heart disease. In: Narula J, Virmani R, Reddy KS, et al, editors. Rheumatic fever. Washington, DC: American Registry of Pathology; 1999. p. 485–97.

83. Carapetis JR. Rheumatic heart disease in developing countries. N Engl J Med 2007;357:439–41.

84. Strasser T. Cost-effective control of rheumatic fever in the community. Health Policy 1985;5:159–64.

85. Manyemba J, Mayosi BM. Penicillin for secondary prevention of rheumatic fever. Cochrane Database Syst Rev 2002;(3):CD002227.

86. Lue HC, Wu MH, Hsieh KH, et al. Rheumatic fever recurrences: controlled study of 3-week versus 4-week benzathine penicillin prevention programs. J Pediatr 1986;108:299–304.

87. Lue HC, Wu MH, Wang JK, et al. Long-term outcome of patients with rheumatic fever receiving benzathine penicillin G prophylaxis every three weeks versus every four weeks. J Pediatr 1994;125:812–6.

88. McDonald M, Brown A, Noonan S, et al. Preventing rheumatic fever: the role of register based programmes. Heart 2005;91:1131–3.

89. Bach JF, Chalons S, Forier E, et al. 10-year educational programme aimed at rheumatic fever in two French Caribbean islands. Lancet 1996;347:644–8.

90. Carapetis JR. Pediatric rheumatic heart disease in the developing world: echocardiographic versus clinical screening. Nat Clin Pract Cardiovasc Med 2008;5: 74–5.

91. Bisno AL, Rubin FA, Cleary PP, et al. Prospects for a group A streptococcal vaccine: rationale, feasibility, and obstacles–report of a National Institute of Allergy and Infectious Diseases workshop. Clin Infect Dis 2005;41:1150–6.

92. Group A streptococcal vaccine development: current status and issues of relevance to less developed countries. Geneva: World Health Organization, Department of Child and Adolescent Health and Development; 2005.

93. McNeil SA, Halperin SA, Langley JB, et al. A double-blinded, randomized, controlled phase II trial of the safety and immunogenicity of a 26 valent group A streptococcus vaccine in healthy adults. The XVIth Lancefield International Symposium on Streptococci and Streptococcal Diseases; 2005:25–29. September 2005; Palm Cove, Australia.

94. Steer AC, Jenney AWJ, Kado J, et al. Invasive group A streptococcal disease in Fiji: prospective surveillance 2005–2007. Emerg Infect Dis 2009;15:216–22.

95. Tewodros W, Kronvall G. M protein gene (emm-type) analysis of group A beta hemolytic streptococci from Ethiopia reveals unique patterns. J Clin Microbiol 2005;43:4369–76.

96. Sabharwal H, Michon F, Nelson D, et al. Group A streptococcus (GAS) carbohydrate as an immunogen for protection against GAS infection. J Infect Dis 2006; 193:129–35.

97. Shet A, Kaplan EL, Johnson DR, et al. Immune response to group A streptococcal C5a peptidase in children: implications for vaccine development. J Infect Dis 2003;188:809–17.

98. Batzloff MR, Hayman WA, Davies MR, et al. Protection against group A streptococcus by immunization with J8-diptheria toxoid: contribution of J8-and diptheria toxoid-specific antibodies to protection. J Infect Dis 2003;187:1598–608.

99. Batzloff M, Yan H, Davies M, et al. Preclinical evaluation of a vaccine based on conserved region of M protein that prevents group A streptococcal infection. Indian J Med Res 2004;119(Suppl):104–7.

100. Davidson M, Bulkow LR, Gellin BG. Cardiac mortality in Alaska's indigenous and non-Native residents. Int J Epidemiol 1993;22:62–71.
101. Schaffer WL, Galloway JM, Roman MJ, et al. Prevalence and correlates of rheumatic heart disease in American Indians (The Strong Heart Study). Am J Cardiol 2003;91:1379–82.
102. Longstaffe S, Postl B, Kao H, et al. Rheumatic fever in native children in Manitoba. Can Med Assoc J 1982;127.
103. Steer AC, Kado J, Wilson N, et al. High prevalence of rheumatic heart disease by clinical and echocardiographic screening among children in Fiji. J Heart Valve Dis 2009;18:327–35.
104. Chun LT, Reddy DV, Yamamoto LG. Rheumatic fever in children and adolescents in Hawaii. Pediatrics 1987;79:549–52.
105. Wannamaker LW, Rammelkamp CH Jr, Denny FW. Prophylaxis of acute rheumatic fever by treatment of the preceding streptococcal infection with various amounts of depot penicillin. Am J Med 1951;10:673–81.
106. Manyemba J, Mayosi BM. Intramuscular penicillin is more effective than oral penicillin in secondary prevention of rheumatic fever–a systematic review. S Afr Med J 2003;93:212–8.

Skin Disorders, Including Pyoderma, Scabies, and Tinea Infections

Ross M. Andrews, PhD, M App Epid, MPH, Dip App Sci (Env Hlth)[a],*,
James McCarthy, MD, FRACP[b,c],
Jonathan R. Carapetis, MBBS, B Med Sc, PhD, FRACP, FAFPHM[a],
Bart J. Currie, FRACP, FAFPHM, DTM+H[a]

KEYWORDS

- Pyoderma • Scabies • Skin diseases
- Streptococcal infections • Staphylococcal infections • Tinea

There are 111 million children believed to have pyoderma with many also co-infected with scabies, tinea, or both.[1] Whilst not differentiated by ethnicity or socio-economic status in high prevalence areas, poverty and overcrowded living conditions are important underlying social determinants.[2] Transmission is primarily through direct skin-to-skin contact. Rarely resulting directly in hospitalization or death, there is a high and largely unmet demand for effective management at the primary health-care level, particularly for pyoderma and scabies. Despite particularly high prevalence in some settings, treatment is not sought for many children, and when sought, the clinical benefit from such consultations is variable.[3] The lack of standard, evidence-based recommendations is of much concern. The current evidence base for clinical diagnosis and treatment of these common childhood skin disorders is highlighted.

COMMON CHILDHOOD SKIN DISORDERS

The 3 most common childhood skin disorders are pyoderma, scabies, and tinea. Pyoderma, also commonly called skin sores, is a generic term used to describe a clinical diagnosis of superficial bacterial skin infection, including impetigo, impetigo contagiosa, ecthyma, folliculitis, Bockhart impetigo, furuncle, carbuncle, tropical ulcer,

[a] Menzies School of Health Research, Charles Darwin University, PO Box 41096, Darwin, Northern Territory 0811, Australia
[b] Queensland Institute of Medical Research, Herston Road, Herston, Brisbane, Queensland 4029, Australia
[c] School of Medicine, University of Queensland, Herston Road, Herston, Brisbane, Queensland 4029, Australia
* Corresponding author.
E-mail address: ross.andrews@menzies.edu.au (R.M. Andrews).

Pediatr Clin N Am 56 (2009) 1421–1440
doi:10.1016/j.pcl.2009.09.002   **pediatric.theclinics.com**

and so forth.[3] There are several other diseases that have specific skin features or occasional or accessory skin features (eg, measles, chickenpox, dengue fever and other arboviral infections, leprosy, endemic treponematoses, and filariasis), but consistent with a recent WHO review,[3] they have not been included here.

The global prevalence of pyoderma has been estimated to exceed 111 million children.[1] Most of these children live in less developed countries, or in economically disadvantaged regions of otherwise wealthy countries, and many of them will also have scabies. Although reported prevalence can vary substantially, people of the Pacific region and Australia's Aboriginal and Torres Strait Islander peoples generally have the highest reported prevalence of pyoderma, often in the range of 40% to 90%, and the highest prevalence of scabies, often from 50% to 80%.[1] In African and Asian countries, the prevalence of pyoderma has been estimated to vary from 1% to 20%, whereas scabies prevalence has been in the range of 1% to 10%.[1] The prevalence of tinea amongst children is estimated to be 7% to 33% and, like pyoderma and scabies, is reported to be most prevalent in tropical developing countries.[3]

Although the skin disease burden is generally lower in other populations, it can still be fairly high within the indigenous populace, particularly those living in the most disadvantaged settings. High rates of pyoderma and scabies were reported amongst American Indian populations in the 1950s and 60s in settings where there had also been outbreaks of acute nephritis.[4] More recently, the hospitalization rate for skin or soft tissue infections amongst Alaska's native population was reported to be 0.5%, but almost 2-fold higher for those who lived in areas where less than 80% of homes had piped "in-home" water services and associated waste water disposal facilities compared with those areas where 80% of homes had such services.[5] The findings of Hennessy and colleagues[5] are consistent with an earlier review of data on primary health-care–seeking behavior within Ontario, Canada,[6] which found presentation rates for skin infections in the first year of life were 157 per 100 person-years for indigenous children in the more remote regions, almost 3 times that of indigenous children in urban regions or nonindigenous children. Similarly, the hospitalization rate for skin infections amongst indigenous Polynesian children in New Zealand has been reported to be 138 per 100,000, almost 4 times that of children from other ethnic groups.[7] In Fiji, where the rates of skin infection are generally much higher than developed country settings, skin infection rates (pyoderma and scabies) were 3 to 5 times higher amongst indigenous Fijians than amongst nonindigenous Fijians.[8]

Acquisition of pyoderma, frequently in association with scabies, has been found to commence very early in life.[6,9] In a recent study in 2 remote Australian Aboriginal communities, Clucas and colleagues[9] found that 69% of children had a clinical diagnosis recorded for pyoderma, and 63% for scabies, before their first birthday. The first presentation for clinical care of these conditions peaked as early as 2 months of age.[9] This high rate of health-care–seeking behavior for skin infections has been reported in a separate study amongst children younger than 7 years from 2 other remote Australian Aboriginal communities.[10] Widespread antibiotic use for treatment of pyoderma undoubtedly contributes to the selection pressure facilitating the spread of antibiotic resistance such as methicillin-resistant *Staphylococcus aureus* (MRSA) in these communities.[11,12]

The interrelationship between these skin disorders, the environmental health conditions, and the potential sequelae of infection/infestation have been described in Australian Aboriginal communities (**Fig. 1**)[13] and amongst Alaskan native populations.[5] A WHO review has highlighted how the relative contribution of proposed risk factors is likely to vary according to the particular skin condition (**Table 1**).[3] It is well recognized,

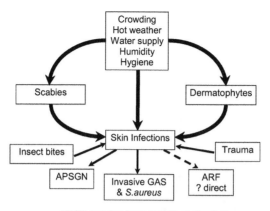

APSGN: Acute Post-Streptococcal Glomerulonephritis
GAS: Group A Streptococcal Disease
ARF: Acute Rheumatic Fever

Fig. 1. Factors affecting skin disease in Australian Aboriginal and Torres Strait Islander communities. (*From* Currie BJ, Carapetis JR. Skin infections and infestations in Aboriginal communities in northern Australia. Australas J Dermatol 2000;41:139.)

however, that action targeting poverty, education, housing, and environmental conditions are important to address the underlying social determinants of poor health.[14] For common childhood skin conditions, there is also an important role for appropriate management and treatment of cases to help minimize the risk of ongoing transmission through direct skin-to-skin contact. A particular issue is community members with scabies hyperinfestation (crusted scabies) who can be "core transmitters" of scabies within family groups or communities.[15]

PYODERMA

Pyoderma (**Fig. 2**) usually manifests as a thick crusted variety or a bullous type.[2] The skin lesions are contagious but usually heal completely without scarring.[16] Although

Table 1
Summary of the estimated strengths of the links between specific skin disorders and the main suspected risk factors

Disorder	Climate	Poor Hygiene	Low Water Use	Overcrowding	Comorbidity with Another Skin Disorder
Pyoderma	+++[a]	+++	++	++	++[b]
Scabies	+[c]	±[d]	−	+++	−
Tinea capitis	?[e]	±[d]	−	++	−

Strengths of links were mainly estimated according to the amount of evidence-based data.
  [a] If hot and humid.
  [b] Mainly scabies, insect bites, traumatic sores.
  [c] Cold season.
  [d] Risk factor for superinfection.
  [e] Superficial mycoses more frequent in a humid/hot climate, but lack of data specific to tinea capitis.
  (*From* World Health Organization: Epidemiology and Management of Common Skin Diseases in Children in Developing Countries. In: Geneva: World Health Organization WHO/FCH/CAH/05.12, 2005.)

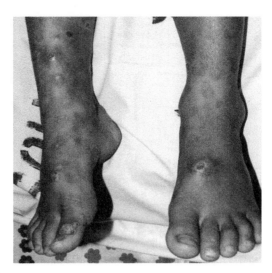

Fig. 2. Pyoderma.

pyoderma can be caused by group A *Streptococcus pyogenes* (GAS) and *S aureus*, boils, furuncles, and carbuncles are usually caused by *S aureus* infections.

In the United States, *S aureus* tends to be the predominant causative organism for pyoderma,[17] whereas GAS has predominated in Australian Indigenous populations until recently.[18,19] Community MRSA (cMRSA) is an emerging pathogen amongst Indigenous Australians in carriage studies[20] and pyoderma surveillance.[11,12] This change in antibiotic sensitivity has significant implications for pyoderma treatment and also highlights the need for ongoing surveillance.[11] It remains to be determined whether cMRSA is just displacing methicillin-sensitive *S aureus* or whether it is also displacing GAS in those tropical settings where GAS has been the predominant pyoderma pathogen.

Pyoderma may lead to serious complications, including sepsis, kidney disease, and heart disease (**Table 2**). The causative organisms, GAS and *S aureus*, can have differing mechanisms of colonization. GAS colonizes the skin by binding directly to epithelial sites exposed by skin trauma, whereas, especially in nontropical locations, *S aureus* has been thought to usually colonize the nasal epithelium first before colonizing the skin. Although GAS does not normally colonize intact skin, in populations where pyoderma is prevalent, GAS may occasionally be recovered from intact skin a few days, or rarely, for up to 1 to 2 weeks before skin lesions develop.[21] The same strain may also appear in the throat (without clinical evidence of pharyngitis) late in the course of the skin infection. GAS strains isolated from pyoderma lesions are often genetically distinct from those associated with pharyngitis, although in tropical settings, particularly in Australian Aboriginal communities, the distinction is much less clear.[12,22] Untreated purulent skin lesions can permit transmission of GAS for weeks. With adequate therapy, the duration of infectiousness is reduced to 48 hours. Similarly, untreated streptococcal pharyngitis can be contagious for 2 to 3 weeks.[23]

Microbiologic Diagnosis of the Pathogens Causing Pyoderma

The identity of a skin pathogen causing pyoderma may be confirmed through culture of a specimen collected from the moist areas below the crusty surface of the lesion. In many cases a microbiologic diagnosis is not necessary, although it may be indicated

Table 2
Possible complications of pyoderma

Sepsis	Pyoderma is the single most important risk factor for GAS and *S aureus* sepsis in Australian Aboriginal peoples.[64] GAS bacteremia in this population has been found to occur 5–8 times more commonly than among non-Aboriginal people living in the same region.[64,65] Sepsis from GAS and *S aureus* can affect any organ (eg, pneumonia, endocarditis, septic arthritis, osteomyelitis) or result in fatal septicemic shock. It is increasingly apparent that infection with some cMRSA strains is more likely to result in systemic sepsis than with others, but the responsible virulence determinants of these strains (and also of those GAS causing severe sepsis) remain to be definitively identified.[11]
APSGN and adult renal disease	Pyoderma caused by GAS is the major precipitant for APSGN,[66] an inflammatory disease of the kidneys. Moreover, pyoderma-related APSGN may lead to chronic renal damage: in one study, APSGN in childhood was associated with a 6-fold increase in the risk of adult renal disease.[67] It seems that only certain GAS strains have the potential to cause APSGN. These so-called nephritogenic strains have traditionally come from a limited range of M protein serotypes (or more recently, emm gene types), but the precise features that distinguish nephritogenic from other GAS strains have not been elucidated.[68]
ARF	The possibility has also been raised that pyoderma caused by GAS may trigger ARF, or in some other way be involved in its pathogenesis.[69–71] It has been suggested that this may occur directly after streptococcal pyoderma or as a consequence of GAS from skin subsequently colonizing the throat, or because recurrent skin infections may in some way "prime" the immune system for rheumatic fever.[70,72,73]

Abbreviations: APSGN, acute poststreptococcal glomerulonephritis; ARF, acute rheumatic fever.

in severe infection; infection not responding to standard therapy (see later discussion); or as part of epidemiologic surveillance.

Prevention of Pyoderma

In endemic areas, mass drug administration programs using topical acaricides (scabies treatments) have also been demonstrated to reduce the prevalence of pyoderma. In Panama, streptococcal pyoderma among children younger than 10 years was reduced from 32% to 2% after mass treatment with topical permethrin cream.[24] Similar programs using topical acaricides have also been successful in other endemic settings in Australia,[25,26] whereas oral ivermectin has been used successfully in the Solomon Islands.[27]

A randomized controlled trial in Pakistan, reported a 34% lower incidence of pyoderma amongst children (aged <15 years) who lived in households with hand-washing promotion and plain soap compared with controls.[28] No added benefit of antibacterial soap over plain soap was observed. As noted earlier, lack of access to in-home sanitation services has been associated with higher rates of pyoderma.[5] An ecological study from Alaska reported higher presentation rates for impetigo amongst indigenous children who lived in regions with fairly low access to in-home sanitation services compared with children who lived in regions with more universal in-home sanitation services, where houses generally had piped potable water and a sewage disposal system.[5] In populations where the prevalence of streptococcal pyoderma is high, it has been proposed that primary prophylaxis with benzathine penicillin may reduce prevalence. However, there are few published studies that have investigated the utility of this approach and the supportive evidence is weak.[2]

SCABIES

Scabies (**Fig. 3**) is an infestation of the skin by the scabies mite *Sarcoptes scabiei*. Damage caused through penetration of the skin by the mite, or the host reaction, or damage from scratching, results in visible papules, vesicles, or tiny linear burrows (these contain the mites and their eggs).[29] Adult *Sarcoptes* mites are 0.4 mm long or less; they cannot fly or jump but can crawl on warm skin. Burrows are typically located on the interdigital spaces of the hand, the flexure surface of the wrist, elbows, genitalia, axillae, umbilicus, belt line, nipples, and buttocks.[29] Scabies can also often involve the head and neck, especially in children and infants in the tropics.[29] The clinical manifestations of scabies in infants may not be easily recognized—the eruption is generalized, involving the head, neck, face, palms, and soles, with an early tendency to pustule formation. Classic burrows may be obscured by secondary infection.[29]

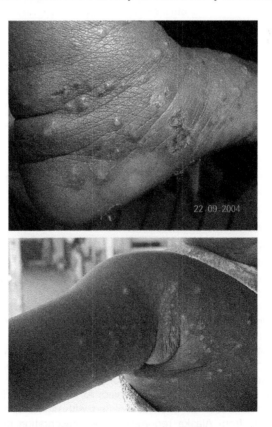

Fig. 3. Scabies.

In scabies-endemic areas, a clinical diagnosis has been demonstrated to be highly sensitive (100%) and specific (96.9%) when based on a case definition of diffuse itching with visible lesions and (1) at least 2 typical locations of scabies; or (2) presence of a household member with itch.[30] A diagnostic algorithm developed in Fiji for the detection of scabies used a simplified clinical diagnosis based on the presence of pruritus and papules (most commonly on the hands, knees, elbows, feet, or trunk).[31]

Confirmation of Scabies

Scabies is usually a presumptive clinical diagnosis based on the features noted earlier, with the finding of classical skin burrows being the most supportive feature.[29] Definitive diagnosis is made by finding the scabies mites or their eggs and fecal pellets (scybala). Several techniques have been described to visualize the mites, including dermatoscopy and the burrow ink test.[29] Parasitologic diagnosis requires the mineral oil scrape technique to collect skin scrapings for microscopic analysis. In tropical regions, the typical skin burrows may not be present, and resources and time for definitive diagnosis are often not available. Hence, most community-based studies do not include microscopy, relying instead on clinical diagnosis alone.[2]

Crusted (Norwegian) Scabies

Although it is rare in pediatric groups, the presence of individuals with crusted scabies in a community constitutes an infection risk for those around them.[2] Crusted scabies can occur in immunodeficient patients, some elderly persons, and patients with human immunodeficiency virus (HIV) and human T-lymphocytic virus type-1 (HTLV-1) infections. Some patients with crusted scabies have had no overt immunodeficiency.[15] Clinical presentation may appear as a generalized dermatitis with extensive scaling and crusting, sometimes in the absence of itching.[29] The mites on a person with crusted scabies are no more virulent or different from those of ordinary scabies. Indeed, most individuals who acquire scabies through contact with a crusted scabies case will themselves develop ordinary scabies lesions.

Scabies and Dogs

There are varieties of the scabies mite that cause mange in animals, but zoonotic infection is rare. Mites from animals cannot reproduce in the human skin, although they can cause transient itching.[29] Therefore, although dog mites can cause transient pruritus, control of scabies epidemics requires emphasis on treating people[25,26] rather than directing resources toward dog programs.

Prevention of Scabies

Available evidence indicates that effective control of endemic scabies requires mass treatment and surveillance of the population, and that opportunistic treatment of individuals or even entire families is likely to be ineffective in controlling endemic disease. The study in Panama,[24] mentioned in the earlier section on pyoderma prevention, included supervised treatment with 5% permethrin cream for all inhabitants of an island and reported reductions in the prevalence of scabies from an overall figure of 33% (78% of those 0–2 years old; 60%, 2–6 years; 54%, 6–10 years; and 22%, 11–50 years) to 2.5% after 1 month. By dealing with the predisposing cause—scabies, in this community—control of endemic streptococcal pyoderma was achieved without the additional use of antibiotics or hygiene and community education programs. Others have similarly reported substantial reductions in scabies prevalence after introducing mass treatment programs with topical permethrin.[25,26] However, a similar regional program involving several remote Aboriginal communities reported no discernible effect on the prevalence of scabies, which a nested study attributed to low levels of treatment use.[32] Although uptake of topical permethrin treatment was low, the odds of remaining scabies-free was almost 6 times greater among individuals belonging to a household where all people reported treatment uptake (odds ratio [OR] 5.9, 95% confidence interval [CI] 1.3, 27.2, $p = .02$).[32]

Ivermectin has been used successfully to control scabies in the Solomon Islands where the prevalence of scabies decreased from 25% to less than 1%, with no adverse reactions reported after 3 years.[27] In an economically disadvantaged fishing village in Brazil, a selective mass treatment study with ivermectin was conducted to control intestinal helminthiasis and parasitic skin disease.[33] Treatment was given to an entire household if 1 member was found to be positive for disease (n = 535). The prevalence of scabies reduced from 3.8% to 1.0% at 1 month and to 1.5% when measured 9 months later.

DERMATOPHYTIC INFECTION (TINEA)

Tinea (**Fig. 4**) is a fungal infection caused by the dermatophytic fungi, mainly anthropophilic species, such as *Trichophyton rubrum*, *T tonsurans*, and *T violaceum*. In addition, infection can be acquired by contact with dogs and cats (eg, *Microsporum* spp). A diagnosis of fungal skin infection is most often made on clinical appearance of the skin rash, especially if there is associated nail disease,[2] but more specific diagnoses are problematic on clinical grounds alone (**Table 3**).

Definitive diagnosis of fungal skin infections requires fungal microscopy of skin scrapings.[2] Where unusual bacterial or fungal skin infections are suspected, culture for the specific organisms is required—either from pus or swabs or, for deeper infections, from a skin biopsy.

More uncommon fungal infections that can involve subcutaneous tissue can sometimes be mistaken for tinea. These are grouped as chromoblastomycosis caused by various organisms. Sporotrichosis is also occasionally seen and requires prolonged therapy. An awareness of the possibility of leprosy remains important, because the skin lesions can be difficult to differentiate from tinea. Occasionally cases of erosive ulcers from *Mycobacterium ulcerans* and other atypical mycobacteria are seen.[13]

MANAGEMENT OF COMMON SKIN CONDITIONS

A practical algorithm for management of common childhood skin conditions has been developed by Steer and colleagues[31] from work conducted in Fiji. The algorithm was

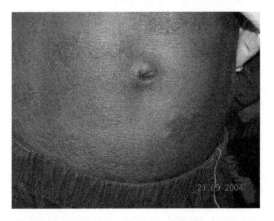

Fig. 4. Tinea.

Table 3 Clinical presentations of common tinea and tinea-like infections	
Tinea corporis (ringworm of the body)	Typically presents as asymmetrically distributed, circular scaly patches, predominantly on the trunk, usually beginning under the belt line. The scale is usually most prominent on the edge of the circular patches. Signs include a spreading edge, scaling, increased pigmentation, and increased skin markings. There may be associated pruritus, especially in sweaty areas. The condition (and secondary infection) is communicable, can be extensive, and often persists for years.[2]
Tinea capitis (ringworm of the scalp)	Often does not have a clear clinical presentation. It can present as scattered areas of white scale with varying degrees of hair loss. Scales can be dandrufflike or thick and adherent
Pityriasis versicolor (tinea versicolor)	A noncontagious, cosmetic condition that is often confused with tinea corporis. Also called "white handkerchief" or "white spot," it is a yeast infection that causes scaly patches of hypopigmentation. It is most common on the upper trunk, upper arms, and neck. It is usually asymptomatic (no itch)
Others	Tinea cruris (groin), tinea unguium (nails), and tinea pedis (foot) are other types of dermatophytic infection

designed to assist nurses and health workers in the clinical diagnosis of common childhood skin conditions and indications for treatment referral, using an Integrated Management of Childhood Illness (IMCI) strategy.[34] The first component of the algorithm involved the initial assessment by IMCI-trained nurses (**Fig. 5**), which was then followed by an algorithm for diagnosis and action. Validated by 2 pediatricians, the diagnosis by the IMCI-trained nurses was shown to be highly sensitive for diagnosing any skin problem (98.7%), but its performance was suboptimal in differentiating between infected and noninfected scabies. **Table 4** shows a modified IMCI algorithm incorporating the authors' suggestion to remove the differentiation of infected/non-infected for scabies[31] and additional detail cross-referencing to the recommendations for treatment that appear later in this article.

TREATMENT OF PYODERMA
Topical Treatments

There is no evidence that topical antiseptic treatment of pyoderma is effective (**Table 5**).[35] A recent Cochrane systematic review concluded that there is evidence that topical antibiotic therapy with sodium fusidate or mupirocin is as effective as oral antibiotics for treatment of pyoderma.[35] However, the review did not include studies from settings where pyoderma is highly prevalent. This was an issue noted by the Cochrane review investigators, in particular that recommendations did not apply to extensive pyoderma.[35] Additionally, concerns were raised about the poor quality of studies of therapy for pyoderma and the potential increasing resistance with the use of topical antibiotics.[35] In the authors' view, topical antibiotic therapy is appropriate for settings where pyoderma occurs sporadically but not in endemic or

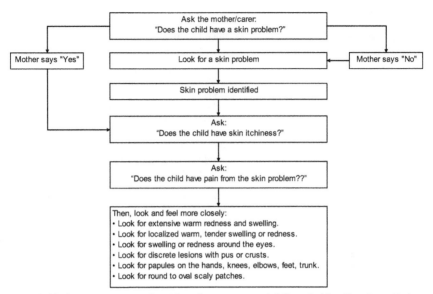

Fig. 5. Child skin assessment algorithm for common childhood skin disorders. (*Adapted from* Steer AC, Tikoduadua LV, Manalac EM, et al. Validation of an Integrated Management of Childhood Illness algorithm for managing common skin conditions in Fiji. Bull World Health Organ 2009;87:173.)

epidemic situations. In settings with high prevalence of pyoderma, the authors advise against widespread use of topical antibiotics, because of lack of evidence supporting their use in these settings and because of the likelihood of emergence of resistance to these topical antibiotics.

Oral Antibiotics

The antibiotics for empiric therapy of pyoderma are directed against GAS ± S aureus (see **Table 5**). With the recent emergence and spread of cMRSA in many regions of the world, it is important to have background regional data on and ongoing surveillance for cMRSA.[11] If empiric therapy fails, then swabs should be taken for culture and antimicrobial sensitivity testing.

Where cMRSA is commonly found in skin lesions, possible oral therapies include sulphamethoxazole/trimethoprim (cotrimoxazole); clindamycin; macrolides, such as erythromycin, roxithromycin, clarithromycin and azithromycin; and doxycycline (children older than 8 years).[36,37] However, the treatment of cMRSA skin and soft tissue infections without antibiotics but with emphasis on drainage of boils and abscesses is being increasingly emphasized.[37]

In many tropical locations where GAS predominates as the primary pathogen for pyoderma, therapy for GAS with penicillin was demonstrated in early studies to have an excellent response, irrespective of the presence of S aureus.[38,39] Bullous impetigo and boils are still more likely to be caused by S aureus than GAS, and drainage of pus should be the initial therapy, as noted earlier, along with appropriate antimicrobial therapy. For treatment of streptococcal pyoderma, when adherence is good, oral phenoxymethyl penicillin (penicillin V) for 10 days is more than 98% effective. It compares favorably with benzathine penicillin G and erythromycin.[16] Even when it was used in pyoderma where only 27% of the lesions had GAS alone or

Table 4
Modified IMCI algorithm to classify common childhood skin conditions

Sign	Diagnosis	Action (Also See Table 5 For Recommended Treatment)
Any general danger sign Extensive warm redness or swelling	Very severe skin infection	• Give first dose of appropriate antibiotic • Refer urgently to hospital
Swelling or redness around eyes	Periorbital or orbital cellulitis	• Give first dose of appropriate antibiotic • Refer urgently to hospital
Localized warm tender swelling and redness	Abscess or cellulitis	• Give first dose of appropriate antibiotic • Refer to hospital[a]
Discrete sores/lesions with pus or crusts	Pyoderma	• Give appropriate oral antibiotic for 7 days • Follow up in 5 days
Itchiness and papules	Scabies	• Provide topical permethrin skin cream • Treat the whole family with permethrin cream • Follow up in 2 weeks
Round-to-oval flat scaly patches, often itchy	Fungal infection	• Give appropriate topical antifungal medication for 2 weeks • Follow up in 2 weeks
If there are not enough signs to classify as any of the above boxes or if other signs present are not found in the above boxes	Other skin conditions	Refer to the doctor or skin clinic

[a] The recommendation of referral to hospital of children with localized warm tender swelling and redness is a guide for primary health workers intended to ensure children receive adequate treatment. Many children with such symptoms can be adequately treated by trained clinical staff (where they are available) without the need to attend hospital.

(*From* Steer AC, Tikoduadua LV, Manalac EM, et al. Validation of an integrated management of childhood illness algorithm for managing common skin conditions in Fiji. Bull World Health Organ 87:173, 2009.)

GAS mixed with staphylococci, phenoxymethyl penicillin given in 3 divided doses for 10 days was 76% effective.[17] However, in many settings where *S aureus* is frequently isolated from pyoderma, with or without GAS, there are concerns that penicillin may not be sufficient. Until further studies are conducted, many clinicians choose to use an oral antibiotic that is effective against GAS and *S aureus*, such as cotrimoxazole, flucloxacillin /dicloxacillin, or a first-generation cephalosporin.

The optimal duration and dosing interval of oral antibiotics for skin infections remains unclear.[35] The recommendation of 10 days of therapy seems to be extrapolated from the old data showing that GAS pharyngitis requires such a duration of penicillin to prevent rheumatic fever. As antibiotic formulations are generally available in 5- to 7-day quantities, completion of a 10-day course through repeat prescription is probably rarely achieved in reality. A meta-analysis of oral penicillin dosing frequency for GAS tonsillopharyngitis showed twice-daily dosing to result in cure rates similar to those when doses were administered 3 to 4 times daily[40]; however, there are little data

Table 5
Treatment of pyoderma, scabies, and dermatophytic infection (tinea)

Medication or Intervention	Recommendation	Grading[74]	Quality of Supporting Evidence[75]
Pyoderma[a]			
Topical antiseptic treatment (eg, chlorhexidine or povidone-iodine)	Not recommended[35]	Strong	Moderate
Topical antibiotic treatment (eg, sodium fusidate or mupirocin)	Recommended only for areas with sporadic pyoderma.[35] Not recommended in areas with high pyoderma prevalence.[35]	Moderate	Moderate
Antistaphylococcal β-lactam antibiotics (flucloxacillin/dicloxacillin, nafcillin, cephalexin)	For treatment in regions where staphylococci are the predominant pathogens (typically bullous pyoderma/boils/carbuncles) or where IM benzathine penicillin is not available or not a preferred option even if GAS is suspected.[36,37]	Strong	High
IM benzathine penicillin G single dose	For treatment in regions where streptococci are the predominant pathogens (typically skin sores/pyoderma/infected scabies).[16,38,39]	Strong	Moderate
Oral phenoxymethyl penicillin (penicillin V) for 10 days	For treatment in regions where streptococci are the predominant pathogens (typically skin sores/pyoderma/infected scabies); and compliance is good.[17]	Strong	Moderate
Sulfamethoxazole/trimethoprim (cotrimoxazole), clindamycin; macrolides, such as erythromycin, roxithromycin, clarithromycin, azithromycin; doxycycline (children older than 8 years)	These oral agents are being increasingly used for cMRSA treatment in regions where staphylococci are the predominant pathogens and there is a high prevalence of cMRSA. However resistance to macrolides and clindamycin is increasing in many locations where cMRSA has become established.[36,37]	Strong	Moderate

	Treatment	Comment	Strength of recommendation	Quality of evidence
Scabies	Topical permethrin cream	For individual treatment of clinical scabies.[47]	Strong	High
	Oral ivermectin	For community treatment of endemic scabies.[24]	Medium	Medium
		For individual treatment of crusted scabies.[15]	Strong	High
		For community treatment of endemic scabies.[27]	Medium	Medium
Tinea	Oral terbinafine	If therapy beyond 2 weeks, then important to monitor full blood count and liver function tests; neutropenia and abnormal liver function can occur.[58,59,62]	Strong	High
	Oral griseofulvin	Griseofulvin is cheaper than terbinafine but inferior as therapy and prolonged treatment courses are often required.[60]	Moderate	High
	Topical therapies (eg, azole creams or topical terbinafine)	Not appropriate for extensive tinea corporis or nail disease	Moderate	Moderate

Abbreviation: IM, intramuscular.

[a] cMRSA is resistant to IM benzathine penicillin, flucloxacillin/nafcillin, and cephalexin. With increasing cMRSA, it is important to have background regional data on and ongoing surveillance for cMRSA. If empiric therapy fails then swabs should be taken for culture and antimicrobial sensitivity testing.

to support twice-daily penicillin for GAS skin infections. Nevertheless, twice-daily penicillin is commonly recommended because of concerns of adherence to more frequent dosing. In another study, a twice-daily dosage regimen of cephalexin over 10 days was shown to be 90.3% effective in achieving bacteriologic eradication in skin and skin structure infections.[41] Because of its prolonged half-life, a shorter course (eg, 5 days) of daily azithromycin has also been successful.[41] However concerns of emerging macrolide resistance warrant caution against unrestrained widespread use of azithromycin for skin and respiratory infections.[37,42]

Parenteral Antibiotics

In Australian Aboriginal populations, a single dose of intramuscular benzathine penicillin has been the drug of choice for empiric therapy of pyoderma (see **Table 5**).[43] The rationale for this management includes incomplete adherence with oral therapy, pyoderma being predominantly due to GAS (even if mixed with staphylococci) and the secondary aim to treat or prevent postinfective complications, including acute poststreptococcal glomerulonephritis (APSGN) and rheumatic fever. Numerous studies, particularly in the 1970s, established the role of benzathine penicillin for treatment of pyoderma, when caused by GAS alone or by a mixture of GAS and staphylococci.[16]

Benzathine penicillin remains the only long-acting parenteral antibiotic for GAS. It is remarkable that no studies have been undertaken in the past 20 years to evaluate the use of benzathine penicillin in pyoderma. It now seems critical that surveillance be undertaken in tropical and other regions where benzathine penicillin has traditionally been used for pyoderma, to ascertain whether the emergence and spread of cMRSA necessitates alternative protocols. Nevertheless, some of the alternative oral regimens that provide antimicrobial activity against cMRSA may not necessarily improve outcomes in pyoderma, and further studies of these regimens are required.[44]

TREATMENT OF SCABIES

Topical permethrin cream is the first-line treatment of choice, except for a few special circumstances,[45] whereas oral ivermectin is a potentially suitable option in other circumstances (see **Table 5**). Although clinical scabies can be managed by the implementation of individual treatment with topical permethrin cream in conjunction with appropriate infection control strategies, a broader approach to identify and treat other family or community members is generally appropriate. Indeed, in most endemic situations, a community-wide strategy is required for effective control.[24–26] Scabies can be treated with a thorough body application of permethrin cream to the whole skin surface, which is left on overnight. Individual patients do not require more than 2 scrupulous applications. In tropical regions and especially for children, the cream should be applied to the neck, head, scalp, and the soles of the feet, with only mucous membranes not covered.[29] Although the need for, and timing of, a second thorough body application of topical acaricide creams is not well studied, it is generally recommended for those with moderate scabies or worse. The second application, if done, should happen 7 to 14 days later to enable killing of all mites hatched from eggs not killed by the first application. Guidelines state that all individuals who have had significant contact with the primary patient should also be treated, because reinfestations can occur if this is not done. There is a paucity of controlled trials that have investigated this and the related issue of bedding and linen cleaning; however, early studies of the lifecycle of the parasite and the interval between primary infection and the first onset of symptoms[46] support the view that occult infection is common in primary disease, and that fomites are not a significant risk for disease transmission, except in the setting of crusted scabies where household cleaning and cleaning of clothing and linen is especially important.

The choices for acaricides in the past has included 1% gamma benzene hexachloride (lindane), benzyl benzoate (Ascabiol), and 5% to 10% sulfur in ointment base. Permethrin cream (5%) has become the treatment of choice for scabies except in a few special circumstances (for example infancy). To be effective, it should be applied to the entire skin surface except the eyes, and it is generally recommended that it be applied in the evening and left on overnight. It is well tolerated, is poorly absorbed across the skin, and the small percentage that is absorbed is rapidly metabolized.[47]

A significant gap in the medical literature is that there are no comparative studies of the safety and efficacy of different treatments for scabies in infants and small children. Available clinical trial data to facilitate selection of the best treatments for individual patients with scabies and communities with endemic scabies are few.[45] Furthermore, most are of a fairly small size, and diagnostic and clinical endpoints are not rigorously defined. On account of theoretical concerns regarding percutaneous absorption of the permethrin in infants, guidelines have generally recommended that crotamiton or a sulfur preparation should be used instead of permethrin in this group. However, given the likely superior efficacy of permethrin[45] and the lack of reports of toxicity, it is being increasingly used in children younger than 1 year. Sensitization to mite antigens is a major factor in the pathogenesis of scabies and has been proposed as the explanation for the persistence of pruritus for some time after effective chemotherapy.

Ivermectin is the only currently available oral medication that can be used to treat scabies. However, the efficacy of ivermectin is not satisfactory unless 2 doses are administered 1 week apart. The safety profile of ivermectin in nonpregnant adults has been well established with over 400 million treatments distributed in Africa through onchocerciasis control programs and with some individuals having received up to 20 annual treatments.[48,49] Although one is advised against the use of ivermectin during pregnancy, reports exist on the inadvertent administration of the drug to pregnant women without adverse fetal outcome.[50,51] However, fatal neurologic toxicity from ivermectin is fairly common in certain breeds of dogs.[52] This neurotoxicity has been attributed to ivermectin transport across the blood-brain barrier, possibly due to an absence of, or functional deficiency in, P-glycoprotein.[53] The immaturity of the blood-brain barrier in infancy provides a reason for caution in the administration of ivermectin to infants and young children. To date, its use for scabies has not been widely studied in pediatric populations. Although a mass drug administration program using ivermectin was found to be very successful for controlling scabies and pyoderma in the Solomon Islands,[27] the major impediment to its use for this purpose includes the paucity of safety data on its use during pregnancy and concerns about administration to small children (<15 kg or 5 years of age).

There are increasing reports of drug resistance in scabies. Treatment failures with lindane[54] crotamiton,[54] and ivermectin[55] have been described. In vitro studies have shown progressively reduced susceptibility to permethrin in mites collected from an indigenous community where mass drug distribution has been deployed.[56,57]

Ivermectin (in multiple doses) is the drug of choice for patients with crusted scabies, given in combination with topical acaricides and topical keratolytic therapy to break down the crusts.[15] Immunologic testing is recommended, including serology for HIV and HTLV-1. Infection control measures should include contact precautions. The burden of disease relating to people with crusted scabies being core transmitters to other community members is not quantified, although it is a likely factor in sustaining endemic transmission.[13]

TREATMENT OF TINEA

Oral terbinafine results in more rapid mycological cure when compared with oral griseofulvin and, where it is affordable, it has become the treatment of choice for extensive tinea corporis and nail disease (see **Table 5**). Topical therapy can still be used for localized tinea.

A systematic review of topical treatments for fungal infections of the skin and nails concluded that topical allylamines, such as terbinafine, cure a few more infections than azoles, such as clotrimazole and miconazole.[58] The review also found no significant differences in efficacy between the individual azoles. A further review recommended topical terbinafine as the treatment of choice for less extensive dermatophytic infections, suggesting that it is more cost-effective than topical miconazole or ketoconazole.[59]

In children, oral terbinafine cures tinea more quickly than griseofulvin and, at a dose of 250 mg (>40 kg) or 125 mg (20–40 kg) for 4 weeks, was 93% effective.[60] A subsequent randomized controlled trial found oral terbinafine had a cure rate of 74% for tinea capitis in children after 1 week of therapy.[61] Occasional cases of severe bone marrow suppression have been observed with oral terbinafine, which has necessitated more stringent follow-up laboratory testing for those continuing terbinafine for more than 2 weeks (liver function, full blood count, electrolytes, and glucose level).[62]

As an alternative to oral terbinafine for extensive tinea corporis, supervised once-weekly oral fluconazole (150 mg) has been shown to be safe, convenient, and effective, with a mean number of 2.6 doses resulting in fungal eradication in 66 of 67 (98.5%) patients with tinea corporis caused by T rubrum.[63] Various pulsed regimens of terbinafine ± oral triazoles, such as fluconazole and itraconazole, are being studied for tinea corporis and nail tinea.

SUMMARY

Pyoderma, scabies, and tinea affect children globally but are especially common in situations of socioeconomic disadvantage that result in overcrowding and poor access to health care and health hardware for hygiene. In such circumstances, these infections are often under-recognized and certainly undertreated, and the potential morbidity and mortality from their sequelae are underappreciated. There are effective therapies for each of them, but recurrent infections are inevitable without addressing the underlying social circumstances and the importance of ongoing transmission, especially between children in these settings. The emergence of cMRSA and resistance to scabicides necessitates ongoing surveillance and further studies to optimize therapeutic regimens.

REFERENCES

1. World Health Organization. The current evidence for the burden of group A streptococcal diseases. vol. WHO/FCH/CAH/05.07. Geneva: World Health Organization; 2005.
2. Couzos S, Currie B. Skin infections. In: Couzos S, Murray R, editors. Aboriginal primary health care: an evidence-based approach. 2nd edition. South Melbourne, Victoria: Oxford University Press; 2003. p. 251–80.
3. World Health Organization. Epidemiology and management of common skin diseases in children in developing countries. vol. WHO/FCH/CAH/05.12. Geneva: World Health Organization; 2005.

4. Anthony BF, Perlman LV, Wannamaker LW. Skin infections and acute nephritis in American Indian children. Pediatrics 1967;39:263–79.
5. Hennessy TW, Ritter T, Holman RC, et al. The relationship between in-home water service and the risk of respiratory tract, skin, and gastrointestinal tract infections among rural Alaska natives. Am J Public Health 2008;98:2072–8.
6. Harris SB, Glazier R, Eng K, et al. Disease patterns among Canadian aboriginal children. Study in a remote rural setting. Can Fam Physician 1998;44:1869–77.
7. Finger F, Rossaak M, Umstaetter R, et al. Skin infections of the limbs of Polynesian children. N Z Med J 2004;117:U847.
8. Steer AC, Jenney AW, Kado J, et al. High burden of impetigo and scabies in a tropical country. PLoS Negl Trop Dis 2009;3:e467.
9. Clucas DB, Carville KS, Connors C, et al. Disease burden and health-care clinic attendances for young children in remote aboriginal communities of northern Australia. Bull World Health Organ 2008;86:275–81.
10. Bailie RS, Stevens MR, McDonald E, et al. Skin infection, housing and social circumstances in children living in remote Indigenous communities: testing conceptual and methodological approaches. BMC Public Health 2005;5:128.
11. Tong SY, McDonald MI, Holt DC, et al. Global implications of the emergence of community-associated methicillin-resistant *Staphylococcus aureus* in Indigenous populations. Clin Infect Dis 2008;46:1871–8.
12. McDonald MI, Towers RJ, Fagan P, et al. Molecular typing of *Streptococcus pyogenes* from remote Aboriginal communities where rheumatic fever is common and pyoderma is the predominant streptococcal infection. Epidemiol Infect 2007;135:1398–405.
13. Currie BJ, Carapetis JR. Skin infections and infestations in Aboriginal communities in northern Australia. Australas J Dermatol 2000;41:139–43.
14. United Nations. The millennium development goals report 2008. New York: United Nations; 2008.
15. Roberts LJ, Huffam SE, Walton SF, et al. Crusted scabies: clinical and immunological findings in seventy-eight patients and a review of the literature. J Infect 2005;50:375–81.
16. Baltimore RS. Treatment of impetigo: a review. Pediatr Infect Dis 1985;4:597–601.
17. Demidovich CW, Wittler RR, Ruff ME, et al. Impetigo. Current etiology and comparison of penicillin, erythromycin, and cephalexin therapies. Am J Dis Child 1990;144:1313–5.
18. Van Buynder PG, Gaggin JA, Martin D, et al. Streptococcal infection and renal disease markers in Australian aboriginal children. Med J Aust 1992;156:537–40.
19. Carapetis J, Gardiner D, Currie B, et al. Multiple strains of *Streptococcus pyogenes* in skin sores of aboriginal Australians. J Clin Monit 1995;33:1471–2.
20. Vlack S, Cox L, Peleg AY, et al. Carriage of methicillin-resistant *Staphylococcus aureus* in a Queensland indigenous community. Med J Aust 2006;184:556–9.
21. Darmstadt GL, Lane AT. Impetigo: an overview. Pediatr Dermatol 1994;11:293–303.
22. Bessen DE, Carapetis JR, Beall B, et al. Contrasting molecular epidemiology of group A streptococci causing tropical and nontropical infections of the skin and throat. J Infect Dis 2000;182:1109–16.
23. Chin J. Control of communicable diseases manual. An official report of the American Public Health Association. 17th edition. Washington, DC: American Public Health Association; 2000.
24. Taplin D, Porcelain SL, Meinking TL, et al. Community control of scabies: a model based on use of permethrin cream. Lancet 1991;337:1016–8.
25. Wong LC, Amega B, Connors C, et al. Outcome of an interventional program for scabies in an Indigenous community. Med J Aust 2001;175:367–70.

26. Carapetis JR, Connors C, Yarmirr D, et al. Success of a scabies control program in an Australian aboriginal community. Pediatr Infect Dis J 1997;16:494–9.

27. Lawrence G, Leafasia J, Sheridan J, et al. Control of scabies, skin sores and haematuria in children in the Solomon islands: another role for ivermectin. Bull World Health Organ 2005;83:34.

28. Luby SP, Agboatwalla M, Feikin DR, et al. Effect of handwashing on child health: a randomised controlled trial. Lancet 2005;366:225–33.

29. McCarthy JS, Kemp DJ, Walton SF, et al. Scabies: more than just an irritation. Postgrad Med J 2004;80:382–7.

30. Mahé A, Faye O, N'Diaye HT, et al. Definition of an algorithm for the management of common skin diseases at primary health care level in sub-Saharan Africa. Trans R Soc Trop Med Hyg 2005;99:39–47.

31. Steer AC, Tikoduadua LV, Manalac EM, et al. Validation of an integrated management of childhood illness algorithm for managing common skin conditions in Fiji. Bull World Health Organ 2009;87:173–9.

32. La Vincente S, Kearns T, Connors C, et al. Community management of endemic scabies in remote aboriginal communities of Northern Australia: low treatment uptake and high ongoing acquisition. PLoS Negl Trop Dis 2009;3:e444.

33. Heukelbach J, Winter B, Wilcke T, et al. Selective mass treatment with ivermectin to control intestinal helminthiases and parasitic skin diseases in a severely affected population. Bull World Health Organ 2004;82:563–71.

34. Gove S. Integrated management of childhood illness by outpatient health workers: technical basis and overview. The WHO Working Group on Guidelines for Integrated Management of the Sick Child. Bull World Health Organ 1997; 75(Suppl 1):7–24.

35. Koning S, Verhagen AP, van Suijlekom-Smit LW, et al. Interventions for impetigo. Cochrane Database Syst Rev 2004;(2):CD003261.

36. Grayson ML. The treatment triangle for staphylococcal infections. N Engl J Med 2006;355:724–7.

37. Stevens DL, Bisno AL, Chambers HF, et al. Practice guidelines for the diagnosis and management of skin and soft-tissue infections. Clin Infect Dis 2005;41: 1373–406.

38. Taplin D, Lansdell L, Allen AM, et al. Prevalence of streptococcal pyoderma in relation to climate and hygiene. Lancet 1973;1:501–3.

39. Kar P, Shah B, Raval R. Use of benzathine penicillin in impetigo in children. Indian J Dermatol Venereol Leprol 1987;53.

40. Lan AJ, Colford JM, Colford JM Jr. The impact of dosing frequency on the efficacy of 10-day penicillin or amoxicillin therapy for streptococcal tonsillopharyngitis: a meta-analysis. Pediatrics 2000;105:E19.

41. Kiani R. Double-blind, double-dummy comparison of azithromycin and cephalexin in the treatment of skin and skin structure infections. Eur J Clin Microbiol Infect Dis 1991;10:880–4.

42. Guchev IA, Gray GC, Klochkov OI. Two regimens of azithromycin prophylaxis against community-acquired respiratory and skin/soft-tissue infections among military trainees. Clin Infect Dis 2004;38:1095–101.

43. Central Australian Rural Practitioners Association. CARPA standard treatment manual. Alice Springs (Australia): Central Australian Rural Practitioners Association; 2003.

44. Elliott DJ, Zaoutis TE, Troxel AB, et al. Empiric antimicrobial therapy for pediatric skin and soft-tissue infections in the era of methicillin-resistant *Staphylococcus aureus*. Pediatrics 2009;123:e959.

45. Strong M, Johnstone PW: Interventions for treating scabies. Cochrane Database Syst Rev 2007;(3):CD000320.
46. Mellanby K. The development of symptoms, parasitic infection and immunity in human scabies. Parasitology 1944;35:197.
47. Franz TJ, Lehman PA, Franz SF, et al. Comparative percutaneous absorption of lindane and permethrin. Arch Dermatol 1996;132:901–5.
48. Basanez MG, Pion SD, Boakes E, et al. Effect of single-dose ivermectin on Onchocerca volvulus: a systematic review and meta-analysis. Lancet Infect Dis 2008;8:310–22.
49. Guzzo CA, Furtek CI, Porras AG, et al. Safety, tolerability, and pharmacokinetics of escalating high doses of ivermectin in healthy adult subjects. J Clin Pharmacol 2002;42:1122–33.
50. Chippaux JP, Gardon-Wendel N, Gardon J, et al. Absence of any adverse effect of inadvertent ivermectin treatment during pregnancy. Trans R Soc Trop Med Hyg 1993;87:318.
51. Gyapong JO, Chinbuah MA, Gyapong M. Inadvertent exposure of pregnant women to ivermectin and albendazole during mass drug administration for lymphatic filariasis. Trop Med Int Health 2003;8:1093–101.
52. Paul AJ, Tranquilli WJ, Seward RL, et al. Clinical observations in collies given ivermectin orally. Am J Vet Res 1987;48:684–5.
53. Edwards G. Ivermectin: does P-glycoprotein play a role in neurotoxicity? Filaria J 2003;2(Suppl 1):S8.
54. Roth WI. Scabies resistant to lindane 1% lotion and crotamiton 10% cream. J Am Acad Dermatol 1991;24:502–3.
55. Currie BJ, Harumal P, McKinnon M, et al. First documentation of in vivo and in vitro ivermectin resistance in Sarcoptes scabiei. Clin Infect Dis 2004;39:e8–e12.
56. Pasay C, Arlian L, Morgan M, et al. The effect of insecticide synergists on the response of scabies mites to pyrethroid acaricides. PLoS Negl Trop Dis 2009; 3:e354.
57. Walton SF, Myerscough MR, Currie BJ. Studies in vitro on the relative efficacy of current acaricides for Sarcoptes scabiei var. hominis. Trans R Soc Trop Med Hyg 2000;94:92–6.
58. Hart R, Bell-Syer SE, Crawford F, et al. Systematic review of topical treatments for fungal infections of the skin and nails of the feet. BMJ 1999;319:79–82.
59. McClellan KJ, Wiseman LR, Markham A. Terbinafine. An update of its use in superficial mycoses. Drugs 1999;58:179–202.
60. Jones TC. Overview of the use of terbinafine (Lamisil) in children. Br J Dermatol 1995;132:683–9.
61. Haroon TS, Hussain I, Aman S, et al. A randomized double-blind comparative study of terbinafine for 1, 2 and 4 weeks in tinea capitis. Br J Dermatol 1996; 135:86–8.
62. Koh KJ, Parker CJ, Ellis DH, et al. Use of terbinafine for tinea in Australian Aboriginal communities in the Top End. Australas J Dermatol 2003;44:243–9.
63. Suchil P, Gei FM, Robles M, et al. Once-weekly oral doses of fluconazole 150 mg in the treatment of tinea corporis/cruris and cutaneous candidiasis. Clin Exp Dermatol 1992;17:397–401.
64. Carapetis JR, Walker AM, Hibble M, et al. Clinical and epidemiological features of group A streptococcal bacteraemia in a region with hyperendemic superficial streptococcal infection. Epidemiol Infect 1999;122:59–65.
65. Norton R, Smith HV, Wood N, et al. Invasive group A streptococcal disease in North Queensland (1996–2001). Indian J Med Res 2004;119(Suppl):148.

66. Kearns T, Evans C, Krause V. Outbreak of acute post-streptococcal glomerulonephritis in the Northern Territory - 2001. NT Dis Control Bull 2001;8:6.
67. White AV, Hoy WE, McCredie DA. Childhood post-streptococcal glomerulonephritis as a risk factor for chronic renal disease in later life. Med J Aust 2001; 174:492–6.
68. Rodriguez-Iturbe B, Musser JM. The current state of poststreptococcal glomerulonephritis. J Am Soc Nephrol 2008;19:1855–64.
69. McDonald M, Brown A, Edwards T, et al. Apparent contrasting rates of pharyngitis and pyoderma in regions where rheumatic heart disease is highly prevalent. Heart Lung Circ 2007;16:254–9.
70. McDonald M, Currie BJ, Carapetis JR. Acute rheumatic fever: a chink in the chain that links the heart to the throat? Lancet Infect Dis 2004;4:240–5.
71. Martin DR, Voss LM, Walker SJ, et al. Acute rheumatic fever in Auckland, New Zealand: spectrum of associated group A streptococci different from expected. Pediatr Infect Dis J 1994;13:264–9.
72. Carapetis JR, Currie BJ, Mathews JD. Cumulative incidence of rheumatic fever in an endemic region: a guide to the susceptibility of the population? Epidemiol Infect 2000;124:239–44.
73. Carapetis JR, McDonald M, Wilson NJ. Acute rheumatic fever. Lancet 2005;366: 155–68.
74. Atkins D, Best D, Briss PA, et al. Grading quality of evidence and strength of recommendations. BMJ 2004;328:1490.
75. Guyatt GH, Oxman AD, Kunz R, et al. Going from evidence to recommendations. BMJ 2008;336:1049–51.

Clinical Management of Type 2 Diabetes in Indigenous Youth

Elizabeth AC. Sellers, MD, MSc, FRCPC[a],*, Kelly Moore, MD, FAAP[b],
Heather J. Dean, MD, FRCPC[a]

KEYWORDS

• Indigenous • Youth • Type 2 diabetes

STATEMENT OF THE PROBLEM

Youth-onset type 2 diabetes is a serious public health problem for indigenous people throughout the world.[1–6] Among Pima Indian youth of southern Arizona, a 2- to 3-fold increase in type 2 diabetes prevalence has been documented over the 30 years before 1996.[3] From 1994 to 2004, the prevalence of diagnosed type 2 diabetes increased by 68% among American Indian (AI) and Alaskan Native (AN) adolescents aged 15 to 19 years who use Indian Health Service health care services.[7] In Canada, type 2 diabetes was diagnosed in 1% of Oji-Cree youth aged 4 to 19 years in 1996 to 1997.[8] Although earlier population-based studies showed a 4% prevalence of diabetes among indigenous adolescent girls in Manitoba[8] and Ontario,[9] the gender distribution has shifted from female predominance to a pattern close to 1:1 in more recent data.[4] In Australia, the prevalence of youth-onset type 2 diabetes almost doubled to 1.3% among a cohort of indigenous Australian youth aged 7 to 18 years surveyed in 1989 and again in 1994.[2,10] Among Maori in Auckland, New Zealand, a clinic-based study of type 2 diabetes trends found type 2 diabetes in 12.5% of new cases of diabetes in youth in the years 1997 to 1999 and 35.7% of new cases in the years 2000 to 2001.[11] Other reports have also demonstrated an increasing rate of diabetes among young Maori.[6,12] Despite the need for more population-based data, the increasing frequency of type 2 diabetes in indigenous youth is well-recognized and prevention should be seen as the foremost strategy.[1–6,13]

Compared with individuals who develop diabetes as middle-aged or elderly adults, indigenous youth who develop type 2 diabetes experience more years of disease

Within this article, the term "youth" will be used to refer to individuals <18 years of age.
[a] Department of Pediatrics and Child Health, University of Manitoba, FE-307, 685 William Avenue, Winnipeg, Manitoba, Canada R3E 0Z2
[b] Centers for American Indian and Alaska Native Health, Mail Stop F800, Nighthorse Campbell Native Health Building, 13055 East 17th Avenue, Room 324, Aurora, CO 80045, USA
* Corresponding author.
E-mail address: esellers@exchange.hsc.mb.ca (E.AC. Sellers).

Pediatr Clin N Am 56 (2009) 1441–1459
doi:10.1016/j.pcl.2009.09.013
0031-3955/09/$ – see front matter © 2009 Elsevier Inc. All rights reserved.

burden and a higher probability of developing serious type 2 diabetes-related complications early in life (see later sections on complications and comorbidities).[1,2,14,15] These complications will threaten life expectancy, reduce quality of life, and lower productivity during the prime years of their lives. The increased frequency of diabetes among young indigenous women of child-bearing age poses an additional risk to future generations, because intrauterine exposure to maternal diabetes places the fetus at risk of future onset of diabetes.[1,14,16,17]

Other factors also contribute to the greater risk of early complications in youth-onset type 2 diabetes. Because of its association with insulin resistance, type 2 diabetes confers additional cardiovascular risk.[18,19] Greater microvascular disease risk may also exist, particularly for diabetic nephropathy.[15,19,20] Because type 2 diabetes in youth may be associated with fewer symptoms than type 1, its treatment is often more problematic with a stronger focus on lifestyle modification and behavioral change. Several factors represent significant challenges to indigenous families and their health care providers in meeting the needs of youth with diabetes: poverty and unemployment; low educational levels; competing priorities and life stresses; limited access to adequate health services, especially in remote and rural locations; limited availability of healthy food choices; fewer options for safe and regular physical activity; lack of appropriate role models with diabetes in the family and community; presence of eating and mood disorders; and specific tribal or culturally held beliefs about diabetes, including a sense of fatalism or despondency about diabetes.[4,14] Often, the result is decreased patient and family adherence.[13,21] To address these issues, strong evidence-based approaches to prevention and treatment of youth-onset type 2 diabetes are an urgent priority for indigenous communities.

Key recommendations for issues relating to type 2 diabetes in indigenous children are summarized in (**Table 1**).

DIAGNOSIS AND CLASSIFICATION OF DIABETES IN CHILDREN

The current criteria for diagnosis of diabetes in children are the same as those used for adults. A random or casual plasma glucose level (meaning at any time of day regardless of the timing of the last meal) of 200 mg/dL (11.1 mmol/L) or more, with the classic symptoms of diabetes of polyuria, polydipsia, and unexplained weight loss is diagnostic of diabetes. A fasting plasma glucose level (meaning no caloric intake for at least 8 hours) of 126 mg/dL (7.0 mmol/L) or more, or a 2-hour plasma glucose of 200 mg/dL (11.1 mmol/L) or more following a 75 g oral glucose load may also be used to diagnose diabetes. In the absence of symptoms and unequivocal hyperglycemia, repeat testing on a different day should be used to confirm hyperglycemia.[22,23]

Classification of type 1 or type 2 diabetes can usually be made based on the patient's clinical presentation.[24] Although most instances of diabetes among indigenous youth is type 2,[3,25] type 1 cases have been reported.[26–28] Diabetic ketoacidosis (DKA) has also been reported in indigenous youth with type 2 diabetes and should not be used to exclude the diagnosis of type 2 diabetes (see later sections on complications).[29] Where the classification is not apparent on clinical grounds, the absence of diabetes-associated autoantibodies can be used to support the diagnosis of type 2 diabetes.[30,31] Fasting C-peptide levels may also be of value after glycemic stabilization, with elevated levels indicating type 2 diabetes. Repeat testing at 1 year or more following diagnosis may be needed for those with normal results.[19] Appropriate classification is important to provide accurate family counseling and education regarding cause, options for treatment, comorbidities, and complications.

Table 1
Screening for diabetes complications and comorbidities in children with type 2 diabetes

Complication/Co-Morbid Condition	Indications and Intervals for Screening	Screening Test
Dyslipidemia	Screening should commence at diagnosis of diabetes and every 1-3 years thereafter, as clinically indicated	Fasting TC, HDL-C, triglycerides, and calculated LDL-C
Hypertension	At diagnosis of diabetes and at every diabetes-related clinical encounter thereafter (at least twice annually)	BP measurement using appropriate-sized cuff
NAFLD	Yearly screening commencing at diagnosis of diabetes	ALT
Nephropathy	Yearly screening commencing at diagnosis of diabetes	• First morning (preferred) or random ACR. • Abnormal ACR requires confirmation at least 1 month later with a first morning ACR, and if abnormal, follow-up with timed, overnight or 24-hour split urine collections for albumin excretion rate. • Repeated sampling should be done every 3–4 months over a 6- to 12-month period to demonstrate persistence.
Neuropathy	Yearly screening commencing at diagnosis of diabetes	Questioned and examined for: • Symptoms of numbness, pain, cramps, and paresthesia • Skin sensation • Vibration sense • Light touch, and • Ankle reflexes
PCOS	Yearly screening commencing at puberty in women with oligo-amenorrhea, acne and/or hirsutism	Androgen levels including DHEAS and free testosterone
Retinopathy	Yearly screening commencing at diagnosis of diabetes	• 7-standard field, stereoscopic-color fundus photography with interpretation by a trained reader (gold standard); or • Direct ophthalmoscopy or indirect slit-lamp fundoscopy through dilated pupil; or • Digital fundus photography

Abbreviations: ACR, albumin to creatinine ratio; ALT, alanine aminotransferase; BP, blood pressure; DHEAS, dehydroepiandrosterone sulfate; HDL-C, high-density lipoprotein cholesterol; LDL-C, low-density lipoprotein cholesterol; NAFLD, nonalcoholic fatty liver disease; PCOS, polycystic ovary syndrome; TC, total cholesterol.
Reproduced from the Canadian Diabetes Association. Clinical Practice Guidelines 2008;32(Suppl 1):S1-20; with permission.

SCREENING AND CASE FINDING

Population-based screening is not recommended, except in research efforts that contribute to the optimal management, diagnosis, and treatment of children with type 2 diabetes.[14,32–36] No randomized controlled trials (RCTs) have been conducted to demonstrate the benefits of early diagnosis through the screening of asymptomatic individuals. Research is needed to determine the cost-benefit of screening for type 2 diabetes in high-risk indigenous youth.

Case finding refers to diagnostic testing in an at-risk population. Early case finding, for example, testing for type 2 diabetes in indigenous youth with identified risk factors, with initiation of appropriate therapy may prevent some sequelae of type 2 diabetes.[14] Testing should be conducted in a clinical setting with adequate interpretation of the results to the patient and family. Follow-up evaluation and treatment should be made available.

Indigenous youth who have entered puberty or who are 10 years of age or older are considered at risk if they have 2 or more of the following risk factors: (1) obesity; (2) family history of type 2 diabetes in a first- or second-degree relative; (3) in utero exposure to diabetes; or (4) a condition associated with insulin resistance, such as acanthosis nigricans, hypertension, dyslipidemia, fatty liver, or polycystic ovarian syndrome.[14,23] These children should be tested every 2 years using a fasting plasma glucose.[14,23] Clinical judgment should be used to test for diabetes in high-risk youth who do not meet these criteria.

PRIMARY PREVENTION

Several studies have demonstrated that lifestyle interventions and pharmaceutical agents can significantly reduce the risk of developing type 2 diabetes in adults with prediabetes.[37] The Diabetes Prevention Program conducted in the United States had 4 centers for the enrollment of AI and AN participants, demonstrating that a lifestyle and a pharmaceutical intervention were effective in the prevention of diabetes in a high-risk adult indigenous population with prediabetes.[38] In youth, the only clear evidence for diabetes prevention relates to breastfeeding.[2] Exclusive breastfeeding for the first 2 months of life has been associated with a 40% reduction in type 2 diabetes among Pima Indians.[39] Studies of Canadian First Nation youth have also shown a lower prevalence of youth-onset type 2 diabetes among those who were breastfed during infancy.[40] Nonetheless, several primary prevention programs for diabetes and its risk factors in indigenous youth populations have been initiated in school settings.[41–47] The Special Diabetes Program for Indians grant programs in the United States have also worked closely with school and community partners to establish policy and environmental changes that support physical activity and healthy eating strategies. Reservation and urban Indian community grant programs have successfully changed school vending machine and wellness policies, increased the availability of school and community physical activity opportunities, increased access to fitness facilities, and built or improved local playgrounds. These programs have created a supportive environment for youth to exercise and eat healthier, helping to lower their risk of developing diabetes.[48] Although much remains to be done to reduce the burden of youth-onset type 2 diabetes in indigenous communities, many tribal and urban indigenous community leaders have recognized this concern and continue to support comprehensive interventions for childhood obesity and diabetes prevention in their communities.

All health professionals play an important role in prevention activities. They can be involved in general community health promotion and health education and advocate for school and community policies that promote regular physical activity and healthier food and drink choices for all youth.[14] In the clinic, physicians and other primary health care professionals can promote universal public health messages that encourage daily physical activity, increased consumption of fruits and vegetables, reduced consumption of sweetened beverages, and reduced screen time (ie, ≤ 2 hours a day) for all youth and families. The early identification of childhood obesity through the universal assessment of body mass index (BMI) is another important clinical activity. Nonjudgmental communication of BMI assessment to parents along with appropriate counseling on nutrition, physical activity, and weight control should occur, especially because evidence has shown that diabetes may be delayed or prevented by lifestyle intervention in at-risk individuals.[14] Monitoring for the comorbidities and complications of type 2 diabetes is a vital secondary prevention activity that will be discussed later in the article.

CLINICAL MANAGEMENT OF TYPE 2 DIABETES IN INDIGENOUS YOUTH

As in primary prevention, the guiding principles of diabetes care for indigenous youth with type 2 diabetes must be individualized, family-centered, interprofessional, and comprehensive, to include care, surveillance, education, advocacy, and psychosocial and emotional support. The focus of diabetes care in indigenous youth is lifestyle modification. Therapeutic plans must be individualized to identify enablers of and barriers to treatment that exist in the physical, emotional, and psychosocial environment of the youth, family, school, and community.

There have been many published consensus statements and review papers on the treatment of type 2 diabetes in children. The clinical report published in 2003 by the American Academy of Pediatrics (AAP) Committee on Native American Child Health and the AAP Section on Endocrinology provides the only guideline that addresses the unique needs of indigenous youth with type 2 diabetes.[14] It was largely based on a previous consensus guideline published by the American Diabetes Association in 2000.[49] The Canadian Pediatric Society Committee on First Nations and Inuit Health published a formal statement on prevention of type 2 diabetes in First Nation children but stopped short of making recommendations on treatment of type 2 diabetes.[50] The Canadian Diabetes Association published a clinical practice guideline in 2008 related to type 2 diabetes in children, with special mention of indigenous youth.[23] The International Society of Pediatric and Adolescent Diabetes published a general consensus guideline regarding the treatment of type 2 diabetes in 2008, but without any specific reference to unique ethnic populations.[51]

There is no systematic review available yet on any treatment modality for type 2 diabetes in youth. This section evaluates the evidence published since the AAP 2003 guidelines to support or challenge the current AAP consensus guidelines on the treatment of type 2 diabetes in youth. This section also explores why there continues to be much opinion on the treatment of type 2 diabetes in youth but very little evidence on which to base therapeutic decisions, including in indigenous youth (see **Table 2**).

GOALS OF THERAPY

The consensus is that the overall goals of therapy for youth with type 2 diabetes should include adequate metabolic control with a target glycated hemoglobin (Hb[A1c]) less than or equal to 7% and prevention of long-term microvascular and macrovascular complications. To achieve these broad goals, the specific goals of therapy should be to promote weight loss and the maintenance of a healthy weight, to normalize

Table 2
Key recommendations for issues relating to type 2 diabetes in indigenous children

Intervention	Recommendation (See Text for Further Explanation)	Recommendation GRADE	Quality of Supporting Evidence
General			
Screening and case finding	Indigenous youth who have entered puberty or who are aged 10 years or older should be screened for type 2 diabetes biannually if they have 2 or more risk factors	Strong	Low[14,23]
Primary prevention	Encourage exclusive breastfeeding for at least the first 2 months of life	Strong	Low[39]
	Promote regular physical activity and healthy food and drink choices	Strong	Low[14,23]
Clinical Management			
Access	In indigenous youth with type 2 diabetes, all youth and their families must have access to diabetes care, education, counseling, and support from diabetes teams with expertise in working with vulnerable adolescent populations with chronic disease	Strong	Low[23,54]
Glycemic control	The use and frequency of blood glucose monitoring should be individualized based on the need for insulin and level of motivation for self-care	Strong	Low[49]
	Lifestyle education with community support should be offered as the focus of self-management. The optimal dose and frequency of daily physical activity is unknown	Strong	Low[54]

For those youth with an A1c in the 7%–9% range, intensive lifestyle modification (without the addition of pharmacologic agents) may be considered	Strong	Low
For those youth with DKA or an A1c level>9%, insulin should be used. The optimum insulin regime must be individualized. The insulin can be discontinued after 2–3 months once metabolic targets are achieved	Strong	Low[60]
For those youth with A1c level 7%–9% at diagnosis, metformin may be the first drug of choice to add to the lifestyle management	Strong	Moderate[62]
Microvascular Complications		
Screen for neuropathy at diagnosis and annually thereafter	Strong	Low[79]
Screen for nephropathy at diagnosis and annually thereafter	Strong	Low[12,82,83]
Screen for retinopathy at diagnosis and annually thereafter	Strong	Low[81,86]

From Canadian Diabetes Association Clinical Practice Guidelines Expert Committee. Canadian Diabetes Association 2008 clinical practice guidelines for the prevention and management of diabetes in Canada. Can J Diabetes 2008;32(suppl 1):S1–201; with permission.

blood glucose levels, to normalize other metabolic abnormalities, and to promote the normal physical and emotional well-being of the youth.

DIABETES EDUCATION FOR THE YOUTH, FAMILY, AND COMMUNITY

The content and delivery system of diabetes education will require customization for each clinical setting and region. Over 10 years ago in obese Pima Indian adults, the "Pima Action" group who were given conventional structured interventions related to physical activity and nutrition were compared with the "Pima Pride" group, given unstructured activities emphasizing Pima history and culture. An important lesson for health professionals, communities, and families is that metabolic outcomes after 12 months were superior in the "Pima Pride" group.[52]

The choice of primary care versus specialty care for indigenous youth with type 2 diabetes depends on the expertise, experience, and comfort level of the primary health care team in the community.[53] The advantages of pediatric specialty care include access to comprehensive surveillance of comorbidities and experience with complex adolescent issues, consistent long-term care, group workshops, multi-media age-appropriate education resources, and case coordination with other pediatric consultants, in disciplines such as nephrology. The pediatric diabetes team usually includes pediatricians, nurse educators, nutrition educators, exercise specialists, social workers, or psychologists. Medical social workers with expertise in working with diverse and vulnerable pediatric populations are essential for indigenous youth with type 2 diabetes, especially those affected by severe poverty and family break-down. The advantages of community-based primary care include culturally appro-priate, family-centered care, liaison with community primary prevention activities, reduced cost of travel, and seamless transition to adult care. Awareness of the chal-lenges of diabetes care by community leaders is highly variable so that a shared care model with outreach pediatric specialty clinics may be optimal, especially when the community primary care staff is consistent and comfortable with treatment of type 2 diabetes. Comprehensive communication systems are required between specialty care, primary care, school, and community groups.

School and community leaders need clear simple messages about lifestyle management of type 2 diabetes, specifically about the importance of frequent unstructured and structured physical activity, healthy eating, and avoidance of sugar-containing beverages.

When possible, an immediate diagnosis and classification of type 2 diabetes using clinical criteria is necessary to avoid confusion and mixed messages about type 1 and type 2 diabetes for the family, community, and staff. Educational content must be adapted to the level of education required for the family, because the content depends on the initial presentation, the comorbidities, and the treatment modality. All families require comprehensive education about intensive lifestyle modification. Some require education at diagnosis about oral diabetes drugs or insulin. All require general educa-tion about oral health and foot care. The girls must receive contraception and precon-ception counseling. Health professionals must allow time for families to share their personal stories about the effect of diabetes on their family. The use of traditional medicines and advice from traditional healers in some communities must be respected.

Annual influenza and pneumococcal vaccine are recommended for adults with type 2 diabetes due to invasive pneumococcal disease, especially pneumonia. However there is no evidence of increased hospitalization or death from influenza- related complications or pneumococcal disease in youth with type 2 diabetes. Because some indigenous youth with type 2 diabetes live in communities where active tuberculosis is found, the diabetes team must be familiar with the local public health tuberculosis surveillance program.

Family-centered care, support, and education must involve parents or guardians, siblings, and in many cases, grandparents, because of the importance of extended families and familial relationships in indigenous communities. In Canada, the importance of family-centered care and education is not always recognized by government agencies responsible for travel grants and escorts for indigenous youth living in remote communities. The diabetes team may need to advocate strongly for family-centered education.

GLYCEMIC MONITORING

Most diabetes consensus statements recommend capillary blood glucose monitoring (BGM) as an integral component of diabetes self-care, specifically for self-monitoring and feedback on progress and for safety in those on insulin or on the oral drugs that cause hypoglycemia. There is no evidence to indicate that BGM motivates adults with type 2 diabetes not requiring insulin to improve self-care.[23] The question must also be asked whether youth with type 2 diabetes managed without drug therapy benefit from monitoring blood glucose levels. Most guidelines indicate individualization of BGM.[23,49]

BODY WEIGHT MANAGEMENT AND LIFESTYLE MODIFICATION

The Indian Health Service, Division of Diabetes Treatment and Prevention, published an excellent Best Practice document in 2006 on the nonpharmacologic treatment and prevention of type 2 diabetes in youth outlining the requirement for a focus on community, health care organizations, delivery systems for health and health care, decision support for families, and clinical informatics systems for tracking outcomes in a chronic disease framework.[54] There is a Cochrane systematic review on the treatment of obesity in children.[55] Most youth with type 2 diabetes are obese and older than 10 years.[49] This section is not an exhaustive review of the treatment of obesity in youth. However, family counseling, psychological support, medical surveillance, and treatment of the obesity in youth with type 2 diabetes must be included in all management strategies.

Experts differ on the benefit of lifestyle alone in achieving glycemic targets in obese youth with type 2 diabetes. The earliest report of improved glycemic control with intensive lifestyle modification in an indigenous youth was in the summer camp environment and was published 20 years ago.[56] Other successful camp experiences have provided evidence of the benefit of intensive lifestyle interventions. The Wellness Camp for Indian youth with diabetes was started in 1991 by the Native American Research and Training Centre of the University of Arizona.[57] The annual weeklong camp accommodates 30 youth aged between 10 and 15 years.[58] Many camp and recreational programs for youth do not allow clinical research, and thus, the long-term outcomes from these community efforts do not appear in the medical literature. There have been many tribal and community-based programs funded by the Indian Health Service in the United States and the Aboriginal Diabetes Initiative of Health Canada that target youth with or at risk of type 2 diabetes and support healthy living programs in the community. The evaluation of these programs is not sufficiently rigorous for publication. There are at least 3 registered clinical trials that specifically address the necessary intensity and frequency of physical activity on type 2 diabetes in youth.[59]

In the absence of ketosis or DKA and an A1c level of 7% to 9% at diagnosis, the optimal duration and intensity of lifestyle modification alone is unknown and must be individualized. The use of lifestyle alone for an A1c level of 7% to 9% at diagnosis will remain controversial until there is more evidence of effectiveness.

PHARMACOLOGIC AND SURGICAL THERAPY OF HYPERGLYCEMIA

In indigenous youth with type 2 diabetes who initially present with ketosis, DKA, and an A1c level greater than 9%, short-term insulin use can be successful.[60] The optimal dose, type, and regimen of insulin are unknown. An experienced pediatric diabetes team will be comfortable in addressing myths about insulin in indigenous families and working effectively with adolescents on realistic short-term timelines and therapeutic goals on insulin. After achieving therapeutic goals on short-term insulin, many youth are able to maintain glycemic targets without further drug therapy for at least a year.[60] In the SEARCH study, 24% or 59 of 257 youth were American Indian and 43% of youth with type 2 diabetes were taking insulin.[61]

In symptomatic indigenous youth with type 2 diabetes and an A1c level of 7% to 9%, metformin is considered by many practitioners as the first drug of choice. Metformin is not approved for use in youth in all countries. The evidence to support metformin is limited to a single international multi-center double-blind randomized placebo-controlled study in youth with type 2 diabetes that showed a reduction in fasting blood glucose of 44 mg/dL (2.4 mmol/L) over 16 weeks.[62] There were many limitations to this study[63]; recruitment was difficult, randomization was offered at diagnosis without assessment of the impact of lifestyle modification, rescue criteria were very stringent, rescue was to metformin without an intention-to-treat analysis, and finally, a greater number of subjects randomized to placebo had a baseline fasting blood glucose greater than 200 mg/dL (11 mmol/L). Adherence has been in the range of 50% in most studies of metformin in youth. There have been no safety concerns. The effect of metformin on blood glucose levels may be delayed by several weeks, and thus, there is theoretical rationale for starting combined therapy with insulin and then weaning the patient off insulin as the fasting blood glucose levels improve.

The Treatment Options for Type 2 Diabetes in Adolescents and Youth (TODAY) study in the USA is the only registered active randomized controlled trial comparing metformin with and without intensive lifestyle modification and rosiglitazone.[64] It includes 17 of 850 (2%) American Indian children. Recruitment is complete and results available in 2011. There is no intensive lifestyle modification alone arm even for subjects with A1c level in the range of 6% to 9%.

Pharmacokinetic data are available to inform future intervention studies of pioglitazone in youth with type 2 diabetes,[68] but there is no clinical trial of this drug in youth with type 2 diabetes currently published or registered. Elevated liver enzyme levels in youth with type 2 diabetes is a relative contraindication and may limit the use of this class of drugs in this age group. As of May 2009, there were other registered clinical trials to study rosiglitazone, orlistat (Xenical), sitagliptin, glyburide, and incretin analogues in youth with type 2 diabetes.[59]

Experience with bariatric surgery in youth with morbid obesity and type 2 diabetes is limited to a few sites with expertise in this procedure. The first retrospective case series of bariatric surgery in 11 adolescents and young adults (<21 years of age, mean 17.8 years) with type 2 diabetes from 5 academic pediatric centers in the United States was recently published.[65] The youth demonstrated significant decrease in BMI from a mean of 50.4 to 33.2 kg/m^2 and A1c level from a mean of 7.33% to 5.58% in follow-up of at least 1 year. These preliminary results are encouraging for the extremely obese cases, but more evidence of efficacy and long-term outcomes is necessary.

There is an active prospective study of surgical outcomes at 5 pediatric centers in the USA (Teen-Longitudinal Assessment of Bariatric Surgery [Teen-LABS], 2009).

There have been no RCTs on the safety or efficacy of traditional medicines or alternative health products. Although several studies have been published in the United States on the use of traditional medicines and traditional healing by AI and AN adults with type 2 diabetes,[66,67] the authors are unaware of any published studies on their use by indigenous youth with type 2 diabetes.

PERSPECTIVES ON THE CHALLENGES OF TREATMENT OF TYPE 2 DIABETES IN INDIGENOUS YOUTH

The reasons for the lack of evidence of effective treatment relate to the major challenges of recruitment and retention of all youth with type 2 diabetes for large clinical trials. The relative rarity of the condition necessitates multi-centre studies to achieve adequate sample size. The frequent presence of metabolic comorbidities, such as fatty liver disease, is a relative contraindication to many oral medications. Unprotected sexual activity and risk of pregnancy is a contraindication to oral diabetes medications in adolescent girls. Practical barriers such as remote place of residence, concomitant chronic illness in the parents or guardians, and other social disrupters may also negatively affect recruitment and retention. The challenges of conducting clinical trials in youth with type 2 diabetes have resulted in the "off-label" use of drugs, further limiting the availability of drug-naïve subjects. The existence of many large robust studies and systematic reviews of the treatment of type 2 diabetes in adults has resulted in an "indication creep" with the use of drug treatment in youth with type 2 diabetes.[68]

However, many pediatricians argue that youth with type 2 diabetes are not small adults with type 2 diabetes and rigorous clinical trials are necessary in this age group. The International Agreement for Harmonization of new drug approval that mandates adequate efficacy studies in children before approval for adults is critical for drugs for type 2 diabetes.[69] The perception of body image and the impact of having type 2 diabetes and chronic disease is different in youth. They do not have measurable cardiovascular outcomes or events, which necessitates the use of surrogate outcomes, such as HbA1c. Youth have dynamic growth and pubertal changes and unique age-related pharmacokinetics. In addition, many indigenous youth have a higher rate of underlying primary renal disease that may further affect pharmacokinetics of the drugs (see later discussion on comorbid conditions).

The clinical approach to type 2 diabetes in youth varies widely.[21,70–72] Strong opinions and biases, different clinical settings and populations, composition and experience of the pediatric team working with youth with type 2 diabetes, and lifestyle interventions are some of the factors that may explain the current wide variation in clinical practice and the initial treatment modalities for youth with type 2 diabetes.

MICROVASCULAR COMPLICATIONS AND COMORBIDITIES

The history of type 2 diabetes in youth is short and thus there is limited data related to short- and long-term complications and associated comorbidities in this population. However, comorbidity is common at diagnosis and long-term microvascular complications have been described at diagnosis and early in the disease course.[73] The Canadian Diabetes Association has recently published screening guidelines for complications and comorbidities in youth with type 2 diabetes (**Table 1**).[23] A recently published systemic review of global complication rates in indigenous people was based primarily on adult populations.[74]

Short-Term Complications

DKA

DKA in youth with type 2 diabetes has been reported with rates of up to 25% at presentation of diabetes.[73] The SEARCH study reported a rate of 9.7% DKA at diagnosis of type 2 diabetes.[75] This report included 56 American Indians. In a Canadian First Nation population, 11% of youth with type 2 diabetes had an episode of DKA, 4.2% of these at diagnosis of diabetes.[29]

Hyperglycemic hyperosmolar state

The hyperglycemic hyperosmolar state (HHS) is an acute life-threatening emergency recently described in children. In pediatrics, HHS is seen as a distinct clinical entity and in combination with DKA. High rates of morbidity and mortality have been reported.[76] HHS in children is associated with significant complications including rhabdomyolysis, shock, pancreatitis, and malignant hyperthermia.[73] Given the relative lack of experience in pediatrics, optimal treatment regimes have not yet been established. Most of the reports of HHS have been in African American or Canadian First Nation youth.[77,78]

Long-Term Complications

Neuropathy

In an Australian population, peripheral neuropathy was seen in 21% of youth with type 2 diabetes (15% of this group with type 2 diabetes were of Aboriginal or Torres Strait Islander descent).[79] In contrast, no cases of neuropathy were detected in a larger cohort of First Nation children with type 2 diabetes, although the prevalence of toenail abnormalities was high.[80] End-stage neuropathy with lower extremity amputation has been described in First Nation young adults diagnosed with type 2 diabetes in childhood.[81]

Nephropathy/albuminuria

Microalbuminuria may be present at the time of diagnosis of type 2 diabetes in youth. At diagnosis of type 2 diabetes, 22% of Pima Indian youth and 14% of Maori youth and young adults (younger than 30 years) had albuminuria.[12,82] In a report by Eppens and colleagues,[79] 28% of youth with type 2 diabetes had microalbuminuria with a median duration of 1.3 years. Fifteen percent of this group was of Australian Aboriginal or Torres Strait Islander descent. Fifty-eight percent of Maori and Pacific Island youth with type 2 diabetes had micro- or macroalbuminuria within 5 year of diagnosis.[11] Progression also seems to be rapid, with 62% of Maori youth progressing to micro- or macroalbuminuria within 10 years of diagnosis. Similarly, 58% of Pima Indians diagnosed with youth-onset type 2 diabetes had microalbuminuria within 10 years.[82] In a Canadian First Nation population, 16% of youth with type 2 diabetes had macroalbuminuria within 8 years of diagnosis.[83]

Many indigenous populations are also at increased risk for nondiabetic, congenital or acquired renal disease.[68,84,85] The relative contribution of nondiabetic renal disease to the development of albuminuria in indigenous youth with type 2 diabetes is not fully understood. In a recent report of Canadian First Nation youth with type 2 diabetes, biopsy results of 10 individuals with macroalbuminuria revealed immune complex disease or glomerulosclerosis in 9 of 10, and in 2 of 10, mild diabetes-related lesions were also seen. Focal segmental glomerulosclerosis, an obesity-related comorbidity, was found in 7 of 10.[83]

Retinopathy

Retinopathy has been reported in youth with type 2 diabetes early in the disease course. In a population of predominantly Maori or Pacific Islander youth and young adults aged 25 years or younger with type 2 diabetes, 4% had background retinopathy and another 4% had sight-threatening retinopathy.[86] In the Pima Indian population, the rate of retinopathy was lower in those diagnosed with type 2 diabetes in childhood compared with those diagnosed as adults. In the Pima, retinopathy was not seen before 20 years of age.[87] However, blindness before 30 years of age has been described in Canadian First Nation young adults with youth-onset type 2 diabetes.[81]

Intrauterine exposure to type 2 diabetes—the next generation
Intrauterine exposure to type 2 diabetes is a determinant, in addition to genetic factors, of youth-onset type 2 diabetes.[88] In the Pima Indian population of the southwestern United States, youth born after their mothers were diagnosed with type 2 diabetes have a greater risk of development of type 2 diabetes at an early age compared with their siblings born before their mother's diagnosis.[88] Similar findings have been reported in Canadian First Nation youth, where intrauterine exposure to pregestational diabetes was identified as a significant predictor of type 2 diabetes before 18 years of age.[40] Thus, the risk of type 2 diabetes in offspring can be considered to be a long-term complication in women diagnosed with youth-onset type 2 diabetes.

Co-morbidities

Dyslipidemia
The incidence of dyslipidemia in youth with type 2 diabetes ranges from 15% to 62.5%[73] and is more frequent than in youth with type 1 diabetes.[89] This wide variance may reflect differences in the definitions of dyslipidemia used in individual reports. Dyslipidemia was reported in 18% of Pima Indian youth at diagnosis of type 2 diabetes, increasing to 30% within 10 years of diagnosis.[82] In a report of New Zealand Maori and Pacific Islander youth with type 2 diabetes, 85% had abnormal lipid levels with a duration of diabetes less than 5 years.[11] In Canadian First Nation youth with type 2 diabetes, an atherogenic profile of increased total cholesterol, triglycerides, and apolipoprotein B was found in 65% to 75% and a decreased high-density lipoprotein cholesterol in 51%.[90]

Hypertension
Hypertension is common in youth with type 2 diabetes.[73] In Maori and Pacific Islander youth with type 2 diabetes of less than 5 years duration, 28% had systolic hypertension.[11] In another report of Maori youth and young adults (diagnosed at <30 years of age), 39% had hypertension within 10 years of diagnosis.[12] In Canadian First Nation youth with type 2 diabetes, 12% had either systolic or diastolic hypertension with a mean duration of diabetes of just over 2 years.[90]

Fatty liver
In a report of 39 youth from San Diego with type 2 diabetes, alanine aminotransferase (ALT) or aspartate aminotransferase (AST) were twice the upper limit of normal in 23% and 3 times the upper limit of normal in 8%.[91] Seven children had liver biopsies (including 3 boys of AI heritage). All 7 had pathologic evidence of fatty liver disease. Elevated transaminase levels were also common among Canadian First Nation youth with type 2 diabetes. In a report of 49 children, ALT was twice the upper limit of normal in 22%, greater than 3 times the upper limit of normal in 16%, and AST and ALT were greater than 3 times the upper limit of normal in 6%.[92]

Polycystic ovarian syndrome
There are several small reports of adolescents with polycystic ovarian syndrome (PCOS) that include 1 or 2 youth with type 2 diabetes.[73] To the authors' knowledge, there are no reports of this comorbidity in indigenous youth.

Psychiatric illness/quality of life

An increased frequency of neuropsychiatric disorders (19.4%) was found at diagnosis in a non-indigenous, mixed ethnic group of 237 youth with type 2 diabetes.[93] In a population of Canadian First Nation youth with type 2 diabetes, an increased frequency of hospital admission was noted compared with youth with type 1 diabetes. This report identified psychiatric illness with suicidal ideation as the most common cause for hospitalization in youth with type 2 diabetes.[94]

Health-related quality of life was lower for youth with type 2 diabetes compared with those with type 1 diabetes in the SEARCH study.[61] American Indians comprised 23.9% of the youth with type 2 diabetes in this report. No ethnic differences in quality of life were reported. In a study of Canadian First Nation youth with type 2 diabetes, youth from northern remote communities and those witnessing diabetes complications in family members had a lower reported health-related quality of life compared with youth without these exposures.[95]

Yeast vaginitis

Type 2 diabetes predisposes adult women to vulvovaginal candidiasis that can be severe.[96] Anecdotally, the authors have seen yeast vulvovaginitis severe enough to precipitate hospital admission in new-onset type 2 diabetes in Canadian First Nation girls.

SUMMARY

Youth-onset type 2 diabetes presents a serious concern to the health of indigenous youth and their families and communities, and it is leading to increased morbidity and mortality during adulthood. Primary prevention efforts are of utmost importance. Secondary prevention with screening of at risk youth and screening for complications and comorbidities in affected youth are important to improve the outcomes of these vulnerable youth.

Treatment of type 2 diabetes in youth is complex. Traditional RCTs may not be the appropriate methodology for evaluating the different modalities of treatment of type 2 diabetes in youth. For complex problems, a single intervention is unlikely to be successful for every individual in every setting. It is likely to require multiple customized context-specific improvement strategies. For this to happen, collaborative efforts involving health care professionals, public health experts, policy makers, community leaders, and affected youth will be necessary.

The challenges that must be addressed by those caring for these youth and their families are (1) the complexity of treatment, (2) the coordination of health care services among many primary and specialty care and community-based health professionals, (3) the motivational skills required to achieve significant changes in health behavior, (4) the lack of a strong evidence base for the prevention and treatment of youth-onset type 2 diabetes, and (5) the provision of cross-cultural health services to indigenous youth and families in a context of extreme poverty and social injustice.

It is hoped that new evidence from clinical trials and the efforts of indigenous community empowerment initiatives around diabetes prevention and living well with diabetes improves the lives of indigenous youth with type 2 diabetes.

REFERENCES

1. Acton KJ, Burrows NR, Moore K, et al. Trends in diabetes prevalence among American Indian and Alaska native children, adolescents, and young adults. Am J Public Health 2002;92(9):1485–90.

2. Alberti G, Zimmet P, Shaw J, et al. Type 2 diabetes in the young: the evolving epidemic: the international diabetes federation consensus workshop. Diabetes Care 2004;27(7):1798–811.

3. Dabelea D, Hanson R, Bennett P, et al. Increasing prevalence of Type 2 diabetes in American Indian children. Diabetologia 1998;41:904–10.

4. Dean HJ, Sellers EAC, Young TK. Type 2 diabetes in youth in Manitoba, Canada, 1986–2002. Can J Diabetes 2003;27(4):449–54.

5. Fagot-Campagna A, Pettitt DJ, Engelgau MM, et al. Type 2 diabetes among North American children and adolescents: an epidemiologic review and a public health perspective. J Pediatr 2000;136(5):664–72.

6. Pinhas-Hamiel O, Zeitler P. The global spread of type 2 diabetes mellitus in children and adolescents. J Pediatr 2005;146(5):693–700.

7. Center for Disese Control. Diagnosed diabetes among American Indians and Alaska Natives aged <35 years - United States. MMWR Morb Mortal Wkly Rep 2006;55(44):1201–3.

8. Dean H, Young T, Flett B, et al. Screening for type-2 diabetes in aboriginal children in northern Canada. Lancet 1998;352:1523–4.

9. Harris SB, Gittelsohn J, Hanley A, et al. The prevalence of NIDDM and associated risk factors in native Canadians. Diabetes Care 1997;20(2):185–7.

10. Braun B, Zimmermann MB, Kretchmer N, et al. Risk factors for diabetes and cardiovascular disease in young Australian aborigines. A 5-year follow-up study. Diabetes Care 1996;19(5):472–9.

11. Hotu S, Carter B, Watson PD, et al. Increasing prevalence of type 2 diabetes in adolescents. J Paediatr Child Health 2004;40(4):201–4.

12. McGrath NM, Parker GN, Dawson P. Early presentation of type 2 diabetes mellitus in young New Zealand Maori. Diabetes Res Clin Pract 1999;43(3):205–9.

13. Mayer-Davis EJ, Bell RA, Dabelea D, et al. The many faces of diabetes in American youth: type 1 and type 2 diabetes in five race and ethnic populations: the SEARCH for Diabetes in Youth Study. Diabetes Care 2009;32(Suppl 2):S99–101.

14. Gahagan S, Silverstein J. Prevention and treatment of type 2 diabetes mellitus in children, with special emphasis on American Indian and Alaska Native children. American Academy of Pediatrics Committee on Native American Child Health. Pediatrics 2003;112(4):e328.

15. Pavkov ME, Bennett PH, Knowler WC, et al. Effect of youth-onset type 2 diabetes mellitus on incidence of end-stage renal disease and mortality in young and middle-aged Pima Indians. JAMA 2006;296(4):421–6.

16. Dabelea D, Knowler WC, Pettitt DJ. Effect of diabetes in pregnancy on offspring: follow-up research in the Pima Indians. J Matern Fetal Med 2000;9(1):83–8.

17. Pettitt DJ, Bennett PH, Saad MF, et al. Abnormal glucose tolerance during pregnancy in Pima Indian women. Long-term effects on offspring. Diabetes 1991; 40(Suppl 2):126–30.

18. Hu FB, Stampfer MJ, Haffner SM, et al. Elevated risk of cardiovascular disease prior to clinical diagnosis of type 2 diabetes. Diabetes Care 2002;25(7): 1129–34.

19. Rosenbloom AL, Baldwin E, Silverstein JH. Type 2 diabetes in children and adolescents: a guide to diagnosis, epidemiology, pathogenesis, prevention, and treatment. Alexandria (VA): American Diabetes Association; 2003.

20. Yokoyama H, Okudaira M, Otani T, et al. High incidence of diabetic nephropathy in early-onset Japanese NIDDM patients. Risk analysis. Diabetes Care 1998; 21(7):1080–5.

21. Dabelea D, DeGroat J, Sorrelman C, et al. Diabetes in Navajo youth: prevalence, incidence, and clinical characteristics: the SEARCH for Diabetes in Youth Study. Diabetes Care 2009;32(Suppl 2):S141–7.
22. American Diabetes Association. Diagnosis and classification of diabetes mellitus. Diabetes Care 2009;32(Suppl 1):S62–7.
23. Canadian Diabetes Association Clinical Practice Guidelines Expert Committee. Canadian diabetes association clinical practice guidelines for the prevention and management of diabetes in Canada. Type 2 diabetes in children. Can J Diabetes 2008;32:S162–7.
24. Dean H. Diagnostic criteria for non-insulin dependent diabetes in youth (NIDDM-Y). Clin Pediatr 1998;37:67–79.
25. Dabelea D, Pettitt DJ, Jones KL, et al. Type 2 diabetes mellitus in minority children and adolescents. An emerging problem. Endocrinol Metab Clin North Am 1999; 28(4):709–29.
26. Craig ME, Femia G, Broyda V, et al. Type 2 diabetes in Indigenous and non-Indigenous children and adolescents in New South Wales. Med J Aust 2007;186(10): 497–9.
27. Search for Diabetes in Youth Study Group. The burden of diabetes mellitus among US youth: prevalence estimates from the SEARCH for Diabetes in Youth Study. Pediatrics 2006;118:1510–8.
28. Moore KR, Harwell TS, McDowall JM, et al. Three-year prevalence and incidence of diabetes among American Indian youth in Montana and Wyoming, 1999 to 2001. J Pediatr 2003;143(3):368–71.
29. Sellers EA, Dean HJ. Diabetic ketoacidosis: a complication of type 2 diabetes in Canadian aboriginal youth. Diabetes Care 2000;23(8):1202–4.
30. Hathout EH, Thomas W, El-Shahawy M, et al. Diabetic autoimmune markers in children and adolescents with type 2 diabetes. Pediatrics 2001;107(6): E102.
31. Sellers E, Eisenbarth G, Young TK, et al. Diabetes-associated autoantibodies in aboriginal children. Lancet 2000;355(9210):1156.
32. Center for Disease Control. The cost-effectiveness of screening for type 2 diabetes. CDC Diabetes cost-effectiveness study group, Centers for disease control and prevention. JAMA 1998;280(20):1757–63.
33. American Diabetes Association. Screening for type 2 diabetes. Diabetes Care 2004;27(Suppl 1):S11–4.
34. Dannenbaum D, Torrie J, Noel F, et al. Undiagnosed diabetes in two Eeyou Istchee (eastern James Bay Cree) communities: a population-based screening project. Can J Diabetes 2005;29(4):397–402.
35. Dean H. What are the screening recommendations for type 2 diabetes in Canadian children. Paediatr Child Health 2009;14(2):73–4.
36. Fagot-Campagna A, Saaddine JB, Engelgau MM. Is testing children for type 2 diabetes a lost battle? Diabetes Care 2000;23(9):1442–3.
37. Gillies CL, Abrams KR, Lambert PC, et al. Pharmacological and lifestyle interventions to prevent or delay type 2 diabetes in people with impaired glucose tolerance: systematic review and meta-analysis. BMJ 2007;334(7588):299.
38. Knowler WC, Barrett-Connor E, Fowler SE, et al. Reduction in the incidence of type 2 diabetes with lifestyle intervention or metformin. N Engl J Med 2002; 346(6):393–403.
39. Pettitt DJ, Forman MR, Hanson RL, et al. Breastfeeding and incidence of non-insulin-dependent diabetes mellitus in Pima Indians. Lancet 1997;350(9072): 166–8.

40. Young TK, Martens PJ, Taback SP, et al. Type 2 diabetes mellitus in children: prenatal and early infancy risk factors among native canadians. Arch Pediatr Adolesc Med 2002;156(7):651–5.

41. Davis SM, Going SB, Helitzer DL, et al. Pathways: a culturally appropriate obesity-prevention program for American Indian schoolchildren. Am J Clin Nutr 1999;69(4 Suppl):796S–802S.

42. Hood VL, Kelly B, Martinez C, et al. A native American community initiative to prevent diabetes. Ethn Health 1997;2(4):277–85.

43. Macaulay AC, Paradis G, Potvin L, et al. The Kahnawake schools diabetes prevention project: intervention, evaluation, and baseline results of a diabetes primary prevention program with a native community in Canada. Prev Med 1997;26(6):779–90.

44. Paradis G, Levesque L, Macaulay AC, et al. Impact of a diabetes prevention program on body size, physical activity, and diet among Kanien'keha:ka (Mohawk) children 6 to 11 years old: 8-year results from the Kahnawake Schools Diabetes Prevention Project. Pediatrics 2005;115(2):333–9.

45. Saksvig BI, Gittelsohn J, Harris SB, et al. A pilot school-based healthy eating and physical activity intervention improves diet, food knowledge, and self-efficacy for native Canadian children. J Nutr 2005;135(10):2392–8.

46. Story M. School-based approaches for preventing and treating obesity. Int J Obes Relat Metab Disord 1999;23(Suppl 2):S43–51.

47. Teufel NI, Ritenbaugh CK. Development of a primary prevention program: insight gained in the Zuni Diabetes Prevention Program. Clin Pediatr (Phila) 1998;37(2):131–41.

48. Available at: www.ihs.gov/medicalprograms/diabetes. Accessed June 1, 2009.

49. American Diabetes Association. Consensus statement: type 2 diabetes in children and adolescents. Diabetes Care 2000;23(3):381–9.

50. First Nations and Inuit Health Committee. Canadian pediatric society. Risk reduction for type 2 diabetes in Aboriginal children in Canada. Paediatr Child Health 2005;10(1):49–52.

51. Rosenbloom AL, Silverstein JH, Amemiya S, et al. ISPAD Clinical Practice Consensus Guideline 2006–2007. Type 2 diabetes mellitus in the child and adolescent. Pediatr Diabetes 2008;9(5):512–26.

52. Narayan KM, Hoskin M, Kozak D, et al. Randomized clinical trial of lifestyle interventions in Pima Indians: a pilot study. Diabet Med 1998;15(1):66–72.

53. Dean HJ, Moffatt M. Care of Aboriginal children with type 2 diabetes: a head-to-head debate regarding the roles of the primary specialty team and the primary health care team. Can J Diabetes 2000;24:28–33.

54. Indian Health Service. Youth and type 2 diabetes. Albuquerque, New Mexico: Indian Health Service; 2006.

55. Oude Luttikhuis H, Baur L, Jansen H, et al. Interventions for treating obesity in children. Cochrane Database Syst Rev 2009;(1):CD001872.

56. Anderson K, Dean HJ. The effect of diet and exercise on a native youth with poorly controlled NIDDM. Beta Release 1990;14:105–6.

57. Joe JR, Frishkopf S. I'm too young for this!: diabetes and American Indian Children. In: Ferreira ML, Lang GC, editors. Indigenous peoples and diabetes: community empowerment and wellness. Durham, North Carolina: Carolina Academic Press; 2006. p. 435–56.

58. Available at: www.nartc.fcm.arizona.edu/diabetes_camp. Accessed June 1, 2009.

59. Available at: www.clinicaltrials.gov. Accessed June 1, 2009.

60. Sellers EA, Dean HJ. Short-term insulin therapy in adolescents with type 2 diabetes mellitus. J Pediatr Endocrinol Metab 2004;17(11):1561–4.
61. Naughton MJ, Ruggiero AM, Lawrence JM, et al. Health-related quality of life of children and adolescents with type 1 or type 2 diabetes mellitus: SEARCH for Diabetes in Youth Study. Arch Pediatr Adolesc Med 2008;162(7):649–57.
62. Jones KL, Arslanian S, Peterokova VA, et al. Effect of metformin in pediatric patients with type 2 diabetes: a randomized controlled trial. Diabetes Care 2002;25(1):89–94.
63. Dean HJ. Dancing with many different ghosts: treatment of youth with type 2 diabetes. Diabetes Care 2002;25(1):237–8.
64. Zeitler P, Epstein L, Grey M, et al. Treatment options for type 2 diabetes in adolescents and youth: a study of the comparative efficacy of metformin alone or in combination with rosiglitazone or lifestyle intervention in adolescents with type 2 diabetes. Pediatr Diabetes 2007;8(2):74–87.
65. Inge TH, Miyano G, Bean J, et al. Reversal of type 2 diabetes mellitus and improvements in cardiovascular risk factors after surgical weight loss in adolescents. Pediatrics 2009;123(1):214–22.
66. Buchwald D, Beals J, Manson SM. Use of traditional health practices among Native Americans in a primary care setting. Med Care 2000;38(12):1191–9.
67. Kim C, Kwok YS. Navajo use of native healers. Arch Intern Med 1998;158(20):2245–9.
68. Pinhas-Hamiel O, Zeitler P. Clinical presentation and treatment of type 2 diabetes in children. Pediatr Diabetes 2007;8(Suppl 9):16–27.
69. International Committee on Harmonization. Clinical investigation of medicinal products in the pediatric population. Available at: www.ich.org/LOB/media/MEDIA487.pdf. Accessed May 25, 2009.
70. Grinstein G, Muzumdar R, Aponte L, et al. Presentation and 5-year follow-up of type 2 diabetes mellitus in African-American and Caribbean-Hispanic adolescents. Horm Res 2003;60(3):121–6.
71. Silverstein JH, Rosenbloom AL. Treatment of type 2 diabetes mellitus in children and adolescents. J Pediatr Endocrinol Metab 2000;13(Suppl 6):1403–9.
72. Zuhri-Yafi MI, Brosnan PG, Hardin DS. Treatment of type 2 diabetes mellitus in children and adolescents. J Pediatr Endocrinol Metab 2002;15(Suppl 1):541–6.
73. Pinhas-Hamiel O, Zeitler P. Acute and chronic complications of type 2 diabetes mellitus in children and adolescents. Lancet 2007;369(9575):1823–31.
74. Naqshbandi M, Harris SB, Esler JG, et al. Global complication rates of type 2 diabetes in Indigenous peoples: A comprehensive review. Diabetes Res Clin Pract 2008;82(1):1–17.
75. Rewers A, Klingensmith G, Davis C, et al. Presence of diabetic ketoacidosis at diagnosis of diabetes mellitus in youth: the Search for Diabetes in Youth Study. Pediatrics 2008;121(5):e1258–66.
76. Rosenbloom AL. Hyperglycemic comas in children: new insights into pathophysiology and management. Rev Endocr Metab Disord 2005;6(4):297–306.
77. Pediatric Death Review Committee: Office of the Chief Coroner of Ontario. Rapid onset of coma and death in the initial presentation of type 2 diabetes in an 11-year old child. Paediatr Child Health 2007;2007(12):41–2.
78. Dean H, Sellers E, Kesselman M. Acute hyperglycemic emergencies in children with type 2 diabetes. Paediatr Child Health 2007;12(1):43–4.
79. Eppens MC, Craig ME, Cusumano J, et al. Prevalence of diabetes complications in adolescents with type 2 compared with type 1 diabetes. Diabetes Care 2006;29(6):1300–6.

80. Chuback J, Embil JM, Sellers E, et al. Foot abnormalities in Canadian Aboriginal adolescents with Type 2 diabetes. Diabet Med 2007;24(7):747–52.
81. Dean H, Flett B. Natural history of type 2 diabetes diagnosed in childhood: long term follow-up in young adult years. Diabetes 2002;51(Suppl 2):A24.
82. Fagot-Campagna A, Knowler WC, Pettit DJ. Type 2 diabetes in Pima Indian children: cardiovascular risk factors at diagnosis and 10 years later. Diabetes 1998; 47(Suppl 1):A155.
83. Sellers EA, Blydt-Hansen TD, Dean HJ, et al. Macroalbuminuria and renal pathology in First Nation youth with type 2 diabetes. Diabetes Care 2009;32(5): 786–90.
84. Bulloch B, Postl BD, Ogborn MR. Excess prevalence of non diabetic renal disease in native American children in Manitoba. Pediatr Nephrol 1996;10(6): 702–4.
85. Hoy WE, Megill DM, Hughson MD. Epidemic renal disease of unknown etiology in the Zuni Indians. Am J Kidney Dis 1987;9(6):485–96.
86. Scott A, Whitcombe S, Bouchier D, et al. Diabetes in children and young adults in Waikato Province, New Zealand: outcomes of care. N Z Med J 2004;117(1207): U1219.
87. Krakoff J, Lindsay RS, Looker HC, et al. Incidence of retinopathy and nephropathy in youth-onset compared with adult-onset type 2 diabetes. Diabetes Care 2003;26(1):76–81.
88. Dabelea D, Hanson RL, Lindsay RS, et al. Intrauterine exposure to diabetes conveys risks for type 2 diabetes and obesity: a study of discordant sibships. Diabetes 2000;49(12):2208–11.
89. Kershnar AK, Daniels SR, Imperatore G, et al. Lipid abnormalities are prevalent in youth with type 1 and type 2 diabetes: the SEARCH for Diabetes in Youth Study. J Pediatr 2006;149(3):314–9.
90. Sellers EA, Yung G, Dean HJ. Dyslipidemia and other cardiovascular risk factors in a Canadian First Nation pediatric population with type 2 diabetes mellitus. Pediatr Diabetes 2007;8(6):384–90.
91. Newfield R, Schwimmer J. Non-alcoholic steatohepatitis in children and adolescents with type 2 diabetes mellitus. Diabetes 2003;52(Suppl 1):A404.
92. Dean H, Sellers E. Steatohepatitis in children with type 2 diabetes mellitus. Diabetes 2001;50(Suppl):A378.
93. Levitt Katz LE, Swami S, Abraham M, et al. Neuropsychiatric disorders at the presentation of type 2 diabetes mellitus in children. Pediatr Diabetes 2005;6(2): 84–9.
94. Coish RMP, Dean HJ. Admissions to hospital of children with type 1 and type 2 diabetes in Manitoba 2004–2006. Paediatr Child Health 2008;13(Suppl A).
95. Allan CL, Flett B, Dean HJ. Quality of life in First Nation youth with type 2 diabetes. Matern Child Health J 2008;12(Suppl 1):103–9.
96. Bohannon BVJ. Treatment of vulvovaginal candidiasis in patients with diabetes. Diabetes Care 1998;21(3):451–6.

Behavioral and Mental Health Challenges for Indigenous Youth: Research and Clinical Perspectives for Primary Care

Michael Storck, MD[a],*, Timothy Beal, MD[b],
Jan Garver Bacon, MSW, PhD[c], Polly Olsen, BA[d]

KEYWORDS

- Indigenous youth • Behavioral and mental health
- Evidence-based practice • Transgenerational trauma
- Community-based participatory research

...I cured with the power that came through me. Of course it was not I who cured...
—Black Elk[1]

The social and political forces that have been exerted on Indigenous communities worldwide for many generations have resulted in profound shifts in Indigenous community structure, family resilience, and overall health. For decades

[a] Division of Child and Adolescent Psychiatry, Department of Psychiatry and Behavioral Sciences, University of Washington School of Medicine, P.O. Box 359300, Seattle, WA 98195, USA
[b] (Cherokee Tribe) Department of Psychiatry, Strong Memorial Hospital, University of Rochester School of Medicine and Dentistry, 300 Crittenden Boulevard, Rochester, NY 14642, USA
[c] Ketron Cottage, Child Study and Treatment Center, Division of Social and Health Services, State of Washington, 8805 Steilacoom Boulevard, SW, Lakewood, WA 98498, USA
[d] (Yakama Tribe) Indigenous Wellness Research Institute, School of Social Work, University of Washington, Box 354900, 4101 15th Avenue NE, Seattle, WA 98195, USA
* Corresponding author. Division of Child and Adolescent Psychiatry, Department of Psychiatry and Behavioral Sciences, University of Washington School of Medicine, P.O. Box 359300, Seattle, WA 98195.
E-mail address: storck@u.washington.edu (M. Storck).

Pediatr Clin N Am 56 (2009) 1461–1479
doi:10.1016/j.pcl.2009.09.015
0031-3955/09/$ – see front matter © 2009 Elsevier Inc. All rights reserved.

now, leading indicators of psychologic distress among Indigenous[e] youth have shown significantly higher rates of such major challenges as suicidality and substance abuse. As Indigenous peoples have struggled to move beyond painful eras of community disintegration and centuries-long governmental policies that have disrupted families some positive changes are occurring within Indigenous communities and within national governmental and health care initiatives.[2] Reflecting some positive trends internationally for Indigenous societies, during the last 20 years the governments of New Zealand, Canada, and Australia have offered formal apologies to its Indigenous and First Nations peoples for past acts of aggression and social disruption. In 2007, several United States Senators drafted a proposal for an official apology to Native Americans from the United States government. This proposal has not yet made it through the United States Congress.

This article balances acknowledgment of profoundly destabilizing pasts for Indigenous communities with presentation of efforts leading to revitalization. Mental and behavioral health variables are essential factors in the substrate and sustenance of health across childhood and in family and community functioning in general. For the primary care clinician, grounded in the "medical home" model (the American Academy of Pediatrics describes the medical home as a model of delivering primary care that is accessible, continuous, comprehensive, family-centered, coordinated, compassionate, and culturally effective care[3]), working with youth and their families on behavioral and mental health issues is often a richly rewarding, although challenging process. The process of creating successful medical homes can be especially arduous and daunting for providers serving Indigenous communities when those communities have historic legacies of mistrust. This original mistrust has been exacerbated by major demographic and geographic shifts that include the youthfulness of the population, history of out-of-home-placements, and forced or coerced urban migration.

The individual primary care clinician has substantially different tasks caring for an Indigenous child depending on the specific ecologic forces at work in the child's life. Their family and community stories are likely compelling, as may be the case for many families. As one works from a medical home relationship outward, the family's and community's constellation of influences and narratives emerge as potent forces in shaping and defining behavioral and mental health symptomatology including severity of distress and dysfunction. A knowledge base of the research literature should help bolster the clinician's readiness for aligning more comfortably with Indigenous youth, their families, and communities.

---

[e] A note regarding nomenclature. In the United States, Indigenous peoples are often referred to as "American Indian/Alaska Native" or "Native Hawaiian" and some prefer the term "Native American." In Canada, "First Nations" is often the preferred term for Indigenous people. Australians most often refer to their first peoples as "Aborigines." Given the historical legacies and related implications and inevitable shifts in naming, there are no perfect answers for common terminology. This effort to clarify naming conventions is offered in part to sensitize the reader to the inherent difficulties in over-generalization and to encourage a spirit of inquiry with Indigenous patients about their own naming stories and preferences. Patients and their communities experience their own dynamic shifts in naming and changes in attributions connected to specific distress and disease terminology. Naming issues can be pivotal communications and treatment variables in the clinician-patient relationship.[81]

For more than two decades in the United States, initiatives have been gathering momentum to establish culturally competent approaches to serving the mental health needs of Indigenous American communities. Many Native American communities have helped direct and been prime beneficiaries of these efforts. Such centers include (and are referenced in more detail later) the American Indian and Alaska Native Mental Health Research Center in Colorado[4]; One Sky Center in Oregon[5]; the Indigenous Wellness Research Institute in Washington state[6]; the national network of the Native American Research Centers for Health (NARCH)[7]; and the US Public Health Service National Epidemiology Program of the IHS (regional centers throughout the United States).[8]

Similar research institutions have emerged in other nations, including the Kulunga Research Network in Western Australia for Aboriginal Australians[9]; the Winnipeg-based First Nations Research Site, a partnership initiative of the First Nations Child and Family Caring Society of Canada and the Center of Excellence for Child Welfare[10]; and Ngā Pae o te Māramatanga, Maori Institute of Excellence, Auckland, New Zealand.[11] The evolution of fully fledged evidence-based research data regarding Indigenous child and adolescent mental health concerns is in the early stages. Most of the research perspectives presented here derive from programs and practices from the United States with additional findings from Canadian and Pacific Rim studies.

Every tribe and Indigenous community has a unique historical legacy and cultural story that shapes the health of its families and children. Each has endured specific challenges and barriers across the generations of sociopolitical forces. "Colonialization" and "expulsion or annihilation" are some of the categories of complex pernicious influence. Other dynamic metacultural pressures that are disruptive, although perhaps less categorically destructive to communities, include "assimilation" and quests for "pluralism." Marger[12] presents a model for understanding how these processes occur when cultures come into contact, then continue to evolve across generations. This brief foray into anthropology is offered not to unduly complicate the reader's experience but to acknowledge the fundamental sociologic and ecologic[13] underpinnings that drive community progression and ultimately shape specific mental health and behavioral signs and symptoms for Indigenous youth.[14–17]

A literary example of an Indigenous teenager trying to make sense of his people's past is presented in the following excerpt from Alexie's *The Absolutely True Diary of a Part-Time Indian*,[18] in which the young narrator "Junior," whose sister had recently died, discusses his experience after having transferred to an "off-reservation" high school.

> *…I was crying for my tribe…I was crying because I knew five or ten or fifteen more Spokanes would die during the next year, and that most of them would die because of booze.*
>
> *I cried because so many of my fellow tribal members were slowly killing themselves and I wanted them to live. I wanted them to get strong and get sober and get the hell off the rez.*
>
> *It's a weird thing.*
>
> *Reservations were meant to be prisons, you know? Indians were supposed to move onto reservations and die. We were supposed to disappear.*
>
> *But somehow or another, Indians have forgotten that reservations were meant to be death camps.*
>
> *I wept because I was the only one who was brave and crazy enough to leave the rez. I was the only one with enough arrogance.*
>
> *I wept and wept and wept because I knew that I was never going to drink and because I was never going to kill myself and because I was going to have a better life out in the white world.*

As Indigenous peoples of the Americas, Australia, New Zealand, and perhaps worldwide have experienced diverse forces of societal upheaval, there have been common processes that have profoundly influenced family health:

- Transgenerational disruptions in family and community life are cardinal variables shaping past, present, and future individual, family, and community mental and behavioral health. This has been conceptualized as "historical trauma" by leading American Indian psychologists including Evans-Campbell,[19] Walters,[16] Duran and Duran,[15] Brave Heart,[20] and Brave Heart and DeBruyn.[21]
- Forced separation of children from families, including generations of boarding school placements (for some communities, notably in Australia in the mid-twentieth century, this included governmental policy-driven kidnapping of children).[22–25]
- Centuries of diminishment of "original instructions" and principles of community guidance, loss of subsistence living pattern, and of traditional healing practices.[16]
- Indigenous peoples have historically embraced more holistic views of health (seeing physical, mental, spiritual health as interwoven) than is routinely offered in allopathic clinics.[26,27] Recently there has been a resurgence of focus on Indigenous constructs of healing and wellness complementing allopathic practices.[6]
- Although many rural tribal populations are growing, in most countries the population of urban Indigenous peoples has now surpassed the rural population.[f] Health care needs for urban Indigenous families may differ greatly from those for rural and reservation families.

RECENT DIAGNOSTIC AND EPIDEMIOLOGIC FINDINGS

The authors of this article share with others the central bias that transgenerational community traumas have greatly influenced the severity of mental health challenges for Indigenous youth. It is nearly a universal theme for Indigenous peoples that disruption, dislocation, disconnection, and at times destruction of kinship ties has occurred. For many the deleterious influences continue to extend across generations. Brave Heart and coworkers[20,21] conceptualize historical trauma as a major generative factor in a multiplicity of emotional, cognitive, and behavioral symptom clusters.

Historical trauma (HT) is cumulative emotional and psychological wounding over the lifespan and across generations, emanating from massive group trauma experiences; the historical trauma response (HTR) is the constellation of features in reaction to this trauma. The HTR often includes depression, self-destructive behavior, suicidal thoughts, and gestures, anxiety, low self-esteem, anger, and difficulty recognizing and expressing emotions. It may include substance abuse, often as an attempt to avoid painful feelings through self-medication.

---

[f] The line between "voluntary" and "involuntary" migrations has often been blurred. For example, in the United States, The Relocation Act of 1956[28] provided funding to establish job training centers for American Indians in various urban centers, and to finance the relocation of individual Indians and Indian families to these locales. It was coupled to a denial of funds for similar programs and economic development on the reservations themselves. Those who availed themselves of the opportunity for jobs represented by the federal relocation programs were usually required to sign agreements that they would not return to their respective reservations to live. The result, by 1980, was a diaspora of Native Americans, with more than half of the 1.6 million Indians in the United States having been scattered to cities across the country. Today, in the United States approximately two thirds American Indians and Alaska Natives live in urban areas.

The research literature is strongest in documenting an increased prevalence of behavioral symptom sets, such as those labeled as "disruptive behavior problems." The term "disruptive behavior" may refer to conduct dysregulation, anxiety responses, attentional and anger management problems, and some substance abuse behaviors. Whitbeck and colleagues[29,30] found a longitudinal increase in prevalence rates of substance abuse and conduct disorders during adolescence among First Nations youth in Canada. They noted that the lifetime conduct disorder rate was twice that of the general population. Interestingly, Whitbeck's study, suggesting transgenerational "transmission," also found that youth whose mothers had higher rates of depression were markedly more likely to have disruptive behavior problems. Andrade and colleagues[31] discovered significantly higher rates of anxiety and depressive disorders for Native Hawaiian youth. Studies by Costello and colleagues,[32,33] Duclos and colleagues,[34] and Beals and colleagues[35,36] provide compelling general prevalence data in line with the preceding studies. Research perspectives looking at the prevalence of common childhood mental health disorders, such as depression, posttraumatic stress disorder, and attention deficit–hyperactivity disorder, however, are lacking with regards to prevalence rates for specific Indigenous and tribal populations.

Indigenous youth, as a composite group, face increased incidences of severe distress including suicidality and substance dependence. The US Public Health Service–Indian Health Service (IHS) has tracked these concerns for decades. The most recent published IHS Trends (2000–2001)[37] depicts strikingly heightened suicide and substance abuse related death rates for Native youth. For American Indian and Alaska Native youth, the suicide rate is 3.3 times the national United States aggregate rate. The alcohol-related death rates for the same comparison groups are 10 times the United States national aggregate. Beautrais and Fergusson[38] report from New Zealand that young Maori males were almost three times more likely and young Maori females were twice as likely to die by suicide as their non-Maori counterparts. Blaire and coworkers[39] and Zubrick and colleagues[40] reporting on the results of the Western Australian Aboriginal Child Health Survey noted that Aboriginal youth were 50% more likely to have "clinically significant emotional or behavioral difficulties" than their non-Aboriginal counterparts. To underscore the added relative risk contributed by generational trauma, the subset of Aboriginal youth, whose primary caregivers as children were forcibly separated from their own natural families, had a rate of severe difficulties that was 50% higher than their Aboriginal cohorts whose primary caregivers did not experience such separation.[41] A hopeful example of community resilience in the face of transgenerational trauma is provided by Costello and colleagues[42] in the Great Smoky Mountain Study. They followed a population of American Indian youth and families across a decade when, because of new tribal enterprises, tribal income and employment dramatically improved. During this interval, a clinically significant decrease in psychiatric symptomatology was noted for youth in families who had moved out of poverty.

This limited database may help give a broad view of the topography of behavioral symptomatology for Indigenous youth. Even if the database were more robust and comprehensive, however, the generalization of findings to diverse tribal communities (and indeed across regions of the world) is problematic. In the United States alone there are over 500 federally recognized tribes, each with its own historical, cultural, demographic, and health risk profiles. For example, regional differences between tribes within the United States for such indicators as suicide rates may vary as much as 400%.[43]

PRIMARY CARE AND COMMUNITY PERSPECTIVES ON RESEARCH

Children of any age or culture cannot be defined or adequately understood by their diagnoses alone (psychiatric or otherwise). Furthermore, evidence is growing regarding the long-term primary health implications of early life psychosocial challenges. For example, Bullock and Bell[44] note the link between early life psychosocial instability and heightened risk in later life for arthritis and cardiovascular disease. Heim and colleagues[45] also delineate, with elegance and precision, the emerging database on the appreciable impact of early life psychosocial challenges on neurophysiologic development. Primary care providers are in a central position to effectively describe and address the complex behavioral health challenges of youth, and as such are likely to have a more holistic view of a child's psychosocial health path. For many children, cultural and specific developmental differences, learning disabilities, dyslexia, autism, and medical problems are deeply interwoven with psychosocial variables. For instance, a child exposed to early life oral health problems, such as baby-bottle tooth decay, are likely at heightened risk for chronic mouth pain, dentition and nutritional problems, and self-image, anxiety, attention regulation and learning difficulties in grade school, and possibly lifelong challenges with inflammatory diseases. Likewise, a teenager with type II diabetes and obesity may be at heightened susceptibility for oppositionality, dysthymia, depression, and substance abuse. A primary care clinician's treatment plan when caring for such a child is of necessity complex. The plan cannot be reduced to a standard set of medical or psychiatric interventions. These kinds of health challenges call for sophisticated collaborations between a variety of health, educational, and social service providers and require solutions that are community-based. Research data for defining and intervening in such health problems is even less developed than for more categorically defined psychiatric problems.

In Indigenous communities, mistrust of the agendas of "researchers from the outside" is a common hurdle to the development of effective research projects. Health providers and academics entering communities with the best intentions still bring their own complex hopes and agendas to such underserved communities. Clinicians eager to support research in the communities in which they practice can find guidance in the American Academy of Pediatrics Policy Statement: "Ethical considerations in research with socially identifiable populations." This document, developed by the American Academy of Pediatrics Committee on Native American Child Health,[46] offers pragmatic suggestions for researchers that underscore the primary importance of appreciating a community's own understandings of potential beneficence and risk for a particular project.

In the last two decades, particularly with the establishment of the Native research centers mentioned previously, Indigenous communities have been offered and now actively initiate roles in defining behavioral and mental health research needs. Many such projects have established new ground in delineating research emphases that combine traditional principles of community organization and Native constructs of health and wellness with current academic research methodologies. To accomplish this fusion, Community-based participatory research (CBPR) has emerged as an often preferred research approach that positions a community team in a leadership role in research that addresses health problems that beset their community.[47–51] CBPR is seen by Indigenous communities as an empowering approach to understanding and addressing their health issues.

CBPR is committed to working from a community's strengths. Its priorities include establishing trust and seeking holistic solutions. This approach challenges academic and community partners to invest in team building, resource sharing, and an exchange of hypotheses related to illness and wellness constructs and criteria for optimal outcomes. For Indigenous communities, CBPR generates data that inform scientists and practitioners and also provides community partners with perspectives that enhance their ability to reduce health disparities and promote health. This approach makes more likely the affirmation of effective traditional practices, the validation of what some tribes call "original" or "first" instructions for health, and their complementary interweaving with Western science-based knowledge.

MANAGEMENT STRATEGIES AND RESOURCES

With historical, prevalence, and community perspectives presented, the call for research-based practice guidelines for pediatric behavioral and mental health for Indigenous youth must be answered. This section provides practical summaries of evidence-based strategies and presents tools for individual practice and community collaboration. The following perspectives are explored: (1) brief review of evidence-based practice (EBP) mental health interventions for child psychiatry, (2) presentation of EBP mental health interventions specific to Indigenous youth, and (3) research centers addressing Indigenous mental health.

EBP is the operative phrase for quality interventions that have scientific support for their effectiveness. As evidence aggregates from multiple research studies, showing efficacy of a particular intervention, the practitioner's confidence in the intervention rises. Applications across various settings, which produce like results and meet statistical or clinical significance, further support practitioners in use of the intervention. This process gradually may be seen as higher order validation of a therapeutic practice when compared with what was offered by past generations of practitioners. Shipman and Taussig[52] describe what constitutes EBP as "well designed, randomized clinical trials using outcomes that are tied to specific treatments." They further state that EBP incorporates as "core nonspecific factors" the importance of the relationship between patient and practitioner, "clinician interpersonal skills, and common codes of good practice and professional ethics."

EBP: General Pediatric Psychiatric Research Literature

Compared with the rest of pediatric practice, the research database for behavioral and mental health interventions for youth is regarded as rather limited. Most child psychiatric practice is not yet well vetted by the EBP literature. Risk assessment issues, informed consent challenges, ethical concerns, and the complexity of variables when studying child mental health are some factors complicating the process of establishing EBPs. McClellan and Werry[53] provide a thoughtful benchmark summary of evidence-based treatments in child and adolescent psychiatry across psychopharmacologic and psychosocial modalities. In their review, very few treatment strategies have risen to a compelling level of evidence. For illustration purposes, several of those that reach the level of "best practices" are (1) use of stimulant medications for treatment of attention deficit–hyperactivity disorder (more than 160 randomized control studies have validated the use of stimulants); (2) use of the serotonin-specific reuptake inhibitors for treating obsessive-compulsive disorder (the US Food and Drug Administration has approved three serotonin-specific reuptake inhibitors for use in pediatric obsessive-compulsive disorder and other anxiety disorders); (3) cognitive-behavioral therapy for depression and anxiety disorders (supported by more than a dozen randomized control trials); (4) parent training interventions for oppositional youth; and (5) multisystemic therapy for conduct disorder.

These strategies, and others described in detail by McClellan and Werry,[53] have the best evidence bases for youth in general. Not incidentally, these are the same treatment strategies that are often recommended and implemented as part of interventions with Indigenous children. McVoy and Findling[54] also provide an extensive up-to-date review of best practices in pediatric psychopharmacology. The American Academy of Child and Adolescent Psychiatry has developed practice parameters for a range of child psychiatric diagnoses and clinical challenges.[55] These tools offer the primary care clinician a guide to multimodal treatment approaches and evidence-based strategies. Additionally, recent EBP literature particularly relevant to addressing the most prominent psychiatric challenges for Indigenous youth includes growing support for the following specific therapeutic approaches: trauma-focused cognitive behavioral therapy[56] (for posttraumatic stress disorder and depression); parent child interactive therapy[52] (for parents overwhelmed by childrearing challenges); dialectical behavioral therapy[57] (for suicidal youth); and motivational interviewing[58,59] (for substance abuse prevention). As of yet, there are no completed studies of the use of these specific modalities with Indigenous youth.

EBP: Indigenous Youth Specific

The database for EBP research treatment strategies for behavioral and mental health problems facing Indigenous youth is quite limited. Gone and Alcantara[60] provide a rich reference point to begin a survey of evidence-based mental health practices for American Indian and Alaska Native populations. In summarizing the existing literature on treatment outcomes for mental health interventions directed specifically toward American Indians and Alaskan Natives children and adults, they reviewed 56 research articles and review chapters, of which only nine studies assessed outcomes under scientifically controlled conditions, and only two studies were deemed as adhering to the standards of an EBP. Their article highlights the dearth of empirically assessed treatments for American Indian and Alaskan native peoples suffering from mental illness and makes a compelling argument for more rigorous evaluations in this population.

Using PubMed, PsycINFO, Google, and other search engine databases the authors gathered available formal research articles regarding interventions with Indigenous youth within the last 25 years. Keywords applied in searches included a range of terms identifying origins of youth, such as Native Americans, Aboriginal, First Nations, American Indian and Alaska Native, Maori, and Indigenous combined with common behavioral, mental health, and substance use disorder terminology. The results are presented in **Table 1**.

DISCUSSION

In the research literature compiled in **Table 1**, only one psychopharmacologic intervention study was identified that selectively focused on Indigenous youth. This study, by Oesterheld and colleagues,[61] assessed the short-term effectiveness and side effects of methylphenidate in treating symptoms of attention deficit–hyperactivity disorder in four American Indian children (5–12 years old) in residential care with documented fetal alcohol syndrome or partial fetal alcohol syndrome. This was a randomized double-blind cross-over study using two placebos and a fixed dose of methylphenidate. Methylphenidate correlated with significant improvement in hyperactivity symptoms but not in some measures of inattentiveness. This study had a commendable EBP design and is consistent with data from the general child and adolescent population but given its very small sample size has limited generalizability to the larger population of American Indian youth.

Table 1
Evidence-based practice: research regarding mental health treatment for indigenous children and adolescents

Focus of Treatment	Intervention	Grading of Recommendation	Quality of Supporting Evidence
For attention deficit–hyperactivity disorder in children with comorbid fetal alcohol syndrome	Methylphenidate	Strong	High (Oesterheld and colleagues, 1998[61])
For adolescent posttraumatic stress disorder and depression	Manualized cognitive behavioral therapy group	Strong	High (Morsette, 2009[62]; Stein, 2003[63])
To prevent substance abuse and dependency	Individual and group skills-based prevention programs	Strong	High (Hawkins, 2004[64]; Gilchrist, 1987[65])
To prevent substance abuse and dependency	Skills-enhancement prevention approaches	Strong	High (Schinke, 2000[66])
To prevent substance abuse and dependency	Health promotion program	Weak	Moderate (Cheadle, 1995[71])
To prevent substance abuse and dependency	Multicultural evidence-based drug prevention curriculum	Weak	Low (Dixon, 2007[67])
For suicide prevention	Risk and protective factor identification	Strong	High (Middlebrook, 2001[68])
To remediate the behavioral and cognitive correlates of suicide	Generalizeable culturally tailored social cognitive development intervention program	Strong	High (LaFromboise and Lewis, 2008[69])
Prevention of antisocial behavior in children	Early intervention program students, teachers, and parents	Strong	Moderate (Diken and Rutherford, 2005[70])
To foster infant mental health	Parent skills training	Strong	Moderate (Walkup, 2009[51])

The search yield for psychosocial intervention studies was more expensive and includes a variety of individual and group interventions. Morsette and colleagues[62] studied a reservation-based cohort of American Indian adolescents who presented with symptoms of posttraumatic stress disorder and depression. These symptoms decreased for three of the four students who completed a 10-week, school-based, manualized cognitive and behavioral therapy group. Stein and colleagues[63] also used a manualized 10-week school-based cognitive behavioral therapy group to treat Hispanic and American Indian sixth graders who presented with symptoms of posttraumatic stress disorder and depression. After 3 months, the intervention group had significantly lower scores on symptoms of posttraumatic stress disorder, depression, and psychosocial dysfunction, but not in acting out, shyness and anxiousness, or learning problems, when compared with a (no intervention) wait-list delayed-intervention group.

In a review article by Hawkins and colleagues,[64] strong support was shown for individual and group skills-based substance abuse prevention programs for American Indian youth, but limited support for community- and peer-based educational efforts, reinforcing the evidence for the effectiveness of skills based practices (eg, cognitive-behavioral therapies). Best practice approaches cited by Hawkins included (1) conceptualizing behavior change and prevention on a continuum and using stage of change interventions, (2) stepped-care based on needs and success of prior interventions, (3) biculturally focused life skills curriculum, and (4) collaboration with communities based on readiness and resources.

Schinke and coworkers[66] developed and tested skills and community-based approaches to prevent substance abuse among American Indian youth. Over the course of this 3.5-year study, increased rates of tobacco, alcohol, and marijuana use were reported by youths across the three arms of the study. Although cigarette use was unaffected by intervention, follow-up rates of smokeless tobacco, alcohol, and marijuana use were lower for youths who received skills intervention than for youth in the control arm. Community intervention components seemed to exert no added beneficial influence on youths' substance use, beyond the impact of skills intervention components alone.

A culturally tailored 10-session skills enhancement program was delivered to American Indian adolescents in reservation and nonreservation settings.[65] At 6-month follow-up, intervention subjects had better knowledge of drug effects; better interpersonal skills for managing pressures to use drugs; and lower rates of alcohol, marijuana, and inhalant use. Intervention subjects were also less likely to consider themselves users of these substances.

The effectiveness of a 5-year community-based health promotion program to reduce the rate of substance use by American Indian adolescents on a reservation was examined by Cheadle and colleagues.[71] Adolescents from other Community Health Promotion Grants Program communities (including a small sample of rural American Indians) were used as a basis for comparison. Use of both alcohol and marijuana declined substantially among adolescents living on the reservation; however, there were similar declines in alcohol use in the comparison groups. Because there was no evidence of a relative increase in exposure to alcohol and drug programs on the reservation, the authors were cautious in attributing the significant declines in substance use to the community-based program.

Dixon and colleagues[67] evaluated effects of a multicultural evidence-based drug prevention curriculum with a sample of urban American Indian youth in the southwest United States. Alcohol and marijuana use increased for all youth but drug use by the American Indian group indicated a steeper rise in the amount and frequency of alcohol and marijuana use compared with the youths with other racial and ethnic identifications.

Middlebrook and colleagues[68] reviewed nine suicide prevention programs serving American Indian and Alaska Native youth. None of the programs reviewed had evidence that the targeted risk factors or protective factors mitigated suicide or suicidal behaviors. Further, only a few programs provided sociodemographic variables that would help identify risk factors. Only one program actually identified a specific research design with comparison group. Three tracked suicide rates. This review highlights the importance of identifying risk factors in indigenous populations that accurately predict morbidity outcomes, such as suicide and parasuicidal behavior.

The Zuni Life Skills Development curriculum, a culturally tailored suicide prevention program, was designed as a model of social cognitive development. This curriculum was offered to students for remediation of behavioral and cognitive correlates of suicide.[72] Assessment of this program showed that students completing the curriculum scored better than the no-intervention group at posttest on suicide probability and hopelessness but not depression.[69] This was considered a model program by the US Substance Abuse and Mental Health Services Administration.

In a 2005 study, Diken and Rutherford[70] examined the effectiveness of the First Step to Success early intervention program with four American Indian students, their teachers, and their parents. The First Step to Success program had a significant positive affect on all participant students' social play behaviors; social play behaviors significantly increased and nonsocial behaviors decreased. Substantial decreases in problem behaviors were also reported by two teachers. All but one parent reported significant changes in problem behaviors of targeted students.

A recent promising study, based on CBPR principles, looked at infant mental health. Walkup and colleagues[51] randomized expectant American Indian women aged 12 to 22 years to one of two paraprofessional-delivered, home-visiting interventions: the 25-visit "Family Spirit" intervention, which addressed prenatal and newborn care and maternal life skills (treatment); and an alternative 23-visit breast-feeding and nutrition education intervention (active control). The interventions began during pregnancy and continued to 6 months postpartum. At 6 and 12 months postpartum, treatment mothers compared with control mothers had greater parenting knowledge gains. At 12-months postpartum, treatment mothers reported that their infants had significantly lower scores on the externalizing domain and less separation distress. No between-group differences were found for maternal involvement; home environment; or mothers' stress, social support, depression, or substance use.

The previously described research represents significant beginnings in contributing to the knowledge base regarding work with Indigenous youth. The strong evidence for the benefits of skills training curricula for youth (who are experiencing a variety of behavioral, mental health, and substance abuse problems) represents a unifying theme of the successful research practices to date.[63,65,66,69,70] Although the scarcity of rigorous EBP reports may lead some to conclude that little is known regarding effective mental health treatment of Indigenous people, there is a relative wealth of information already extant in descriptive, cross-sectional, and ethnographic publications. Although EBP is limited, there are nonetheless rich and clinically useful experience-based practice perspectives available from many authors including allopathic and traditional Indigenous medicine practitioners, and from others who have made it their life's work to know and participate in the life of Indigenous communities both in rural and urban settings.[27,73–75] Although participation in traditional Native healing practices and ceremonies is prevalent alongside biomedical services in many tribal communities, there have not yet been any research studies published that assess outcomes for Indigenous youth engaged in such practices.[76]

Specific Research Programs Dedicated to Indigenous Health

To address the need for more evidence-based research (including for traditional healing methods) for American Indian and Alaskan Native and other Indigenous populations worldwide, the last two decades have witnessed the establishment of many research consortiums, epidemiologic centers, and academic institutions dedicated to improving Indigenous mental health. Many states and regions sponsor programs that have given rise to health promotion and disease prevention programming. Also, in the last decade the IHS inaugurated a network of epidemiology centers focused on advancing health research. There are now 12 centers nationwide.[7] Also, many states have launched their own centers for biobehavioral health and prevention research and have sponsored projects to improve Indigenous health. One example of this is the Zuni Health Lifestyles program supported by the state of New Mexico and the IHS.[77] There are well-established institutes worldwide to help clinician-scientists appreciate current Indigenous health research programming and projects.[9–11] A brief description of several nationally prominent programs in the United States is offered next.

The NARCH established in 2002, is a collaborative research program coordinated by the IHS and the National Institute of General Medical Sciences of the US National Institutes of Health.[7] NARCH initiative supports partnerships between tribally based health institutions and academic centers that conduct biomedical, behavioral, and health services research. Current NARCH efforts regarding pediatric populations include juvenile justice, youth suicide prevention, tobacco prevention and pulmonary diseases, prenatal alcohol exposure, CBPR, contextual issues in traditional healing, and the development of an ethnomedical encyclopedia.

The National Center for American Indian and Alaska Native Mental Health Research,[4] based at the University of Colorado, is one of four minority mental health research centers sponsored by the US National Institute of Mental Health. Its mission includes research, training, information dissemination, and technical assistance. Since 1987, The National Center has sponsored a professionally refereed scientific journal, *American Indian and Alaska Native Mental Health Research: The Journal of the National Center*. National Center consultants have provided technical assistance and research mentorship for the US Substance Abuse and Mental Health Services Administration Circles of Care program since its inception. Through the Circles of Care program[78] 19 American Indian and Alaska Native communities have designed and implemented their own community-specific projects bringing sophisticated research methodologies to bear on community-identified community-wide behavioral and mental health challenges. Many grantees have used CPBR principles. The entire edition of its April 2004 journal is devoted to describing the Circles of Care projects.[79]

The One Sky Center at the Oregon Health Sciences University[5] is a national resource center whose mission is to improve prevention and treatment of mental health and substance abuse problems and services among Native people. The One Sky Center guides the development of projects, publications, and training manuals for model programs serving Native communities (eg, the recently published on-line training manual "Motivational Interviewing: Enhancing Motivation for Change-A Trainer's Manual for the American Indian/Alaska Native Counselor").[80]

The Indigenous Wellness Research Institute[6] (IWRI) is a research and program development partnership between the Schools of Social Work and Public Health at the University of Washington and with national and international Indigenous health organizations. IWRI has a leadership role in the International Network of Indigenous Health Knowledge and Development Program. IWRI's vision statement, "To support the inherent rights of Indigenous peoples to achieve full and complete health and wellness by collaborating in decolonizing research and knowledge building and sharing," is exemplified by their recently completed HONOR project, which surveyed the impact of historical trauma on the health and wellness of Native lesbian, gay, transgendered, and "two-spirited" men and women.

Box 1
Orientational strategies

Strategies for thriving as a scientist-practitioner

1. Learn the tribal community's story (including subtexts)

2. Locate the nearby research support centers (include urban Indian centers, state departments of health, and so forth)

3. Appreciate the resource structure of the local community (find out how health, education, welfare, cultural, religious, and political organizations work)

4. Think ethnographically and ecologically[81,82]

5. Investigate historical and modern community strengths and wellness practices

6. Take a long-term view; appreciate how difficult it can be for patients, families, and communities to change

Resilience strategies for the participant-observer

1. Patiently learn the local "language" for greetings, social discourse, signs of respect, and taboos

2. Establish partnerships with community mentors and outside advisors (allopathic, traditional, and complementary)

3. Seek to appreciate the complex kinship grids to which your patients belong, such as generational roles including expectations and obligations; multiple current affiliation zones, which particularly apply to adolescents, including peer cohort (eg, traditional, school, church, sports, "gang") and family, clan, and tribe; other person-specific social kinships; and your own kinship experiences

4. Work to find out "what matters most" for your patients, your coworkers, and yourself; cultivate healing zones that allow context to emerge and narratives to flow

5. Be aware that providers and patients have different vantage points from which to view clinical truths and presenting concerns; through "the eye of the beholder," seek to understand special attributions and meaning offered by patient, family, and community team[83,84]

6. Value and pursue full coinvestigator partnerships with patients

7. Be available to be invited to meetings, powwows, naming ceremonies, potlatches, and more; in keeping with maintaining your own serenity, show up

8. Continue what you already know are your own effective self-care practices[85]

9. Take breaks (step back)

Although the preceding listing is not all-inclusive, it does provide options for Web entry and inquiry points to guide the clinician to up-to-date action zones for national, regional, and local research and best-practice implementations for Indigenous communities. Awareness of the offerings from these centers should complement EBP perspectives and boost practitioners' momentum for medical home-centered practice for individual children and families.

PRACTICAL APPLICATIONS

Clinicians serving Indigenous youth, families, and communities are at once scientist-practitioners and participant-observers, and must also be primary stewards of their own resilience. Maintaining teamwork and clinical focus when providing complex medical home (including mental health) supports for youth and families can be a rewarding and daunting process. The following guide-points (**Box 1**) may largely be self-evident but nonetheless are offered as summary orientational strategies for the clinical calling that is medical practice in Indigenous communities.

In closing, a return to Junior's narrative[18]:

> *...I realize that I might be a lonely Indian boy, but I was not alone in my loneliness. There were millions of other Americans who had left their birthplaces in search of a dream.*
>
> *I realized that, sure, I was a Spokane Indian. I belonged to that tribe. But I also belonged to the tribe of American immigrants. And to that tribe of basketball players and that tribe of bookworms....*
>
> *And that tribe of teenage boys.*
> *And the tribe of small town kids...*
> *And the tribe of tortilla chips-and-salsa lovers.*
> *And the tribe of poverty.*
> *And the tribe of funeral-goers.*
> *And the tribe of beloved sons.*
> *And the tribe of boys who really missed their best friends.*
> *It was a huge realization.*
> *And that's when I knew I was going to be okay.*
> *But it also reminded me of the people who were not going to be okay...*
>
> —Junior, the narrator

SUMMARY

Addressing the mental health and substance abuse health problems of children and adolescents lies at the heart of any healthy modern community. Given the pervasiveness and complexity of health and identity challenges for contemporary Indigenous youth, their families, and communities the need for redoubled efforts is truly and tragically urgent for Indigenous peoples worldwide. Failure to confront these difficulties perpetuates the hindrances to community well-being for the present population and also for generations to come. The sort of community-based sea change that is needed is evolving but cannot be successfully accomplished by any single provider group, governmental policy, or single generation of programs or people.

Clinicians of many backgrounds, substance abuse professionals, traditional healers, tribal leaders, educators, religious leaders, many other groups, and, most importantly, the youth and their families themselves must together solve these health care dilemmas and challenges. Essential to this mission is the enduring pursuit of multidisciplinary community-specific evidence-based research practices and promising approaches. Primary health care providers, for each child and for the community as a whole, serve from the core of this quest.

> *I think I have told you, but if I have not, you must have understood, that a man who has a vision is not able to use the power of it until after he has performed the vision on earth for the people to see.*
>
> —Black Elk[1]

ACKNOWLEDGMENTS

The authors gratefully acknowledge the editorial assistance of Susan Storck, MD, and Victor Storm, MD.

REFERENCES

1. Neihardt JG. Black Elk speaks: being the life story of a holy man of the Oglala Sioux. Albany (NY): State University of New York Press; 2008. p. 163.
2. Theirry J, Brenneman G, Rhoades E, et al. History, law, and policy as a foundation for health care delivery for American Indian and Alaska Native children. Pediatr Clin North Am 2009;56(6):1539–59.
3. American Academy of Pediatrics. Available at: http://www.medicalhomeinfo.org/. Accessed May 15, 2009.
4. American Indian and Alaska Native Mental Health Research Center. Available at: http://aianp.uchsc.edu/ncaianmhr/ncaianmhr_overview.htm. Accessed May 15, 2009.
5. One Sky Center. Available at: http://www.oneskycenter.org/. Accessed May 15, 2009.
6. Indigenous Wellness Research Center. Available at: http://www.iwri.org. Accessed May 31, 2009.
7. Native American Research Centers for Health (NARCH). Available at: http://www.ihs.gov/medicalprograms/research/narch.cfm. Accessed May 31, 2009.
8. Listing of the 12 national Indian Health Service Epidemiology Centers. Available at: http://www.npaihb.org/epicenter/other_epicenters/. Accessed June 2, 2009.
9. The Kulunga Research Network in Western Australia for Aboriginal Australians. Available at: http://www.ichr.uwa.edu.au/kulunga/research/current_research. Accessed June 9, 2009.
10. First Nations Research Site (FNRS) is a partnership initiative of the First Nations Child & Family Caring Society of Canada and the Centre of Excellence for Child Welfare. Available at: http://www.fncfcs.com/projects/FNRS.html. Accessed June 9, 2009.
11. Maori youth research: Ngā Pae o te Māramatanga, Maori Institute of Excellence, Auckland, New Zealand. Available at: http://www.maramatanga.co.nz. Accessed June 9, 2009.
12. Marger MN. Race and ethnic relations: American and global perspectives. 3rd Edition. Belmont (CA): Wadsworth; 1994.
13. Bronfenbrenner U, editor. Making human beings human: bioecological perspectives on human development. Thousand Oaks (CA): Sage Publications; 2005.
14. Langford RA, Ritchie J, Ritchie J. Suicidal behavior in a bicultural society: a review of gender and cultural differences in adolescents and young persons of Aotearoa/New Zealand. Suicide Life Threat Behav 1998;28(1):94–106.
15. Duran E, Duran B. Native American postcolonial psychology. Albany (NY): State University of New York Press; 1995.
16. Walters KL. Historical trauma, Dis-placement, Dis-ease and well-being of indigenous women. Fourth Annual Women's Symposium International Women's Day, March 6, 2007, Fordham Institute for Women & Girls, New York, New York, Fordham University.
17. Walters KL, Simoni JM. Decolonizing strategies for mentoring American Indians and Alaska Natives in HIV and mental health research. Am J Public Health 2009;99(Suppl 1):S71–6 [Epub 2009 Feb 26].
18. Alexie S. The absolutely true diary of a part-time Indian. New York: Little Brown; 2007. p. 226–7.
19. Evans-Campbell T. Historical trauma in American Indian/Native Alaska communities: a multilevel framework for exploring impacts on individuals, families, and communities. J Interpers Violence 2008;23(3):316–38.
20. Brave Heart MY. The historical trauma response among natives and its relationship with substance abuse: a Lakota illustration. J Psychoactive Drugs 2003;35(1):7–13.

21. Brave Heart MY, DeBruyn LM. The American Indian Holocaust: healing historical unresolved grief. Am Indian Alsk Native Ment Health Res 1998; 8(2):56–78.
22. Australian Human Rights Commission. Bringing them home: the stolen children report 1997. Available at: http://www.hreoc.gov.au/social_justice/bth_report/index.html. Accessed July 14, 2009.
23. Dinges NG, Duong-Tran Q. Suicide ideation and suicide attempt among American Indian and Alaska Native boarding school adolescents. Am Indian Alsk Native Ment Health Res Monogr Ser 1994;4:167–82 [discussion: 182–8].
24. Robin RW, Rasmussen JK, Gonzalez-Santin E. Impact of childhood out-of-home placement on a Southwestern American Indian tribe. J Hum Behav Soc Environ 1999;2(1–2):69–89.
25. Child B. Boarding school seasons: American Indian families, 1900–1940. Lincoln (NE): University of Nebraska Press; 1998.
26. Roubideaux Y. Cross-cultural aspects of mental health and culture-bound illness. In: Galloway JA, Goldberg BW, Alpert JA, editors. Primary care of native Americans: diagnosis, therapy and epidemiology. Boston: Butterworth; 1999. p. 269–72.
27. Peete WF. Native healing: four sacred paths to health. Tucson (AZ): Rio Nuevo; 2002.
28. The U.S. Relocation act of 1956. Available at: http://www.coppercountry.com/article_97.php. Accessed June 15, 2009.
29. Whitbeck LB, Johnson KD, Hoyt DR, et al. Prevalence and comorbidity of mental disorders among American Indian children in the Northern Midwest. J Adolesc Health 2006;39:427–34.
30. Whitbeck LB, Yu M, Johnson KD, et al. Diagnostic prevalence rates from early to mid-adolescence among indigenous adolescents: first results from a longitudinal study. J Am Acad Child Adolesc Psychiatry 2008;47(8):890–900.
31. Andrade NN, Hishinuma ES, McDermott JF Jr, et al. The National Center on indigenous Hawaiian behavioral health study of prevalence of psychiatric disorders in native Hawaiian adolescents. J Am Acad Child Adolesc Psychiatry 2006;45(1): 26–36.
32. Costello EJ, Angold A, Burns BJ, et al. The Great Smoky Mountains Study of Youth: goals, design, methods, and the prevalence of DSM-LH-R disorders. Arch Gen Psychiatry 1996;53(12):1129–36.
33. Costello EJ, Farmer EMZ, Angold A, et al. Psychiatric disorders among American Indian and White Youth in Appalachia: the Great Smoky Mountain Study. Am J Public Health 1997;87:827–32.
34. Duclos CW, Beals J, Novins DK, et al. Prevalence of common psychiatric disorders among American Indian adolescent detainees. J Am Acad Child Adolesc Psychiatry 1998;37(8):866–73.
35. Beals J, Piasecki J, Nelson S, et al. Psychiatric disorder among American Indian adolescents: prevalence in Northern Plains youth. J Am Acad Child Adolesc Psychiatry 1997;36(9):1252–9.
36. Beals J, Novins DK, Whitesell NR, et al. Prevalence of mental disorders and utilization of mental health services in two American Indian reservation populations: mental health disparities in a national context. Am J Psychiatry 2005;162(9): 1723–32.
37. IHS Trends 2000–2001. Available at: http://www.ihs.gov/nonmedicalprograms/IHS_stats/index.cfm?module=hqPub&option=t00. Accessed June 8, 2009.
38. Beautrais AL, Fergusson DM. Indigenous suicide in New Zealand. Arch Suicide Res 2006;10(2):159–68.

39. Blair EM, Zubrick SR, Cox AH. WAACHS Steering Committee. The Western Australian Aboriginal Child Health Survey: findings to date on adolescents. Med J Aust 2005;183(8):433–5.
40. Zubrick SR, Silburn SR, Lawrence DM, et al. The Western Australian aboriginal child health survey: the social and emotional wellbeing of Aboriginal children and young people. Perth: Curtin University of Technology and Telethon Institute for child Health Research; 2005.
41. WAACH. Available at: http://www.ichr.uwa.edu.au/files/user17/Volume2_Chapter7.pdf. Accessed May 15, 2009.
42. Costello EJ, Compton SN, Keeler G, et al. Relationships between poverty and psychopathology: a natural experiment. JAMA 2003;290(15):2023–9.
43. IHS regional differences in Indian health 1998–99. Available at: http://www.ihs.gov/publicinfo/publications/trends98/RD_98c.pdf. Accessed May 30, 2009.
44. Bullock A, Bell RA. Stress, trauma, and coronary heart disease among Native Americans. Am J Public Health 2005;95(12):3–4.
45. Heim C, Newport CJ, Mletzko T, et al. The link between childhood trauma and depression: Insights from HPA axis studies in humans. Psychoneuroendocrinology 2008;33:693–710.
46. American Academy of Pediatrics Committee on Native American Child Health, American Academy of Pediatrics Committee on Community Health Services. Ethical considerations in research with socially identifiable populations. Pediatrics 2004;113(1 Pt 1):148–51.
47. Viswanathan M, Ammerman A, Eng E, et al. Community-based participatory research: assessing the evidence. Evidence report/technology assessment no. 99 (Prepared by RTI—University of North Carolina Evidence-based Practice Center under Contract No. 290-02-0016). AHRQ Publication 04-E022-2. Rockville (MD): Agency for Healthcare Research and Quality; 2004.
48. Novins D, Freeman B, Thurman PJ, et al. Principles for participatory research with American Indian and Alaska Native communities: lessons from the circles of care initiative. Poster Presented at the 2006 Conference indigenous suicide prevention research and programs in Canada and the United States: setting a Collaborative Agenda, Albuquerque, New Mexico. February 7–9, 2006. Sponsored by the National Institutes of Health, the Substance Abuse and Mental Health Services Administration, the Indian Health Service, Health Canada, and the Canadian Institutes of Health Research.
49. Novins DK. Participatory research brings knowledge and hope to American Indian communities. J Am Acad Child Adolesc Psychiatry 2009;48(6):585–6.
50. Thurman PJ, Allen J, Deters P. The circles of care evaluation: doing participatory evaluation with American Indian and Alaska native communities. Am Indian Alsk Native Ment Health Res 2004;11(2):139–54.
51. Walkup JT, Barlow A, Mullany BC, et al. Randomized controlled trial of a paraprofessional-delivered in-home intervention for young reservation-based American Indian mothers. J Am Acad Child Adolesc Psychiatry 2009;48(6):591–601.
52. Shipman K, Taussig H. Mental health treatment of child abuse and neglect: the promise of evidence-based practice. Pediatr Clin North Am 2009;56(2):417–28.
53. McClellan JM, Werry JS. Evidence-based treatments in child and adolescent psychiatry: an inventory. J Am Acad Child Adolesc Psychiatry 2003;42(12):1388–400.
54. McVoy M, Findling R. Child and adolescent psychopharmacology update. Psychiatr Clin North Am 2009;32(1):111–33.

55. Available at: http://www.aacap.org/page.ww?section=Practice+Parameters& name=Practice+Parameters. Accessed June 21, 2009.

56. Silverman WK, Ortiz CD, Viswesvaran C, et al. Evidence-based psychosocial treatments for children and adolescents exposed to traumatic events. J Clin Child Adolesc Psychol 2008;37(1):156–83.

57. Jones C, Chancey R, Walsh E, et al. An overview of the use of dialectical behavior therapy with adolescents for primary care physicians. Adolesc Med State Art Rev 2009;20(1):243–52.

58. Sindelar HA, Abrantes AM, Hart C, et al. Motivational interviewing in pediatric practice. Curr Probl Pediatr Adolesc Health Care 2004;34(9):322–39.

59. Suarez M, Mullins S. Motivational interviewing and pediatric health behavior interventions. J Dev Behav Pediatr 2008;29(5):417–28.

60. Gone JP, Alcántara C. Identifying effective mental health interventions for American Indians and Alaska Natives: a review of the literature. Cultur Divers Ethnic Minor Psychol 2007;13(4):356–63.

61. Oesterheld JR, Kofoed L, Tervo R, et al. Effectiveness of methylphenidate in Native American children with fetal alcohol syndrome and attention deficit/hyperactivity disorder: a controlled pilot study. J Child Adolesc Psychopharmacol 1998;8(1):39–48.

62. Morsette A, Swaney G, Stolle D, et al. Cognitive behavioral intervention for trauma in schools (CBITS): school-based treatment on a rural American Indian reservation. J Behav Ther Exp Psychiatry 2009;40(1):169–78.

63. Stein BD, Jaycox LH, Kataoka SH, et al. A mental health intervention for schoolchildren exposed to violence: a randomized controlled trial. JAMA 2003;290(5):603–11.

64. Hawkins EH, Cummins LH, Marlatt GA. Preventing substance abuse in American Indian and Alaska native youth: promising strategies for healthier communities. Psychol Bull 2004;130(2):304–23.

65. Gilchrist LD, Schinke SP, Trimble JE, et al. Skills enhancement to prevent substance abuse among American Indian adolescents. Int J Addict 1987;22(9):869–79.

66. Schinke SP, Tepavac L, Cole KC. Preventing substance use among Native American youth: three-year results. Addict Behav 2000;25(3):387–97.

67. Dixon AL, Yabiku ST, Okamoto SK, et al. The efficacy of a multicultural prevention intervention among urban American Indian youth in the southwest U.S. J Prim Prev 2007;28(6):547–68.

68. Middlebrook DL, LeMaster PL, Beals J, et al. Suicide prevention in American Indian and Alaska Native communities: a critical review of programs. Suicide Life Threat Behav 2001;31(1 Suppl):132–49.

69. LaFromboise T, Lewis HA. The Zuni life skills development program: a school/community-based suicide prevention intervention. Suicide Life Threat Behav 2008;38(3):343–53.

70. Diken IH, Rutherford RB. First step to success early intervention program: a study of effectiveness with Native-American children. Educ Treat Children 2005;28(4):444–65.

71. Cheadle A, Pearson D, Wagner W, et al. A community-based approach to preventing alcohol use among adolescents on an American Indian reservation. Public Health Rep 1995;110(4):439–47.

72. LaFromboise T, Howard-Pitney B. The Zuni life skills development curriculum: description and evaluation of a suicide prevention program. J Couns Psychol 1995;42(4):479–86.

73. Duran E. Healing the soul wound: counseling with American Indians and other Native peoples. New York: Teachers College; 2006.

74. O'Nell TD. Disciplined hearts: history, identity, and depression in an American Indian community. Berkeley (CA): University of California Press; 1996.
75. Gone JP. Psychotherapy and traditional healing for American Indians: exploring the prospects for therapeutic integration. The Counseling Psychologist, Doi: 10.1177100110000008330831. [Epub ahead of print].
76. Novins DK, Beals J, Moore LA, et al. AI-SUPERPFP Team. Use of biomedical services and traditional healing options among American Indians: sociodemographic correlates, spirituality, and ethnic identity. Med Care 2004;42(7):670–9.
77. Zuni healthy lifestyles. Available at: http://hsc.unm.edu/chpdp/projects/shtzunip. htm. Accessed June 15, 2009.
78. SAMHSA circles of care (technical assistance provided by AIANP). Available at: http:// aianp.uchsc.edu/coc/coc_overview.htm. Available at: http://www.systemsofcare. samhsa.gov/ResourceDir/circleshome.aspx. Accessed May 30, 2009.
79. Monograph on the circles of care program. Am Indian AIsk Native Ment Health Res April 2004. Available at: http://aianp.uchsc.edu/ncaianmhr/journal/pdf_files/ 11(2).pdf. Accessed May 30, 2009.
80. Motivational interviewing: enhancing motivation for change - a trainer's manual for the American Indian/Alaska Native counselor. Available at: http://www.oneskycenter. org/education/documents/AmericanIndianTrainersGuidetoMotivationalInterviewing. pdf. Accessed May 30, 2009.
81. Kleinman A, Benson P. Anthropology in the clinic: the problem of cultural competency and how to fix it. PLoS Med 2006;3(10):e294. Available at: http://www. plosmedicine.org. Accessed June 15, 2009.
82. Storck MG, Vanderstoep A. Fostering ecologic perspectives in child psychiatry. Child Adolesc Psychiatr Clin N Am 2007;16:133–63.
83. Fisher PA, Storck M, Bacon JG. In the eye of the beholder: risk and protective factors in rural American Indian and Caucasian adolescents. Am J Orthop 1999;69(3):294–304.
84. Levin SJ, Like RC, Gottlieb JE. ETHNIC: a framework for culturally competent ethical practice. Patient Care 2000;34(9):188–9.
85. Epstein RM. Mindful practice. JAMA 1999;282(9):833–9.

Oral Health of Indigenous Children and the Influence of Early Childhood Caries on Childhood Health and Well-being

Robert J. Schroth, DMD, MSc[a,b,*],
Rosamund L. Harrison, DMD, MSc, MRCD(C)[c,d],
Michael E.K. Moffatt, MD, MSc, FRCPC[a,b,e]

KEYWORDS

- Dental caries • Early childhood caries • Health services
- Indigenous • North America • Health promotion • Indians

Dental caries in Indigenous children is a child health issue that is multifactorial in origin and strongly influenced by the determinants of health. The evidence, although generally of a lower quality, suggests that extensive dental caries has an effect on health and well-being of the young child. Although counseling about dietary practices and tooth brushing and interventions involving fluoride show promise in reducing the severity of early childhood caries (ECC), the level of evidence for each is variable. Combined approaches are recommended. This article focuses on ECC as an overall proxy for Indigenous childhood oral health, because decay during early life sets the foundation

[a] Department of Pediatrics & Child Health and Department of Oral Biology, University of Manitoba, 507–715 Mc Dermot Avenue, Winnipeg, Manitoba R3E 3P4, Canada
[b] The Manitoba Institute of Child Health, 507–715 Mc Dermot Avenue, Winnipeg, Manitoba R3E 3P4, Canada
[c] Division of Pediatric Dentistry, University of British Columbia, 2199 Wesbrook Mall, Vancouver, British Columbia V6T 1Z3, Canada
[d] Child and Family Research Institute, 950 West 28th Avenue, Vancouver, British Columbia V5Z 4H4, Canada
[e] Division of Research and Applied Learning, Winnipeg Regional Health Authority, 4th Floor, 650 Main Street, Winnipeg, Manitoba R3B 1E2, Canada
* Corresponding author. Department of Pediatrics & Child Health and Department of Oral Biology, University of Manitoba, 507–715 Mc Dermot Avenue, Winnipeg, Manitoba R3E 3P4, Canada.
E-mail address: umschrot@cc.umanitoba.ca (R.J. Schroth).

Pediatr Clin N Am 56 (2009) 1481–1499
doi:10.1016/j.pcl.2009.09.010
0031-3955/09/$ – see front matter © 2009 Elsevier Inc. All rights reserved.

pediatric.theclinics.com

for oral health throughout childhood and adolescence. Strategies should begin with community engagement and always include primary care providers and other community health workers.

CURRENT STATE OF ORAL HEALTH AMONG INDIGENOUS CHILDREN

Despite advances in prevention and treatment, many children still experience elevated rates of dental disease. Recent evidence from the National Health and Examination Surveys (NHANES) in the United States indicates that the prevalence and severity of tooth decay among preschool children has risen significantly over the last two decades.[1] Higher rates of dental disease are often exhibited among at-risk populations including ethnic and cultural groups and those economically challenged. Indigenous children also bear an unfair burden of dental disease. The numerous life-challenges they face place them at higher risk for decay.

The etiology of ECC or decay in the primary teeth of infants and preschool-aged children is complex and multifactorial.[2,3] Apart from the traditional etiologic triad for caries (ie, host resistance or tooth integrity, oral flora [eg, *Streptococcus mutans*], and diet), many more lifestyle factors (eg, oral health literacy, oral hygiene) and environmental factors (eg, fluoride exposure, water fluoridation, community support, socioeconomic status, geographic isolation) exert influence.[4,5] Similar to other chronic diseases (see the article on diabetes in Indigenous children elsewhere in this issue), social determinants play a critical role in susceptibility.

This article focuses on ECC as an overall proxy for Indigenous childhood oral health because decay during early life sets the foundation for oral health throughout childhood and adolescence. A rampant subtype of ECC, called severe early childhood caries (S-ECC), afflicts many and frequently requires rehabilitation (restorations or extractions) under general anesthesia (GA). This dental surgery merely treats the signs or outcomes of the disease, but has little impact on slowing the disease process.

Children who experience ECC frequently face dental challenges as they mature. New "cavities" are surprisingly common within months of rehabilitation under GA and for many, retreatment requiring another GA is necessary.[6–8] Children with a history of ECC are at increased risk for future dental decay in their permanent teeth.[9,10] In addition, the premature loss of primary teeth may contribute to future malocclusion of the permanent teeth requiring expensive orthodontic treatment, which is often out of reach.[11]

Canada

Indigenous Canadians are referred to as "Aboriginal." This term encompasses several groups including First Nations (FN), who are either Status or non-Status Indians, the Métis, and the Inuit. Of these groups, only registered FN and recognized Inuit have access to dental benefits through the Non-Insured Health Benefits (NIHB) Program offered by Health Canada.[12] It is no surprise that data are unavailable on the oral health status of Métis children.

The oral health of Canadian Aboriginal children is a public health concern. Their prevalence and rates of caries are substantially greater than reported in the general population.[13–15] Although this disparity is most apparent for children from remote FN and Inuit communities, it also applies to those residing in urban centers.[16–20] In some communities, the prevalence of ECC exceeds 90%.[17,18] Experience of dental caries in the primary dentition can be designated as the "deft" or "dmft," which is a cumulative score of decayed, extracted or missing, and filled primary teeth. The total score possible is 20. Some reported mean deft rates range from 1.8 in Keewatin Inuit children less than 3 years of age; to 4.8 in FN 5 years olds in Manitoulin, Ontario; to as high as 13.7 in 3 to 5 year olds in a northern FN Manitoba community.[17,19,21] Unfortunately, only one third of children less than 4 years of age with NIHB dental benefits have a yearly dental visit.[12] Dental surgery under GA remains the most common surgical day care procedure at many pediatric hospitals in Canada and demand for this service continues to grow.[22]

The only regular national marker of the oral health of Aboriginal Canadians is dental service use data from the NIHB program.[23] Despite evidence of the poor state of Aboriginal children's oral health, however, less than 10% of the total NIHB budget is dedicated toward oral health promotion activities.[23] The only true national data available on FN preschool oral health comes by the FN Regional Longitudinal Health Survey (RHS).[24] This survey was administered by and for FN and is based on a holistic perspective that addresses all determinants of health. Data were collected by questionnaires administered to on-reserve FN in 238 communities across Canada. Although clinical examinations were not done, the value of the RHS data collected should not be dismissed because self-reported measures of oral health have been shown to be associated with clinical dental needs.[25] Not surprisingly, the RHS revealed many FN children to be affected by ECC.[24]

United States of America

There are two main groups of Indigenous people in the United States: American Indians and Alaska Natives (AI-AN). Like their counterparts in Canada and the developed world, AI-AN face more economic hardship and educational disparities, and are younger than the general population.[26,27] The Indian Health Service (IHS) is the branch within the US Department of Health and Human Services responsible for providing health services to AI-AN.[27] Over 1.4 million individuals were recipients of IHS services in 2004.[27] Although the tracking of dental services may not be entirely accurate and may underestimate the true proportion of dental users, it seems as though only a minority of AI-AN receive dental care within a given fiscal year, just like their Canadian counterparts.[27] Despite this underuse, the IHS spent $125 million on dental health services in 2007.[28]

Oral Health in America: a Report of the Surgeon General stated in 2000 that the oral health of young AI-AN has declined over the last several decades.[29] Results of the 1999 IHS oral health survey indicate that 79% of 2663 AI-AN preschool children surveyed had ECC.[30,31] Specifically, dental caries in the primary dentition has risen significantly over time, although caries in the permanent dentition has fallen.[29] Further, caries rates among AI-AN 2 to 4 year olds are five times that of non-Indigenous children.[29] What is of more concern is that the rate of untreated primary tooth decay is nearly three times greater than in the general population.[29]

Native Hawaiians tend to be a forgotten Indigenous group who comprise 10% of the population of Hawaii and have some of the highest caries rates in the Hawaiian Islands.[32,33] Although there is no evidence on the true prevalence of ECC using the recognized case definition,[3] 14% of Native Hawaiian 5 year olds have been identified as having three or more primary maxillary anterior teeth affected by decay.[32] An earlier publication reported that the caries surface rate for Native Hawaiian preschoolers participating in Head Start was three times higher (11.9 $\pm$ 14.7 dfs) than rates among participating Native American children (3.9 $\pm$ 6).[34]

Australia

Aboriginals and Torres Strait Islanders comprise the Indigenous peoples of Australia.[35,36] On the national level, Indigenous children represent less than 5% of the overall pediatric population.[35] Some regions, like the Northern Territory, have a greater proportion of Indigenous children.[35] Overall, about half of Indigenous children reside in urban areas.[37] Compared with their non-Indigenous peers, Indigenous preschool children from rural Australia are significantly more likely to have ECC and display more severe manifestations of caries.[38] ECC is also common among urban Indigenous children.[39]

A recent report on the oral health of Aboriginal and Torres Strait Islander children revealed that ECC affects over 60% of the population with mean deft rates considerably higher than non-Indigenous children.[36] Dental treatment under GA also serves as an indicator for the burden of caries in the very young. A review of GA statistics over a 10-year period revealed higher rates of dental GA for Indigenous children.[40] When tooth extractions were considered, rates were 46% greater for Indigenous children.[40] Further, hospitalization rates because of dental disease are three times greater for Aboriginal infants.[41]

New Zealand

The Maori, the Indigenous people of New Zealand and Maori children, have significantly higher caries rates than non-Maori children.[42] The recent National Child Nutrition Survey revealed that Maori children were significantly more likely to have had a dental restoration as a result of caries and significantly more likely to have experienced dental pain at night than children from other ethnic groups.[43] This is despite the fact that New Zealand has a School Dental Service that provides dental care for all children.

Structural reforms to the welfare state within New Zealand during the early 1990s negatively impacted the oral health of Maori children.[44] Data from 1995 to 2000 revealed that more than 50% of 5-year-old Maori children had ECC.[44] Further, they had greater odds for caries (OR = 2.94) and had caries rates 2.2 times that of other New Zealand children.[44] Linear trending at the end of the 6 years of analysis revealed that the severity of ECC for Maori children was 40% greater than for New Zealand children of European origin compared with only 5% higher in 1995.[44]

School-age Children and Youth

The alarmingly high prevalence of ECC in Indigenous preschool children is worthy of increased attention. The oral health of Indigenous school-aged children and youth also bears consideration. Most modern surveys of older children have focused on dental caries, but other oral health issues including malocclusion, periodontal disease, and oral disease related to tobacco use should not be overlooked.

The 2002 to 2003 RHS collected data on the oral health of Canadian children 0 to 11 years by proxy reports from parents and through self-reports of youth 12 to 17 years.[24] Of the 6657 children 0 to 11 years, 69.1% had received some form of dental care in the previous year, whereas 79% of the 4983 youth had received care in the same period; these rates of care were actually equivalent to the general Canadian population.[24] Youth from isolated FN communities, however, were significantly less likely to report receiving care. Overall, 19.1% of FN youth reported a recent episode of dental pain.[24]

The most recent national survey of Aboriginal children in Canada was in 1996 to 1997.[45] Similar to the RHS survey, FN living in urban areas were excluded. Overall, the survey included 21% of the age 6 and age 12 Aboriginal population living on-reserve and in the Yukon and Northwest territories. About 95% of 6 years olds and 91% of 12 year olds had experienced one or more dmft.[45] For the same time period, about 50% of non-Aboriginal children in industrialized countries experienced decay. These results are similar to 1988 data for FN children living in the Pacific region of Canada.[46] Although the caries experience for the children had steadily improved over the preceding 8 years, it was still high compared with non-FN children of comparable ages.[46]

Recent IHS data for on-reserve AI-AN children and youth mirror Canadian data; 87% of 6 to 14 years olds and 91% of 15 to 19 year olds had a history of tooth decay.[31,47] Previous declines in decay rates had not been maintained. Comparisons with other national data revealed that although 46% of AI-AN children had untreated decay, the national rate from NHANES-III was 11%.[31] Similarly, 68% of Native American teenagers had untreated decay in permanent teeth compared with 24% of other American teenagers.[31]

A survey of over 11,000 Australian Aboriginal children conducted between 2000 and 2003 demonstrated their dental health to be consistently worse than non-Indigenous children.[36] This tendency was a reversal of the trend before the 1980s. The mean dmft in 6-year-old Indigenous children was 2.4 times the mean dmft of non-Indigenous children (3.7 vs 1.5, respectively). Similarly, Indigenous 12 year olds had 1.7 times the number of affected permanent teeth than non-Indigenous children. Irrespective of metropolitan or rural location, Indigenous Australian children experienced more decay.

Oral disease is more than dental caries, but recent surveys are limited on other aspects of oral health. In the twenty-first century, a healthy smile with straight teeth is important for self-esteem. Current data on malocclusion in Indigenous groups, however, are limited. A report on Canadian FN children in the Pacific region of Canada demonstrated improvement in some aspects of dental malocclusion between 1980 and 1988.[48] The prevalence of severe malocclusion in youth 13 to 15 years of age had not improved, however, and compared with other children, FN children had a much higher prevalence of various types of malocclusion. Not surprisingly, significantly fewer FN than non-FN children received comprehensive orthodontic treatment. About 50% of children in the 1996 to 1997 national survey of FN in Canada had some form of malocclusion, with nearly 20% demonstrating a serious problem.[45] Both the IHS 1999 survey[31] and the Australian survey[36] were silent on malocclusion in Indigenous youth.

Healthy supporting tissues (ie, the periodontia) are essential for longevity of the dentition. Data from South Australian children demonstrated that bleeding on probing of gingival tissues was higher for Indigenous than non-Indigenous children but more non-Indigenous children had calculus (calcified plaque).[36] Canadian data from 1996 to 1997 revealed that over half of Aboriginal children examined had some gingival bleeding on probing.[45]

Finally, given the relationship between tobacco use and oral cancer and the fact that habitual tobacco use is strongly associated with periodontal disease, use of tobacco in children and youth should be mentioned. Overall, 23% of AI-AN 15 to 19 year olds used tobacco with over half smoking daily.[31] Self-reports from the Canadian RHS data demonstrated an overall prevalence of smoking in 12 to 17 year olds of 37.8%.[24]

The overall picture on oral health in Indigenous infant, children, and youth in Canada, the United States, Australia, and New Zealand is one of increased prevalence of dental caries, which often remains untreated. Other concerns are malocclusion and poor periodontal health. Analyzing the associations between oral health and other aspects of systemic health is imperative. "Rotten teeth," however, are inherently unacceptable for any child and are a grave child health problem that does not need a connection to other pediatric health issues before action is taken. Every child deserves a healthy smile.

RELATIONSHIP BETWEEN ECC AND CHILDHOOD HEALTH AND WELL-BEING

Continuing with ECC as a proxy for overall oral health, the association of ECC with three key areas of childhood health and well-being are reviewed next: (1) growth and development, (2) common pediatric illnesses and conditions, and (3) quality of life (QoL). Although not a formal systematic review, relevant investigations of associations are discussed. Unfortunately, few studies relating ECC to childhood health involve Indigenous children, but results from studies with other children can be extrapolated to Indigenous children, because these same connections are also biologically plausible for Indigenous children. Overall, the evidence for these associations is of low quality.

A few words about associations between diseases or symptoms and characteristics of patients and diseases are timely. Associations are measured by correlations, odds ratios, and risk ratios, sometimes referred to as "relative risk." When there is a study of adequate design that finds a significant association between two variables, the relationship could be simply that one variable is a risk marker for the other if there is no causal relationship or a risk factor if one variable is a link in the chain of causation of the other. Determining causation (ie, whether a particular exposure is part of the cause of a disease) is quite complex, but causation is important in deciding appropriate policy and clinical action. Sir Austin Bradford Hill identified nine criteria of causation[49]:

Strength of association
Consistency
Specificity
Temporality
Biologic gradient
Plausibility
Coherence
Experiment
Analogy

Although an in-depth discussion of causation is beyond the scope of this article, no simple formula exists for putting all these criteria together. The only criterion that must be met each time is temporality (ie, the cause must precede the outcome). There is often a lack of clarity in the literature about whether associations are causal or simply risk markers. With this in mind, the literature on several conditions that have been reported to be associated with ECC is reviewed.

Growth and Development

Speech development

Parents and practitioners are often concerned that premature loss of primary maxillary incisors results in speech problems; however, little published evidence exists. Two studies examined the association between the loss of primary maxillary incisors because of ECC and speech development.[50,51] The first involved speech and articulation assessments revealing that 40% had some form of speech distortion with those having extractions between 2 and 4 years of age having more severe speech problems.[50] The second reported that 36.5% of parents indicated their child had difficulty speaking and learning to speak as a result of premature tooth loss.[51] Unfortunately, poor study design, small sample size, and low parental response rates disallowed further generalizations.

A recent cross-sectional study of 349 young children from the Inuvik region of Northern Canada revealed a trend toward increasing speech difficulties with increasing severity of caries; however, this relationship was not significant ($P = .19$).[52] The aggregated evidence suggests a plausible association, but the existing evidence is of low quality.

Height

The first published study to examine the effect of extensive dental decay on height was a case control study that compared 3- to 5-year-old children with S-ECC with those cavity-free. The latter children were significantly taller than those with caries (101.5 ± 14.2 cm vs 97.7 ± 16.6 cm; P<.05).[53] Of interest, no statistically significant differences were found in mean head circumference between groups (P>.05).[53] A cross-sectional study of 1344 Chinese children 3 to 5 years of age found increased caries rates among children who had low height for age (P<.05).[54]

Logistic regression analysis of a nationally representative sample of United Kingdom preschool children was unable to support an association between age-adjusted height and ECC (P = .41).[55] Further, the NHANES III with 4236 preschool children revealed no significant association between caries prevalence, caries rates, and short stature for age.[56]

Finally, recent research from Brazil examined this relationship using World Health Organization Child Growth Standards for height-for-age.[57] Z-scores for children were generated and cutoffs used to denote excessive height or inadequate height, but neither was found to be associated with the presence of ECC.[57] The results of epidemiologic surveys that involved impressive sample sizes suggested no relationship between the presence of ECC and stature.

Weight and body mass index

The understanding of a putative relationship between ECC and childhood weight comes from observational studies that compare caries-free children with children with caries and from cohort studies that compare children before and after oral rehabilitation under GA. The earliest report examining this relationship compared 1105 children (5.9 ± 2.2 years) who had primary teeth extracted under GA with 527 control children who received dental care but had no extractions.[58] An extraction was considered a "proxy" for the severity of ECC. Statistically significant differences in children's weights were reported; children requiring extractions weighed significantly less (P<.001).[58] When examining age-specific mean weights, however, the only significant differences were found in 4 years olds (16.4 ± 2.1 kg vs 17.4 ± 2 kg; P<.01) and 5 years olds (17.9 ± 2.5 kg vs 19 ± 2.3 kg; P<.001), but not younger children.[58]

A retrospective chart review contrasted weights of children undergoing sedation or GA for the treatment of decay with matched controls without signs of gross decay.[59] The mean weight for those with S-ECC was significantly less than controls (15.2 ± 2.7 kg vs 16.2 ± 3.1 kg; P<.005).[59] Further, a larger proportion with S-ECC weighed less than 80% of their ideal weight (8.7% vs 1.7%; P<.01) and nearly 20% were less than or equal to the tenth percentile for weight compared with only 7% among the comparison group (P<.01).[59] A Turkish case control study reported that caries-free children weighed significantly more than their S-ECC peers (P<.05) and fewer weighed less than 80% of their ideal weight than those with rampant decay (0.7% vs 7.1%; P<.02).[53]

National studies with large sample sizes from Taipei (Three-year-old Health Survey) and the United States (NHANES III), however, have failed to support any association between body mass index (BMI) and caries status. Rates of primary tooth decay among 5133 Taipei participants did not differ significantly between the various percentiles of BMI (P = .25) and the difference in mean BMI between the ECC and caries-free groups was not significant (16 ± 1.6 vs 16.1 ± 1.6; P = .21).[60] Further, the mean caries rates did not significantly differ by BMI percentile (P = .17).[60] Likewise, data on 4236 American preschoolers found no relationship between BMI adjusted for age and caries experience (P>.05).[56] To confound the understanding even further, a recent report involving a convenience sample of 276 Hispanic children between 12 and 35 months attending a Women, Infants, and Children Supplemental Feeding program in South Texas concluded that those with higher caries experiences had significantly higher BMIs than those with lesser degrees of decay.[61]

The most recent evidence of a possible association comes from a cross-sectional study of 1018 Brazilian children 12 to 59 months of age, randomly enrolled at immunization visits.[57] Inadequate weight-for-age but not excessive weight-for-age was significantly associated with dental caries placing children at 2.8 times greater risk ($P = .038$).[57] Likewise, inadequate weight-for-height was associated with an increased risk (OR = 4.1; $P = .002$), but not excess weight-for-height.[57] Inadequate BMI was significantly associated with increased caries prevalence (OR = 3.2; $P = .007$), however, whereas excess BMI was associated with reduced likelihood of caries (OR = 0.6; $P = .046$).[57] Final logistic regression modeling revealed that children with low BMI-for-age were significantly more likely to have caries (OR = 3.2; $P = .011$), whereas those having BMI-for-age above two Z-scores were less likely to experience decay (OR = 0.58; $P = .036$).[57]

There are also reports on the effect rehabilitative dental treatment for S-ECC has on body weight. A case series report of preschoolers with S-ECC diagnosed with failure-to-thrive based on weight or height percentiles and failure to maintain growth patterns (ie, below the fiftieth percentile before 12 months of age) reported accelerated weight gains exceeding the fifth percentile following dental surgery.[62]

A case control study that recruited children from hospital dental clinics contrasted weights of preschool children with S-ECC with age, gender, and socioeconomic status matched cavity-free controls.[63] The sample size was low, but significant differences in baseline weights were observed between the S-ECC and comparison group (14.7 ± 2.3 kg vs 16.9 ± 2.9 kg; $P<.001$) and significant differences in percentile weights at baseline. Children with S-ECC weighed significantly less than caries-free children ($P<.001$). Further, 14% of the S-ECC group met failure-to-thrive weight criteria at baseline; none in the comparison group met these criteria ($P<.03$).[63] Children receiving complete treatment for ECC in one session were invited for the follow-up assessment. Children who had their teeth repaired experienced significant increases in their age-adjusted percentile weights ($P<.01$).[63] At the end of the observational period, no significant differences in weight remained between the groups. Overall, children treated under GA displayed catch-up growth and increased growth velocities.[63] Another group of investigators tried to replicate these results and found an increase in the mean percentile weight postoperatively, but observed that the increase was not statistically significant.[64]

The relationship between extensive dental decay and childhood growth and development is not entirely clear. No conclusions can be drawn related to speech; however, extensive caries in young children may contribute to low weight.

Common Pediatric Illnesses and Conditions

Otitis media

The literature reporting a link between otitis media (OM) and ECC has been mixed. A recent case control study on 71 children with ECC and 56 caries-free children ages 2 to 5 years found no relationship between caries and the presence of OM, although those children with ECC who had ear infections had a higher number of episodes of OM.[65] Meanwhile, a cohort study using Medicare databases from Michigan found that children who had a visit for OM or a respiratory infection during the first year of life were 29% more likely to develop ECC (as measured by a visit for dental care) in the subsequent period up to age 3.[66] When OM diagnoses were separated from respiratory infections, the increased risk for children with an OM history was only 11%.[66] Both of these studies were looking at ECC as a possible outcome of OM early in life. The relationship is not strong, and certainly there is no justification for thinking of OM as a risk factor for ECC. It may be a risk marker, but not a very specific one. The plausibility of a causal relationship is usually based on the possibility that infections result in enamel hypoplasia in children. It is also possible that socioeconomic environment leaves children at risk for both OM and ECC.

Respiratory tract infections

The data are similar for respiratory infections. A database cohort study showed an increased risk of 34% for ECC in children who had reported respiratory infections in the first year of life.[66] A 1989 case control study of risk factors for ECC found no association with respiratory infections, although it did report that 44% had respiratory infections.[67] Again, the picture is mixed; evidence of a causal relationship is lacking at present, and the use of frequent or repeated respiratory infections as a marker of risk for ECC is not very specific.

Eating patterns

It is logical to make the assumption that children with poor teeth have difficulty eating and that these children do better once their teeth are repaired. A study of 77 children in Montreal, Canada, undergoing GA for dental surgery asked caregivers to complete a questionnaire on the day of surgery and again 1 to 2 months postoperatively.[68] A significant improvement in their child's ability to eat was noted following treatment; 97% had no problems eating certain foods compared with 43% before surgery ($P<.001$).[68] More than half of the children who had problems eating before GA now had improved appetites and ate better than before rehabilitation.[68] Three similar American studies also reported that 69% of parents of children who underwent rehabilitative dental surgery under GA noted improvements in their child's eating behaviors[69] and noticeable reductions in chewing difficulties (8% postoperatively versus 60% pretreatment; $P<.05$).[64] Further, a study assessing both parental and child ratings of oral health suggested that ECC had significant negative effects on chewing behaviors.[70] Results from a cohort study of children with ECC suggested that only a minority had difficulty eating and chewing following extraction of their primary upper incisors.[51] Again, poor study design and small sample size limited the statistical analysis; neither did the survey tool clarify the consistency or texture of their diets. Finally, a more recent survey of 349 Inuit children in northern Canada reported that as the severity of caries increased, so did parental concerns about their child's ability to chew.[52] Overall, 14% of parents with children with severe caries were dissatisfied with their child's ability to chew compared with less than 1% of parents whose children were caries-free ($P<.001$).[52]

Iron deficiency

Two groups of investigators have examined the relationship between iron deficiency with or without anemia and ECC. The first studied 146 disadvantaged Hispanic and African American children and found no relationship between ECC (of any degree) and iron deficiency (unclear how this was defined).[71] The other involved 45 Canadian children undergoing dental surgery for S-ECC and found that 28% had low hemoglobin levels; 80% had iron depletion (ie, low serum ferritin); and 11% had iron deficiency anemia.[72] This result suggests that S-ECC may be a risk marker for iron deficiency.[72] No causal implications can be attributed from these cross-sectional studies, but a most likely explanation is that children with S-ECC are also disadvantaged in other ways. It may be worthwhile checking a complete blood count on children presenting with S-ECC.

Quality of Life

QoL extends to several levels including functional, psychosocial, and economic.[29] Pain and discomfort, sleep disturbances, and behavior troubles that may arise as a result of dental problems during the early childhood years are reviewed.

Pain

Chronic pain can influence QoL.[29] Assessing pain among children with ECC is a challenge because of their young age, limited ability to communicate, and absence of a suitable instrument to measure dental pain in young children.

Most reports on pain and ECC are observational. The Montreal study of 77 preschool children (mean age 44 months) investigated the influence of S-ECC on QoL.[68] Before their GA for dental surgery, 48% of the cohort complained about pain of dental origin, but 98% of these children no longer complained of pain 4 to 8 weeks after treatment.[68] Overall, there was a statistically significant reduction in dental pain following rehabilitative surgery (P<.001).[68] Another study surveyed 223 parents regarding their satisfaction with their preschool child's dental surgery under GA in Washington, DC.[69] Parents overwhelmingly indicated that the most improved domain of QoL for their child was a reduction in pain; 86% reported improvements.[69] Similar findings were also observed in Florida as parents reported significant improvements following surgery; specifically, only 2% had complaints of dental pain postoperatively compared with 56% before rehabilitation (P<.05).[64] Most parents (84%) of 45 healthy 24 to 60 month olds from North Carolina who required dental surgery under GA reported their child was pain-free following treatment and that the elimination of pain was a significant predictor of overall parental satisfaction with GA.[73] Likewise, both parents and children in another study reported significantly less pain following surgery.[70]

Meanwhile, a cross-sectional study of preschool oral health among 482 Head Start Center participants in Maryland investigated pain slightly differently. The main caregivers completed a survey that included questions about their child's complaints and crying because of dental pain.[74] Overall, 55% of children had ECC but only 10% of caregivers indicated that their child had complained of dental pain.[74] Among those with ECC, this frequency was 17%; 9% of children with ECC were reported to have cried from toothaches.[74] Only one identified study has reported on ECC and dental pain in Aboriginal children.[52] Parents of 2- to 6-year-old Inuit children with S-ECC were significantly more likely to report that their child experienced pain than those cavity-free (P = .003).[52]

Sleep

Sleep disturbances in children are a concern for today's parents. Three case-control studies suggest that children with severe forms of decay have difficulty sleeping. Researchers in the American Northwest contrasted children with S-ECC with caries-free children.[75] They reported that those with S-ECC (N = 104) were significantly more likely to have reported night waking episodes (1.2 episodes vs 0.7; P<.01), fewer hours of sleep each night (9 hours vs 9.6; P<.05), and slept through the night nearly 1 day less per week (5.6 days vs 6.5; P<.001) than caries-free controls.[75] Five percent of this ethnically diverse group were AI.[75] A second group of investigators in New Jersey found that significantly more children with ECC had difficulties sleeping than age- and gender-matched cavity-free controls (58.3% vs 4.2%; P = .05).[76] The most recent study in Columbus, Ohio, used a validated instrument, the

Child Behavior Checklist, to assess differences in responses to 100 questions on childhood behavior for participants with ECC (N = 60) and without ECC (N = 60).[77] Caregiver responses revealed that children with ECC were significantly more likely to have sleep problems (P = .049) because they reported statistically higher scores on this question of the Child Behavior Checklist.[77]

Other observational studies have reported significant improvements in sleeping habits of children with S-ECC following dental treatment.[68,69] The study at Montreal Children's Hospital found that before treatment 35% of children had sleeping problems, either manifesting as waking up often, not sleeping through the night, or taking a long time to fall asleep.[68] Following treatment, parents reported improved sleeping patterns (P<.001).[68] Another study in Washington, DC, surveyed parents of children who underwent treatment under GA.[69] Forty-one percent of parents reported that their child's sleeping had improved after treatment.[69] A third study examined the effects of treatment on children and found a significant reduction in the proportion with sleeping problems following dental surgery (30% before GA vs 4% post-GA; P<.05).[64] Other parent satisfaction surveys have also reported improvements in duration of sleeping following treatment.[73]

Behavior

Several studies have assessed the behavior of children with ECC and of children who had GA for oral rehabilitation. The study assessing parental perceptions of the effect of extraction of their child's primary "front teeth" found that 21.2% noticed behavior changes in their child following extractions, 12% of children showed signs of shyness or abnormal behavior, and 13.5% had problems making friends after treatment.[51] The Montreal Children's Hospital study, however, reported that only 5% of children had negative behavior before surgery; only half of these children report improvements in behavior.[68] This finding was not statistically significant.[68] Both studies had small sample sizes and were observational in nature.

QoL assessments among parents whose children underwent GA to resolve S-ECC concluded that treatment resulted in a significant reduction in behavioral problems (32% pre-GA versus 0% post-GA).[64] Similarly, other researchers had parents complete a 10-item QoL survey following GA.[73] Improvements in social aspects related to their child's smiling, attentiveness in school, and sociability were reported.[73] Logistic regression analysis further emphasized increased social interaction of preschool children postoperatively.[73] Meanwhile, the Child Behavior Checklist administered to parents of children with and without ECC found that those with caries had significantly higher scores for anxiety and depression, aggressive behavior, externalizing problems, and attention deficit–hyperactivity problems.[77] Another QoL study found that ECC affected playing habits and school performance.[70]

Although the evidence to support the associations that have been described is in many cases limited and of low grade, it suggests that severe dental caries may indeed have an impact on the health and well-being of young children. This scarcity of high-quality evidence should be a call to action for more focused research on the impact of ECC on childhood health.

PREVENTION OF ECC AND PROMOTION OF EARLY CHILDHOOD ORAL HEALTH
Oral Health Promotion Research

This section focuses on the prevention of ECC and the promotion of oral health in young children. Because dental caries is the most prevalent dental disorder in young Indigenous children, this section is limited to strategies aimed to prevent ECC.

Unfortunately, a universally effective, caries-prevention program with predictable long-term results has yet to be found.

ECC is a complex disease that is multifactorial in origin; any preventive program must include a variety of strategies.[78] There is no "magic bullet." The spread of the microorganisms implicated in the initiation of caries is usually from mother to child; the fidelity of the transmission seems to be related to maternal oral health status, diet, and oral hygiene practices.[79,80] Improving the oral health of expectant and new mothers is an important oral health promotion strategy.

Encouraging remineralization of tooth enamel with fluoride is another essential caries-prevention strategy. Regular brushing with fluoride toothpaste is crucial once an infant's teeth begin to erupt. Although water fluoridation is the most cost-effective and equitable way of preventing decay, the remoteness, small size, and lack of infrastructure in many communities usually means that water fluoridation is neither realistic nor economic.[81] Results of a recent unpublished study performed in Alaskan communities suggests, however, that water fluoridation should be pursued. A reduction in caries by 30% to 50% with community fluoridation "even when other risk factors were accounted for" was reported (Michael Bruce, Arctic Investigations Program, Centers for Disease Control and Prevention, Alaska, personal communication; 2009). Another means to introduce fluoride is fluoride varnish, an agent ideally suited for infants and toddlers because of ease of use, acceptability, and low risk of overingestion of fluoride. In many jurisdictions, varnish may be applied by "nondental" community workers and health professionals. Recent reviews on fluoride varnish substantiate its effectiveness; evidence-based guidelines recommend a biannual application regimen for high-risk populations, including FN children.[82,83]

Dietary modification is also a fundamental ECC prevention strategy. Bottle use while sleeping, constant daytime sipping from a bottle or sippy cup containing anything other than water, and frequent snacking between meals are practices linked to the development of extensive caries and increase caries risk.[84]

Most caries-prevention strategies targeting young children require that parents change an existing behavior (eg, bottle feeding) or adopt a new one (eg, regular tooth brushing). Providing knowledge alone (eg, traditional anticipatory guidance), however, rarely leads to long-term changes in preventive behaviors.[85] Behavioral approaches developed by and for Indigenous communities that structure and assist parents in the process of change are more likely to lead to lasting behavior change.

When interventions with Indigenous communities are tested in the framework of a research project, the process must be based on consultation, strong community participation, respect of Indigenous ways of knowing, and responsiveness to the communities and their concerns.[86] Randomized controlled trials, which by their nature withhold an intervention from some communities, may be viewed with mistrust by Aboriginal communities. Early and meaningful community involvement and allowing the community to run the trial have been suggested as useful strategies for successful outcomes.[87] To date, relatively few community-based research initiatives to improve the oral health of young Indigenous children have been undertaken[20,88] and scant few have been conducted as randomized controlled trials.[89]

A community-based ECC prevention program in 12 AI-AN communities demonstrated a 25% decrease in ECC after 3 years.[88] In five communities that continued the program for an 8-year period, the overall decrease was 38% ($P<.001$), whereas in the communities where the program was discontinued, the rate began to increase.[88] Another demonstration project, designed and implemented by a committee of mothers and local community workers, in a Canadian FN community also reported promising results.[20] Traditional child-rearing practices, such as a cradle loan project, and one-on-one counseling by the community health nurse were offered.[20] Positive yet insignificant reductions in caries rates were reported in these 30-month-old children.[20] These projects, however, have shortcomings: none of them randomly assigned communities or families to an intervention and volunteer bias may have contributed to successful outcomes. In addition, lack of rigor in the evaluation protocols was a concern and fluoride applications were not part of either program.

A randomized controlled trial conducted with 1275 young Aboriginal children in the Sioux Lookout region of Ontario, Canada, enhanced the positive trends of these earlier observational studies.[89] Fluoride varnish, offered at least twice per year in conjunction with caregiver counseling, conferred an 18% reduction in the 2-year mean net increment in caries surface rates in participating Aboriginal children.[89] Certainly, community-based strategies that include fluoride fn addition to counseling show promise to positively affect lifestyle factors contributing to decay.

Guidelines for the Primary Care Provider About Promoting Oral Health

Decreasing the incidence of tooth decay in Indigenous children has proved challenging and primary care providers struggle with "how to help." Only with consideration of the "up-stream" and "down-stream" factors that collectively lead to poor oral health will this serious problem in Indigenous children ever be improved.

The evidence to support the best strategies for primary care providers to use in their efforts to improve Indigenous child dental health is wanting. This lack of evidence is unfortunate given that primary care providers are uniquely situated to play a pivotal role in ECC prevention. The evidence for the effectiveness of various physician interventions has been recently reviewed.[90] High-quality evidence for the effectiveness of three traditionally recommended, primary care provider interventions (screening, referral, and counseling) was found to be lacking. Furthermore, only fair evidence was available for the effectiveness of physician-initiated fluoride-based interventions (fluoride supplements and varnish). It should be noted, however, that a recent systematic review of fluoride supplementation commissioned by the America Dental Association concluded that the evidence for a caries-preventive effect of fluoride supplements (drops, tablets, lozenges) on primary teeth is weak and inconsistent.[91] Supplements do help to prevent caries in permanent teeth, but as with any medication, compliance with administration is an ongoing challenge.

The America Academy of Pediatrics recently updated their policy statement and developed evidence-based recommendations for preventive oral health interventions by primary care pediatric practitioners.[92] Although assessment of caries-risk is essential, the America Academy of Pediatrics correctly states that caries-risk assessment is "very much a work in progress." Given their demonstrated prevalence of caries, however, it is reasonable to assume that most young Indigenous children are at high caries risk.

The dental home concept, endorsed by the America Academy of Pediatrics, refers to a continuing relationship between provider and child, beginning no later than 12 months of age, where the child's access to comprehensive and coordinated oral health care and prevention is the central focus and tailored to the needs of the child.[93] Unfortunately, for many Aboriginal children, a dental home is simply not attainable. Residence in remote regions, parents whose own experience of dentistry has been unpleasant, and local practitioners who choose not to see young children are just some of the barriers to establishing a dental home. Models of care, such as the pediatric oral health therapist recently introduced to remote AN villages, however, provide a much-needed opportunity for early establishment of a dental home. Dental therapists have worked in selected Canadian FN and Inuit communities for decades.[94]

	Quality of Evidence	Strength of Recommendation
Table 1 **Preventive strategies**		
Guideline		
Dietary counseling for optimal oral health as an intrinsic component of general health counseling	Low	Strong
Supervised use of fluoride toothpaste for all children with teeth	High	Strong
Regular application of fluoride varnish by primary health care providers or other personnel for children who do not have a dental home	Moderate	Strong
Collaborative relationships with local dental professionals to optimize the availability of a dental home	Low	Strong

Primary care providers who see Indigenous children should collaborate with community health staff, such as dental hygienists, public health nurses, and community health representatives, to develop their own community-specific version of the dental home.

Although mindful of the inadequacies of oral health counseling,[90] anticipatory guidance during well-child visits is understood by primary care providers to be an effective way to inform parents about maintaining their child's health.[92] Oral health anticipatory guidance should be considered. General preventive strategies as recommended by the American Academy of Pediatrics for preschool Aboriginal children as part of oral health anticipatory guidance are listed in **Table 1**.[92]

Although not a specific recommendation of any professional organization, all health professionals have a role in the wider community as advocates for Indigenous children and their families. Collectively, health professionals should lobby policymakers and government for improvements to housing, access to safe water, availability of regular dental services, and economic opportunities for Indigenous families.

SUMMARY

Dental caries in Indigenous children is a child health issue that is multifactorial in origin and strongly influenced by the determinants of health. The evidence, although generally of a lower quality, suggests that extensive dental caries has an effect on health and well-being of the young child. Although counseling about dietary practices and tooth brushing and interventions involving fluoride show promise in reducing the severity of ECC, the level of evidence for each is variable. Combined approaches are recommended. Strategies should begin with community engagement and always include primary care providers and other community health workers. Health professionals' role as advocates for improvements in the social determinants of oral health in Indigenous communities is also significant.

ACKNOWLEDGMENTS

The authors thank Eleonore Kliewer for her assistance with manuscript preparation.

REFERENCES

1. Dye BA, Tan S, Smith V, et al. Trends in oral health status: United States, 1988–1994 and 1999–2004. Vital Health Stat 11 2007;1–92.

2. American Academy of Pediatric Dentistry. Definition of early childhood caries (ECC). Pediatr Dent 2008;30:13.
3. Drury TF, Horowitz AM, Ismail AI, et al. Diagnosing and reporting early childhood caries for research purposes. A report of a workshop sponsored by the National Institute of Dental and Craniofacial Research, the Health Resources and Services Administration, and the Health Care Financing Administration. J Public Health Dent 1999;59:192–7.
4. Selwitz RH, Ismail AI, Pitts NB. Dental caries. Lancet 2007;369:51–9.
5. Mouradian WE, Wehr E, Crall JJ. Disparities in children's oral health and access to dental care. JAMA 2000;284:2625–31.
6. Almeida AG, Roseman MM, Sheff M, et al. Future caries susceptibility in children with early childhood caries following treatment under general anesthesia. Pediatr Dent 2000;22:302–6.
7. Graves CE, Berkowitz RJ, Proskin HM, et al. Clinical outcomes for early childhood caries: influence of aggressive dental surgery. J Dent Child (Chic) 2004;71:114–7.
8. Schroth R, Smith W. A review of repeat general anesthesia for pediatric dental surgery in Alberta, Canada. Pediatr Dent 2007;29:480–7.
9. Li Y, Wang W. Predicting caries in permanent teeth from caries in primary teeth: an eight-year cohort study. J Dent Res 2002;81:561–6.
10. Peretz B, Ram D, Azo E, et al. Preschool caries as an indicator of future caries: a longitudinal study. Pediatr Dent 2003;25:114–8.
11. Robke FJ. Effects of nursing bottle misuse on oral health: prevalence of caries, tooth malalignments and malocclusions in North-German preschool children. J Orofac Orthop 2008;69:5–19.
12. Non-insured health benefits program annual report 2006/2007. 3005, 1–100. Ottawa (Canada): First Nations and Inuit Health Branch, Non-Insured Health Benefits Directorate. Health Canada; 2008.
13. Schroth RJ, Harrison R, Lawrence H, et al. Oral health and the aboriginal child: a forum for community members, researchers and policy-makers. J Can Dent Assoc 2008;74:429–32.
14. Schroth RJ, Moffatt ME. Determinants of early childhood caries (ECC) in a rural Manitoba community: a pilot study. Pediatr Dent 2005;27:114–20.
15. Weinstein P, Smith WF, Fraser-Lee N, et al. Epidemiologic study of 19-month-old Edmonton, Alberta children: caries rates and risk factors. ASDC J Dent Child 1996;63:426–33.
16. Schroth RJ, Moore P, Brothwell DJ. Prevalence of early childhood caries in 4 Manitoba communities. J Can Dent Assoc 2005;71:567.
17. Schroth RJ, Smith PJ, Whalen JC, et al. Prevalence of caries among preschool-aged children in a northern Manitoba community. J Can Dent Assoc 2005;71:27.
18. Lawrence HP, Romanetz M, Rutherford L, et al. Effects of a community-based prenatal nutrition program on the oral health of aboriginal preschool children in Northern Ontario. Probe 2004;38:172–90.
19. Peressini S, Leake JL, Mayhall JT, et al. Prevalence of early childhood caries among First Nations children, District of Manitoulin, Ontario. Int J Paediatr Dent 2004;14:101–10.
20. Harrison R, White L. A community-based approach to infant and child oral health promotion in a British Columbia First Nations community. Can J Community Dent 1997;12:7–14.
21. Young TK, Moffatt ME, O'Neil JD, et al. The population survey as a tool for assessing family health in the Keewatin region, NWT, Canada. Arctic Med Res 1995; 54(Suppl 1):77–85.

22. Schroth RJ, Morey B. Providing timely dental treatment for young children under general anesthesia in a government priority. J Can Dent Assoc 2007; 73:241–3.

23. A statistical profile on the health of First Nations in Canada. Ottawa (Canada): Her Majesty the Queen in Right of Canada, represented by the Minister of Health Canada; 2005. HC.Pub.No.: 3056. p. 1–101.

24. First Nations Centre. First nations regional longitudinal health survey (RHS) 2002/ 03. Results for adults, youth and children living in first nations communities. Ottawa (Canada): First Nations Centre; 2005. p. 1–312.

25. Jamieson LM, Thomson WM, McGee R. An assessment of the validity and reliability of dental self-report items used in a National Child Nutrition Survey. Community Dent Oral Epidemiol 2004;32:49–54.

26. Trends in Indian health. 2000–2001 edition. Washington, DC: US Government Printing Office, US Department of Health and Human Services, Indian Health Service; 2004. p. 1–242.

27. US Department of Health and Human Services, Indian Health Service. Regional differences in Indian health 2002–2003 edition. Washington, DC: US Department of Health and Human Services. Government Printing Office; 2008. p. 1–109.

28. US Department of Health and Human Services Indian Health Service. Indian Health Service Annual Report 2007. Washington, DC: US Department of Health and Human Services Indian Health Service; 2007. p. 1–43.

29. US Department of Health and Human Services. Oral health in America: a report of the Surgeon General. Rockville (MD): US Department of Health and Human Services, National Institute of Dental and Craniofacial Research, National Institutes of Health; 2000. p. 1–308.

30. Jones C, Phipps K, Reifel N, et al. The oral health status of American Indian/Alaska Native preschool children: a crisis in Indian Country. IHS Primary Care Provider 2001;26:133–7.

31. Indian Health Service. The 1999 oral health survey of American Indian and Alaska Native dental patients: findings, regional differences and national comparisons. Rockville (MD): Indian Health Service, Division of Dental Services; 2002. p. 1–107.

32. Greer MH, Tengan SL, Hu KI, et al. Early childhood caries among Hawaii public school children, 1989 vs. 1999. Pac Health Dialog 2003;10:17–22.

33. Greer MH, Tendan SL. Early childhood dental caries in Hawai'i. Hawaii Dent J 1998;29:10, 14.

34. Louie R, Brunelle JA, Maggiore ED, et al. Caries prevalence in Head Start children, 1986–87. J Public Health Dent 1990;50:299–305.

35. Jamieson LM, Bailie RS, Beneforti M, et al. Dental self-care and dietary characteristics of remote-living Indigenous children. Rural Remote Health 2006;6:503.

36. Australian Institute of Health and Welfare, Dental Statistics and Research Unit, Jamieson LM, et al. Oral health of Aboriginal and Torres Strait Islander children. AIHW cat. no. DEN 167. Canberra (Australia): Australian Institute of Health and Welfare; 2007. (Dental Statistics and Research Series No. 35). p. 1–123.

37. Jamieson LM, Armfield JM, Roberts-Thomson KF. Indigenous and non-indigenous child oral health in three Australian states and territories. Ethn Health 2007;12:89–107.

38. Kruger E, Dyson K, Tennant M. Pre-school child oral health in rural Western Australia. Aust Dent J 2005;50:258–62.

39. Seow WK, Amaratunge A, Sim R, et al. Prevalence of caries in urban Australian aborigines aged 1–3.5 years. Pediatr Dent 1999;21:91–6.

40. Jamieson LM, Roberts-Thomson KF. Dental general anaesthetic trends among Australian children. BMC Oral Health 2006;6:16.
41. Tennant M, Namjoshi D, Silva D, et al. Oral health and hospitalization in Western Australian children. Aust Dent J 2000;45:204–7.
42. Thomson WM. Ethnicity and child dental health status in the Manawatu-Wanganui Area Health Board. N Z Dent J 1993;89:12–4.
43. Jamieson LM, Koopu PI. Associations between ethnicity and child health factors in New Zealand. Ethn Dis 2007;17:84–91.
44. Thomson WM, Williams SM, Dennison PJ, et al. Were NZ's structural changes to the welfare state in the early 1990s associated with a measurable increase in oral health inequalities among children? Aust N Z J Public Health 2002;26: 525–30.
45. Health Canada. Report on the 1996–1997 oral health survey of First Nation and Inuit children in Canada aged 6 and 12. Ottawa (Canada): Minister of Public Works and Government Services Canada; 2000. p. 1–71.
46. Harrison RL, Davis DW. Caries experience of Native children of British Columbia, Canada, 1980–1988. Community Dent Oral Epidemiol 1993;21:102–7.
47. Reifel N, Phipps K, Skipper B. The 1999 oral health survey of American Indian and Alaska Native dental patients: children and adolescents. IHS Prim Care Provid 2001;26:145–50.
48. Harrison RL, Davis DW. Dental malocclusion in native children of British Columbia, Canada. Community Dent Oral Epidemiol 1996;24:217–21.
49. Hill AB. The environment and disease: association or causation? Proc R Soc Med 1965;58:295–300.
50. Riekman GA, el Badrawy HE. Effect of premature loss of primary maxillary incisors on speech. Pediatr Dent 1985;7:119–22.
51. Koroluk LD, Riekman GA. Parental perceptions of the effects of maxillary incisor extractions in children with nursing caries. ASDC J Dent Child 1991;58:233–6.
52. Leake J, Jozzy S, Uswak G. Severe dental caries, impacts and determinants among children 2–6 years of age in Inuvik Region, Northwest Territories, Canada. J Can Dent Assoc 2008;74:519.
53. Ayhan H, Suskan E, Yildirim S. The effect of nursing or rampant caries on height, body weight and head circumference. J Clin Pediatr Dent 1996;20:209–12.
54. Li Y, Navia JM, Bian JY. Caries experience in deciduous dentition of rural Chinese children 3–5 years old in relation to the presence or absence of enamel hypoplasia. Caries Res 1996;30:8–15.
55. Williams SA, Kwan SY, Parsons S. Parental smoking practices and caries experience in pre-school children. Caries Res 2000;34:117–22.
56. Dye BA, Shenkin JD, Ogden CL, et al. The relationship between healthful eating practices and dental caries in children aged 2–5 years in the United States, 1988–1994. J Am Dent Assoc 2004;135:55–66.
57. Oliveira LB, Sheiham A, Bonecker M. Exploring the association of dental caries with social factors and nutritional status in Brazilian preschool children. Eur J Oral Sci 2008;116:37–43.
58. Miller J, Vaughan-Williams E, Furlong R, et al. Dental caries and children's weights. J Epidemiol Community Health 1982;36:49–52.
59. Acs G, Lodolini G, Kaminsky S, et al. Effect of nursing caries on body weight in a pediatric population. Pediatr Dent 1992;14:302–5.
60. Chen W, Chen P, Chen SC, et al. Lack of association between obesity and dental caries in three-year-old children. Zhonghua Min Guo Xiao Er Ke Yi Xue Hui Za Zhi 1998;39:109–11.

61. Reifsnider E, Mobley C, Mendez DB. Childhood obesity and early childhood caries in a WIC population. J Multicult Nurs Health 2004;10:24–31.

62. Acs G, Lodolini G, Shulman R, et al. The effect of dental rehabilitation on the body weight of children with failure to thrive: case reports. Compend Contin Educ Dent 1998;19:164–8, 170–1.

63. Acs G, Shulman R, Ng MW, et al. The effect of dental rehabilitation on the body weight of children with early childhood caries. Pediatr Dent 1999;21:109–13.

64. Thomas CW, Primosch RE. Changes in incremental weight and well-being of children with rampant caries following complete dental rehabilitation. Pediatr Dent 2002;24:109–13.

65. Nelson S, Nechvatal N, Weber J, et al. Dental caries and ear infections in preschool-aged children. Oral Health Prev Dent 2005;3:165–71.

66. Alaki SM, Burt BA, Garetz SL. Middle ear and respiratory infections in early childhood and their association with early childhood caries. Pediatr Dent 2008;30:105–10.

67. Srkoc O, Bajan M, Stilinovic D. [Etiology of nursing caries]. Acta Stomatol Croat 1989;23:159–65 [in Croatian].

68. Low W, Tan S, Schwartz S. The effect of severe caries on the quality of life in young children. Pediatr Dent 1999;21:325–6.

69. Acs G, Pretzer S, Foley M, et al. Perceived outcomes and parental satisfaction following dental rehabilitation under general anesthesia. Pediatr Dent 2001;23:419–23.

70. Filstrup SL, Briskie D, da Fonseca M, et al. Early childhood caries and quality of life: child and parent perspectives. Pediatr Dent 2003;25:431–40.

71. Ramos-Gomez FJ, Weintraub JA, Gansky SA, et al. Bacterial, behavioral and environmental factors associated with early childhood caries. J Clin Pediatr Dent 2002;26:165–73.

72. Clarke M, Locker D, Berall G, et al. Malnourishment in a population of young children with severe early childhood caries. Pediatr Dent 2006;28:254–9.

73. White H, Lee JY, Vann WF Jr. Parental evaluation of quality of life measures following pediatric dental treatment using general anesthesia. Anesth Prog 2003;50:105–10.

74. Vargas CM, Monajemy N, Khurana P, et al. Oral health status of preschool children attending Head Start in Maryland, 2000. Pediatr Dent 2002;24:257–63.

75. Shantinath SD, Breiger D, Williams BJ, et al. The relationship of sleep problems and sleep-associated feeding to nursing caries. Pediatr Dent 1996;18:375–8.

76. Marino RV, Bomze K, Scholl TO, et al. Nursing bottle caries: characteristics of children at risk. Clin Pediatr (Phila) 1989;28:129–31.

77. Williamson R, Oueis H, Casamassimo PS,, et al. Association between early childhood caries and behavior as measured by the child behavior checklist. Pediatr Dent 2008;30:505–9.

78. Tinanoff N, Kanellis MJ, Vargas CM. Current understanding of the epidemiology mechanisms, and prevention of dental caries in preschool children. Pediatr Dent 2002;24:543–51.

79. Li Y, Caufield PW. The fidelity of initial acquisition of mutans streptococci by infants from their mothers. J Dent Res 1995;74:681–5.

80. Wan AK, Seow WK, Purdie DM,, et al. Oral colonization of Streptococcus mutans in six-month-old predentate infants. J Dent Res 2001;80:2060–5.

81. Ehsani JP, Bailie R. Feasibility and costs of water fluoridation in remote Australian Aboriginal communities. BMC Public Health 2007;7:100.

82. Marinho VC, Higgins JP, Logan S, et al. Fluoride varnishes for preventing dental caries in children and adolescents. Cochrane Database Syst Rev 2002;(3): CD002279.
83. Azarpazhooh A, Main PA. Fluoride varnish in the prevention of dental caries in children and adolescents: a systematic review. J Can Dent Assoc 2008;74:73–9.
84. American Academy of Pediatric Dentistry. Policy on use of a caries-risk assessment tool (CAT) for infants, children, and adolescents. Pediatr Dent 2008;30: 29–33.
85. Benitez C, O'Sullivan D, Tinanoff N. Effect of a preventive approach for the treatment of nursing bottle caries. ASDC J Dent Child 1994;61:46–9.
86. Cochran PA, Marshall CA, Garcia-Downing C, et al. Indigenous ways of knowing: implications for participatory research and community. Am J Public Health 2008; 98:22–7.
87. Andersson N. Afterword: directions in Indigenous resilience research. Pimatisiwin: A Journal of Aboriginal and Indigenous Community Health 2008;6:201–8.
88. Bruerd B, Jones C. Preventing baby bottle tooth decay: eight-year results. Public Health Rep 1996;111:63–5.
89. Lawrence HP, Binguis D, Douglas J, et al. A 2-year community-randomized controlled trial of fluoride varnish to prevent early childhood caries in Aboriginal children. Community Dent Oral Epidemiol 2008;36:503–16.
90. Bader JD, Rozier RG, Lohr KN, et al. Physicians' roles in preventing dental caries in preschool children: a summary of the evidence for the US Preventive Services Task Force. Am J Prev Med 2004;26:315–25.
91. Ismail AI, Hasson H. Fluoride supplements, dental caries and fluorosis: a systematic review. J Am Dent Assoc 2008;139:1457–68.
92. Preventive oral health intervention for pediatricians. Pediatrics 2008;122: 1387–94.
93. American Academy of Pediatric Dentistry. Policy on the dental home. Pediatr Dent 2008;30:22–3.
94. Bolin KA. Assessment of treatment provided by dental health aide therapists in Alaska: a pilot study. J Am Dent Assoc 2008;139:1530–5.

Early Child Development and Developmental Delay in Indigenous Communities

Matthew M. Cappiello, BA, Sheila Gahagan, MD, MPH*

KEYWORDS

- Child development • Health disparities • American Indian
- Indigenous • Fetal alcohol syndrome

Early childhood developmental delay is commonly identified in developed countries including the United States, Canada, Australia, and New Zealand. Developmental delay is defined as late acquisition of developmental milestones. Children who achieve their developmental milestones two or more standard deviations later than the mean age of acquisition are considered delayed. Developmental delays require further assessment, as some are the result of normal variation and others herald problems, including cerebral palsy, sensory impairments, cognitive impairment, and autism. Child health professionals can expect 8% of their patients to experience significant developmental or behavioral problems by the age of 6 years. Furthermore, approximately 15% of children in the United States receive special education services, suggesting that some developmental disorders are not ascertained before school.[1,2] Developmental delays stem from a variety of causes including adverse perinatal factors such as prematurity, genetic conditions, prenatal exposure to alcohol or drugs, social deprivation, or brain injury from trauma or infection (**Box 1**). Like children from other cultural, ethnic, socioeconomic, and geographic groups, some indigenous children experience developmental delays. Unfortunately, published prevalence studies of developmental delay in indigenous populations are lacking. Nonetheless, it is possible that the prevalence of developmental delays is higher in indigenous communities than in other settings because of poverty, lack of resources, lower parental education, and other "upstream determinants" of health and developmental outcomes. Increased rates of developmental delays could result from four possible

---

Division of Child Development and Community Health, University of California at San Diego, 9500 Gilman Drive, Dept. 0927, La Jolla, CA 92093-0927, USA
* Corresponding author.
E-mail address: sgahagan@ucsd.edu (S. Gahagan).

Pediatr Clin N Am 56 (2009) 1501–1517
doi:10.1016/j.pcl.2009.09.017
0031-3955/09/$ – see front matter © 2009 Elsevier Inc. All rights reserved.

Box 1
Risk factors for developmental delay

Genetics

Perinatal factors

    Prematurity

    Prenatal alcohol and drug exposure

    Social deprivation

    Brain injury from trauma or infection

    Micronutrient deficiencies

Exogenous exposures

    Environmental toxins—lead, methylmercury, etc

Social context

    Poverty

    Resources for children with developmental delay

    Child rearing as related to social status within group or within country

    Cultural concern about developmental delay

    Low parental education

---

mechanisms known to relate to health disparities: (1) social stratification within countries, (2) differential exposure to conditions that increase risk for developmental delay, (3) differential vulnerability to certain causes of developmental delay, and (4) differential consequences of developmental delay.[3]

"Social context" connotes societal factors measured at the group level rather than the level of the individual child or family. Social context includes the structure, culture, and function of a social system and can influence child development. Exposures to risk and protective factors are distributed and clustered within populations and social systems. Therefore, developmental delay is also distributed and clustered according to social context. In other words, social systems can contribute to cause or prevention of developmental delay.[4–6] For example, societies that embrace the care and health of the pregnant mother promote a variety of factors that reduce prematurity. On the other hand, some social systems tolerate alcohol consumption during pregnancy, thereby acting as an upstream determinant of fetal alcohol syndrome (FAS). In fact, social behaviors within a culture can be transmitted from "affected" individuals to "susceptible" individuals much as contagious diseases pass from one person to another. In addition to between-group and within-group social determinants, there are powerful national and global drivers that differentially distribute power, wealth, and risks. Labor policies, racial discrimination, systems of education, health care, and political representation can influence health outcomes, including child development. These systems determine available resources that modify risks for developmental delay in different socially, culturally, or geographically defined groups. Social position and the magnitude of inequality at the national or international level can determine group-level health outcomes. Many indigenous groups have low social position within their own countries and even lower status on a worldwide basis. All of these factors could increase risk for developmental delay compared with children who have access to more resources.

Exposures to health risks and protective factors differ by social structure, culture, and geography. Examples of differential exposure to health risks include high rates of alcohol abuse and exposure to environmental toxins in some communities. Alcoholism is prevalent and associated with increased risk for FAS, child neglect, accidents, and injuries in many indigenous societies. Developmental delay can result directly or indirectly. Some indigenous communities are located near environmental contaminants and provide examples of the influence of geography. There is reason to be concerned about potentially adverse effects of environmental chemicals on child development. Theoretically, the risks are higher for individuals exposed in utero and during infancy when there is rapid growth and central nervous system development. Parts of the Navajo reservation, Canada, and aboriginal-controlled lands in Australia and the Marshall Islands are proximate to a variety of toxins such as uranium and nuclear waste from weapons testing.[7-10] While there may be reason for concern, systematic research is lacking. In addition, low-income communities are at increased risk for creating opportunities for toxic exposure. Storage and transport of toxic metals such as lead, mercury, organophosphates, and polychlorinated biphenyls can be enticing to indigenous communities as sources of revenue. These activities could pose potential risks to child development and health.[11,12]

Indigenous people living in Arctic regions experience regular exposure methylmercury, lead, and polychlorinated biphenyls through their marine diet.[13] While little rigorous evaluation exists regarding the effect of toxins on child development in these communities, one cohort of 150 Inuit children in the Nunavik region of northern Quebec is involved in a longitudinal study of neuropsychological status. At preschool age, levels of methylmercury and polychlorinated biphenyls were related to alterations of visual evoked potentials.[14] Methylmercury concentrations were also related to tremor amplitude, a finding previously noted in adults.[15] In addition, blood lead concentrations were correlated with impulsivity and high activity.[16] Blood lead levels were also associated with a variety of neuropsychological variables including reaction time, sway oscillations, alternating arm movements, and action tremor. For some of these outcomes, neuromotor effects of lead exposure were observed at blood concentrations less than 10 μg/dl.

Differential vulnerability explains some excess risk for developmental delay in indigenous groups. Indigenous populations may have differential vulnerability to health-damaging exposures related to prior illness, nutritional status, or cultural practices. Under consideration are sensitive periods of development combined with community-level risks, and genetic causes of developmental delay. Exposures during sensitive periods of development cause pathology even though the same exposure outside of that developmental period is not known to be harmful. One example involves iron deficiency anemia which is associated with irreversible impairment in cognitive and behavioral functioning if experienced during infancy.[17,18] Iron deficiency later in life does not result in similar problems. Iron deficiency anemia continues to be an important problem in North American indigenous children. One study of the prevalence of iron deficiency anemia in Aboriginal children found rates eight times higher than in comparable populations in urban Canada and was especially high among Inuit children.[19] Genetic disorders causing developmental delay are known in some indigenous communities. For example, the Artemis gene prevalent in Navajo and Apache individuals causes an autosomal recessive form of severe combined immunodeficiency syndrome.[20,21] These infants can present with developmental delay because of the severity of their systemic illness. Navajos and some indigenous Alaskan groups have increased rates of metachromatic leukodystrophy, a progressive degenerative disease which presents with delay and loss of milestones. Another example of increased vulnerability to a disease resulting in developmental delay is genetically determined encephalitis and leukoencephalopathy in the Cree.[22–24]

Social and economic consequences of ill health vary by culture. In the case of developmental delay, social consequences may be less adverse in some indigenous groups that are more accepting of individuals with physical handicaps and cognitive impairment than other western societies.[25] Some indigenous cultures define human worth based on holistic and spiritual value rather than on physical or cognitive ability. In societies in which economic survival depends more on the family group than on the individual, developmental disability may be seen as less of a burden. On the other hand, access to needed services for children with developmental delay may be severely curtailed by impoverished schools and geographic isolation. The combination of more acceptance and fewer resources could adversely affect long-term outcomes for affected children.

Many indigenous groups experience high rates of poverty. In the United States, low socioeconomic status has been directly related to a wide variety of developmental delays. Children from families with low socioeconomic status show higher rates of growth retardation, low birth weight, and congenital anomalies than children from more advantaged families.[26,27] Neurobehavioral development during prenatal life and infancy is influenced by poverty-related micronutrient deficiencies. In addition to iron deficiency, deficiencies in folate, zinc, and cadmium could play a role.[28,29] Other factors related to low socioeconomic status, such as cigarette smoking, also influence the in utero availability of micronutrients. Family income and parent education also relate to eventual intellectual attainment. Advantaged socioeconomic groups may have greater access to child developmental activities that stimulate cognitive development in comparison to groups with fewer economic resources including poorer indigenous groups. Programs that promote economic development in addition to nutrition and early childhood educational programs can decrease the rate of developmental delay in low-income groups.[30]

Poverty also shows a clear association with poorer scores on mental health assessments. In the United States, children raised in low-income families score lower on assessments of cognitive development, school achievement, and emotional well-being than children from higher-income families.[31–35] Information about white, African American, and Hispanic American children is available from nationally representative studies. Yet, little is known about how American Indian children compare with other race or ethnic groups.

Family income acts as a determinant of child developmental outcomes in a generic manner. However, family-specific and culture-specific characteristics can modify these relationships. With this in mind, pediatric providers who care for indigenous children may apply their knowledge of the culture and contexts in which they work. This could lead to improved understanding of how child developmental pathways reflect or differ from those of the other cultural groups. One important question is whether the association between poverty and child development is due to income per se, or whether family or societal conditions occurring with poverty determine the developmental pathways. Such family conditions could include single-parent households, young parents, or parents with low educational levels. Societal-level conditions could include unsafe neighborhoods, homelessness, schools with fewer resources, or a culture that does not value or promote child cognitive and language development. If the determinant is not poverty per se, poverty might be associated with conditions that result in lower levels of child development such as poorer conditions for housing and nutrition, or the absence of stimulating toys and books. Some children experience brief periods of poverty while others experience more sustained poverty. Data from the national Longitudinal Survey of Youth showed that children who experienced persistent poverty scored six to nine points lower on tests of child development compared with children who had never lived in poverty. Children who lived transiently below the poverty level also scored two to six points lower on child development tests compared with children who had never been poor.[36] As previously stated, the authors are unaware of studies comparing groups of indigenous children to other developmental cohorts.

SURVEILLANCE, SCREENING, AND ASSESSMENT

Early identification of children with developmental delay allows for diagnosis of conditions that respond to medical or educational intervention. In 2006, the American Academy of Pediatrics recommended that child health providers systematically assess infants and toddlers for developmental delay using a combination of surveillance and standardized developmental screening tools, followed by developmental evaluation for those who exhibit signs of delay.[37] Developmental surveillance is a process of attending to parental concern and direct observation of the child's development at each health care maintenance visit during the first 3 years. While surveillance is an important component for finding children with developmental delay, administration of standardized screening tools increases ascertainment of developmental problems (**Table 1**). Recommended screening takes place at 9, 18, and 30 months. These are important opportunities for assessing sensory, motor, language, and social development. Among many standardized screening tools, the Ages and Stages Questionnaire[38] and the Parents' Evaluation of Developmental Status (PEDS)[39] are efficient, inexpensive, and translated into a number of languages. In addition, a specific tool to assess risk for autism should be included at 18 and 30 months.[40] When developmental delay is suspected based on surveillance or screening, a medical evaluation for diagnosis of possible genetic, motor, or central nervous system conditions is warranted. In addition, most children with suspected developmental delay benefit from a multidisciplinary evaluation by therapists in speech, fine motor and gross motor development, and a developmental psychologist. Referral to early intervention services is possible in the United States as all states have some early education services accessible from birth to 3-years.

EARLY DEVELOPMENTAL MILESTONES IN SPECIFIC CONTEXTS OF INDIGENOUS LIFE
The First Laugh: A Developmental Milestone with Cultural Significance

Different cultures celebrate developmental milestones with a variety of approaches. A particularly interesting celebration of a developmental milestone is the Navajo "first laugh" celebration. Infants laugh aloud at approximately 4-months old. In Navajo culture, this developmental milestone is celebrated as the moment when the child's soul becomes firmly attached to the body. At a time when infant mortality was high, many infants did not survive the first 4 months. As the family celebrated the attachment of the child's soul to the body, the family and the community also acknowledged their attachment to the child. This wonderful symbolic celebration is very alive today. As currently practiced, the person who causes the child to laugh aloud for the very first time is honored to host the feast. The celebration includes symbolic gifts from the infant to the guests. These gifts often represent the family's clan affiliation, such as salt from a special salt mine from an infant born into the Salt Clan.

Cradleboard: A Cultural Practice That Influences Infant Behavior and Development

Early experience can affect later development. The cradleboard is an excellent example of a culturally determined, child-rearing practice that influences social

Table 1
Developmental screening tools for use in primary care

Screening Tool	Age	Duration	Time for Scoring	Requirements	Scoring	Languages	Cost
ASQ: Ages and Stages Questionnaire	4 mo–5 y	10–15 min	3 mins	Age-specific parent questionnaires that test intellectual and motor skills	Score quantified by level of risk in 5 developmental areas.	English Spanish French Korean	$199.95 Brookes Publishing http://www.agesandstages.com (21 questionnaires and scoring sheets for copying and CD-ROM with printable PDFs)
PEDS: Parents' Evaluation of Developmental Status	Birth to 8 y	2–10 min	****	Non-age-specific parental interview. Initial screen for developmental and behavioral problems, with further referral recommended.	Score quantified by level of risk. Algorithm helps to determine whether to refer for evaluation.	English Spanish French Portuguese Laotian Thai Malaysian Arabic Vietnamese Swahili Chinese Taiwanese Indonesian	$30.00 http://www.pedstest.com (Brief Administration & Scoring Guide, 50 PEDS Response Forms, 50 PEDS Score & Interpretation Forms)

development and interaction. Used by many indigenous groups in North America, the cradleboard is a variation of swaddling in which the baby is strapped to a board (**Fig. 1**). Wrapping an infant in a blanket, sheet, or in bands to restrict movement has been practiced widely around the world, especially in temperate climates. This practice continues in the immediate neonatal period in North America, Europe, and Asia. Many societies believe that swaddling reduces spontaneous startles and helps babies to remain calm or asleep. In 1978, Chisholm[41] observed 150 Navajo mother-infant dyads every 2 months for 1 year as part of an ethological study. The infants spent approximately 15 to18 hours per day in the cradleboard during the first 3 months, followed by a gradual decrease to 6 to 9 hours per day at one year. The cradleboard was used mostly to let the infant sleep, although not necessarily at night. The mothers perceived that the cradleboard helped the infants maintain longer sleep, for they did not jerk and wake themselves up. This study showed that these infants spent more time in drowsy or sleep states compared with other infants in the United States who were not swaddled, although no causality was inferred. Chisholm observed that the use of the cradleboard influenced mother-infant interaction in that both were less responsive to each other when the infant was on the cradleboard. This may have been because the cradleboard itself helped the infants to stop crying and to achieve sleep. On the other hand, the cradleboard seemed to promote maternal-child proximity, as the cradleboard was often held or placed supine or upright within 3 ft of the mother.

It is often assumed that the restriction of infant motor movements can delay the onset of walking. Especially in cultures that highly value independence, walking is considered the most important gross motor developmental milestone. In contemporary western societies, children walk independently when they are approximately 13-months old, with 97% taking their first step between 9 and 18 months. While it is clear that restriction of motor activity in children can delay the onset of walking, the

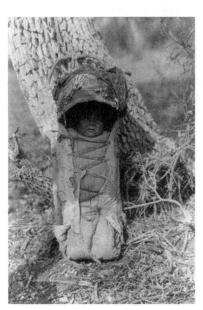

Fig. 1. Apache child in cradleboard. (*Courtesy of* Edward Curtis Collection, Library of Congress.)

cradleboard as practiced by the Navajo does not delay the onset of walking. The average age of independent walking in Chisholm's group of 150 infants was 13.9 months, well within the normal range for North American infants. As practiced by the Navajo, the cradleboard allowed ample time for motor development, leading to walking at the typical developmental age. Therefore, the cultural practice of using the cradleboard for sleep, comfort, and soothing influenced infant behavior but not motor development.

LANGUAGE: INFLUENCE ON DEVELOPMENT

Cultural differences in language development may relate to how adults speak to children. In all studied language groups, children learn nouns before verbs, at least for the first 20 words. Soon thereafter, the categories of new words may diverge according to how caregivers speak to young children in each language. Word development in children with English-speaking caregivers differs from that in children with Mandarin-speaking caregivers. Research by Tardif and colleagues[42] showed that English-speakers emphasized nouns over verbs and Mandarin-speakers emphasized verbs over nouns. When children's spontaneous word production was studied, the children cared for by English-speaking caregivers produced more nouns and those cared for by Mandarin-speaking caregivers produced relatively more verbs. Getner and Boroditsky's[43] work explores the effect of the Navajo language on child language development. In Navajo, verbs are relatively important. For example, there are more verb bases than noun bases, and many nouns are derived from verbs. Furthermore, Navajo verbs are semantically complex, as they can incorporate features of the subject noun and can stand alone as sentences. Finally, verbs often occur in the sentence-final position. In a study of five Navajo monolingual children ages 18 to 26 months, the investigators found that object terms predominated at the beginning of expressive language development. In addition, terms for animate beings were especially common in this context. The proportion of verbs increased with vocabulary size, reflecting their importance. This research suggests that language itself may influence development. Boroditsky[44] is taking this idea a step further and exploring whether language might influence the way that people think, see the world, and live their lives. The Kuuk Thaayorre from Pormpuraaw, a small Aboriginal community on the western edge of Cape York in northern Australia, use cardinal-direction terms—north, south, east, and west—to define space, rather than words that define space relative to the observer such as left, right, forward, and backward.[45] The Kuuk Thaayorre have remarkable navigational ability even in unfamiliar terrain, suggesting that there is an association between language and brain functioning. Pediatric providers in indigenous communities may benefit from greater understanding of the local language and how it might influence a child's development and relationship with the world.

Many indigenous children grow up in bilingual households. Others may speak their native language at home in early childhood and learn another language when they begin school. Language development follows the same sequence for children who acquire two languages simultaneously as for monolingual children. Bilingual children may begin to speak slightly later than monolingual children, but this delay is not associated with later problems.[46] Furthermore, vocabulary development proceeds at a normal rate in bilingual children.[47] It was once believed that bilingual children had lower cognitive abilities, but early acquisition of two languages may in fact enhance "cognitive flexibility," verbal abilities, and spatial perception.[48,49] While bilingualism per se is not related to speech and language delay, socioeconomic status is highly correlated with language development. The risk for language delay in bilingual indigenous households may be related to conditions associated with poverty. Therefore, indigenous children who are living in impoverished circumstances may have higher rates of language delay compared with children in more advantaged settings. It is, therefore, all the more important to systematically screen for language delay in low-income indigenous settings.

Pediatric providers may find it challenging to adequately screen bilingual children or children who speak indigenous languages for language delay. Screening tools that rely on a parental report such as the Ages and Stages Questionnaire[37] may be used as long as there is an appropriate translator and the concepts tested are culturally and geographically appropriate. For example asking a child for their address is not helpful in a setting where there are no street names and house numbers. Another screening tool, the PEDS, has the advantage of relying on parental concern about development rather than focusing on specific milestones.[39,50] To date, this tool has not been systematically tested in an indigenous setting. However, it has been shown to be valid in lower income groups and in urban and rural settings in the United States. Eliciting parental concern seems to be all the more important in low-income settings as these parents are less likely to spontaneously share their concern than parents that are more affluent. The use of a brief informational video in a low-income setting has been shown to lead to more information being shared during the pediatric visit.[51] The Parents' Evaluation of Developmental Status—Developmental Milestones (PEDS-DM) is a tool that can be used in conjunction with the PEDS for review of specific milestones (**Fig. 2**A, B). If the child fails a screening assessment or if the parents are concerned about the child's speech, a comprehensive speech and language assessment is needed. This presents an important challenge as there are few speech pathologists who speak indigenous languages. Rather than assess the child solely in their non-native language, the speech pathologist may work with a skilled translator.

In summary, new research suggests that languages frame thought in interesting ways. Children who speak indigenous languages may develop differently because of the influence of their language and the impact of their culture. An additional consideration is bilingualism. Because research is lacking, it is challenging to identify language delay in indigenous children. Nonetheless, they are at increased risk for language delay from a variety of factors. Therefore, it is important to develop effective screening strategies. Finally, training speech therapists who can evaluate and treat children in their own languages could begin to eliminate some disparities in outcomes.

AUTISM: LANGUAGE AND SOCIAL DEVELOPMENTAL DELAY

Autistic spectrum disorders (ASD) are a group of developmental disorders characterized by speech delay, impaired communication, and social impairment with unusual behaviors and interests. Over the last decade, it has become clear that there is a wide spectrum of impairment for each of the core characteristics. Approximately 70% of autistic children have cognitive impairment. However, some autistic individuals have high IQ and some have significant strengths in music, drawing, memory, or spatial relationships. While ascertained prevalence has gone up dramatically in the United States over several decades, it remains unclear whether this reflects an actual increase or improved ascertainment. Current estimates of the prevalence of ASD in the United States are 1 per 150 children. ASD is four times more likely in boys than girls. The CDC reports that ASD occurs in all ethnic groups. Exciting new research is revealing that many autistic disorders are genetically determined. In addition, some environmental conditions seem to increase risk for autistic behaviors. Children who were premature have an increased incidence of ASD, which suggests that brain injury can contribute to this condition. Furthermore, there is co-occurrence of FAS and ASD. Because both disorders are relatively common, this could occur by chance alone. However, it is also possible that brain injury resulting from alcohol toxicity could sometimes lead to symptoms of ASD.

To date, the documented prevalence of ASD in aboriginal people is low. While it is conceivable that the ASD is uncommon in these populations, it is also possible that ascertainment is poor. For example, cognitively impaired children with ASD may be identified only by their cognitive impairment and without a dual diagnosis. It is also possible that higher functioning children with ASD are accepted within their families and cultures and not labeled as having a disability. Some Native American and Native Hawaiian groups facilitate acceptance of individuals with social and communication impairment and assist their integration into the family and society.[25,52] In other cultural settings, a child with ASD may be viewed as representing past parental misdeeds (Mojave) or the outcome of witchcraft (Navajo).[52] Such beliefs are not uniformly accepted throughout any aboriginal group.

While it was once believed that ASD could only be diagnosed after a child's third birthday, it is now accepted that ASD can be diagnosed during the second year of life. Furthermore, there are often clues even earlier. Early diagnosis is based on speech and language delay and early delays in social development. One of the most marked early social impairments is the absence of joint attention. Typically developing children

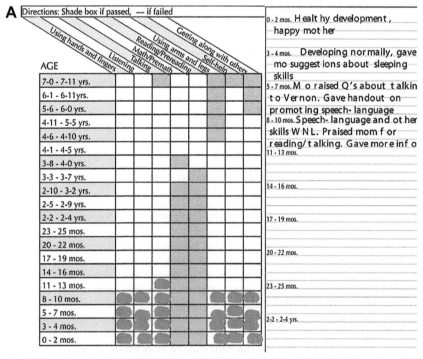

Fig. 2. (A) Sample page from PEDS-DM. (B) Sample page from PEDS-DM. (*Reprinted from* Glascoe FP, Robertshaw NS. PEDS: Developmental Milestones. http://pedstest.com/dm/files/casestudy-2_vernon.pdf. Accessed October 23, 2009.)

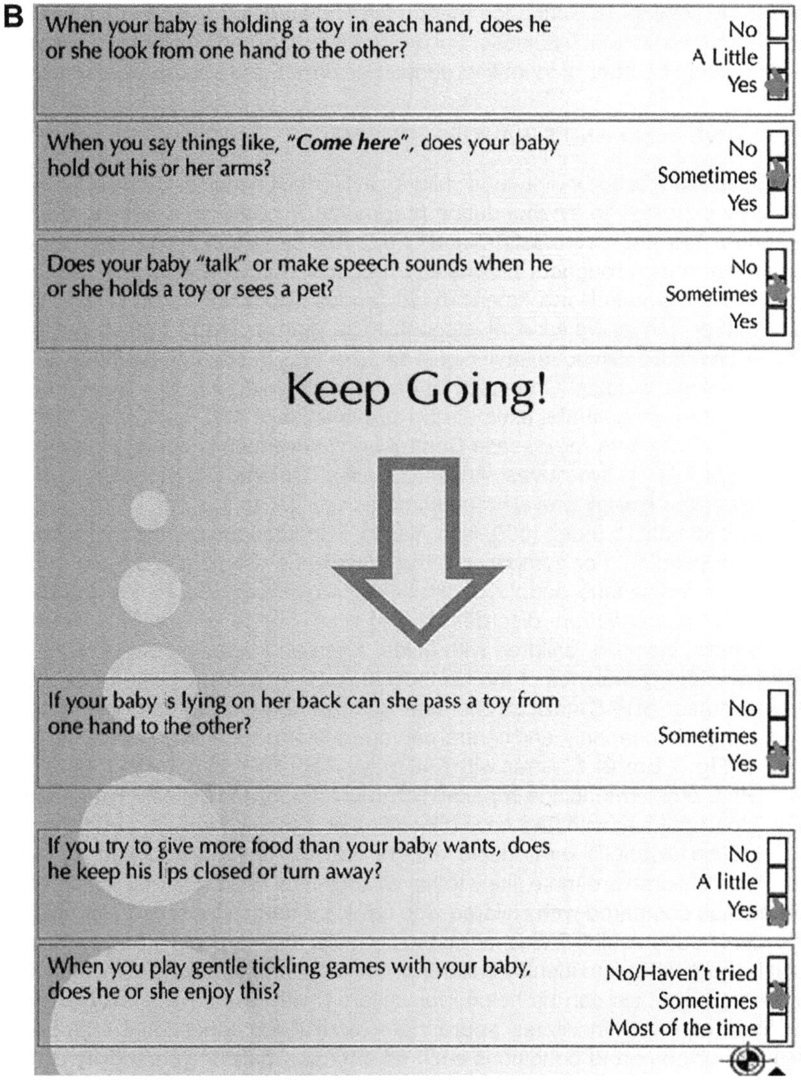

B

| When your baby is holding a toy in each hand, does he or she look from one hand to the other? | No ☐ A Little ☐ Yes ■ |

| When you say things like, **"Come here"**, does your baby hold out his or her arms? | No ☐ Sometimes ■ Yes ☐ |

| Does your baby "talk" or make speech sounds when he or she holds a toy or sees a pet? | No ☐ Sometimes ■ Yes ☐ |

Keep Going!

| If your baby is lying on her back can she pass a toy from one hand to the other? | No ☐ Sometimes ☐ Yes ■ |

| If you try to give more food than your baby wants, does he keep his lips closed or turn away? | No ☐ A little ☐ Yes ■ |

| When you play gentle tickling games with your baby, does he or she enjoy this? | No/Haven't tried ☐ Sometimes ■ Most of the time ☐ |

Fig. 2. (*continued*)

can understand that another person can experience the same thing that they are experiencing. For example, an 18-month old easily understands that he can look at a light and that his mother can look at the same light and see the same thing. In addition, toddlers begin to check to see if their caregivers are watching them during the second year of life. Pediatric providers can assess for lack of joint attention and other early signs of autism using the Modified Checklist for Autism in Toddlers at the 18-month health care maintenance visit.[40] Toddlers who exhibit risk on a screening test should be referred for complete evaluation by a developmental specialist. The Autism Diagnostic Observation Schedule[53] is used for diagnosis.

Identification is important because very early intervention can improve social development and language development. Programs for children with autism include training in social skills that typically developing children learn by observation and imitation. In addition, early speech and language therapy can advance communication and aid in the development of school readiness. Children with autism should also have screening for the increasing number of identified genetic disorders associated with autism.

FAS: COGNITIVE DELAY AND BEHAVIOR PROBLEMS

FAS has been identified in indigenous children in North America since the 1970s. FAS is caused by exposure to alcohol during pregnancy. To date, a safe level of alcohol consumption has not been determined. Furthermore, alcohol can have adverse effects on the fetus throughout pregnancy. It is commonly believed that the prevalence of FAS is higher in North American indigenous populations than in other populations because the prevalence of alcoholism is high in many tribes. Indigenous Australians are also believed to have higher rates of FAS but to date there are few reliable epidemiologic studies. One study of indigenous children in the Top End of the Northern Territory in Australia estimated a prevalence of 1.87 to 4.7 per 1000 live births.[54] The US Centers for Disease Control and Prevention is conducting a prevalence study of FAS in five states: Arizona, Alaska, Colorado, Wisconsin, and New York. To date, the overall prevalence estimates are 0.2 to 1.5 per 1000 live births. The highest estimate, 1.5 per 1000, is in Alaska.[55] Indigenous people make up 22% of Alaska's population. For comparison, the prevalence estimate is 0.3 per 1000 for Arizona where indigenous people comprise approximately 7% of the population. Like ASD, FAS is a spectrum disorder ranging from mild to severe. The prevalence of FAS disorder, including children with milder brain and behavior effects is likely to be three times the prevalence of the full form of FAS.

The presentation of FAS includes characteristic dysmorphic features, growth impairment including microcephaly, and central nervous system problems including cognitive impairment (**Fig. 3, Box 2**). Children with FAS may present with hyperactivity or difficulty learning. Other problems include impaired communication, and deficits in attention and memory. Many children with FAS have difficulties processing tactile or auditory stimulation. Because alcohol's teratogenic effects can disrupt development in various organs, these children are more likely to have congenital heart defects, renal defects, and strabismus compared with children who have not been exposed to alcohol.

While identification of full FAS is facilitated by facial dysmorphism and growth retardation, it is more difficult to identify children with milder presentations of the spectrum. Nonetheless, diagnosis can be helpful for children with less severe involvement as identification of FASD facilitates appropriate referral for educational support and assessment for comorbid conditions such as attention-deficit/hyperactivity disorder

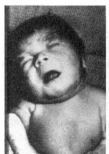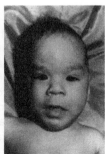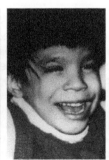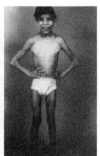

Fig. 3. Indigenous boy, born to alcoholic mother, shown at birth, 8 months, 4 years, and 8 years. (*Courtesy of* Ann Streissguth, PhD, University of Washington Fetal Alcohol and Drug Unit, Seattle.)

Box 2
Phenotype of FAS

Growth

    Prenatal growth deficiency

    Postnatal growth deficiency

    Microcephaly

Performance

    Developmental delay

    Fine-motor dysfunction

    Behavioral problems

Face

    Maxillary hypoplasia

    Short palpebral fissures

    Long, smooth philtrum

    Thin vermilion border of upper lip

(ADHD). In addition, it is helpful for the child and the family to understand the child's behavioral phenotype. Furthermore, a diagnosis helps the family to anticipate a likely lifelong developmental trajectory related to this disability. In addition, early identification has been found to improve prognosis related to social adaptation.

When assessing a child with social or cognitive developmental delay, FASD should be considered as part of the differential diagnosis. The evaluation for FASD begins with a careful prenatal history addressing exposure to tobacco, alcohol, medications, or illicit drugs. When taking an alcohol history, it is useful to assess the mother's pre-pregnancy alcohol-consumption pattern, followed by determination of when she became aware of her pregnancy. This is followed by assessing whether she changed her alcohol intake related to the pregnancy. Frequently, the alcohol-exposed child is out of the mother's care, making a diagnosis more difficult. The authors have been successful obtaining maternal alcohol histories with the help of social service

---

Box 3
The T-ACE Questionnaire

The T-ACE questions

T Tolerance: How many drinks does it take to make you feel high?

A Annoyance: Have people annoyed you by criticizing your drinking?

C Cut down: Have you ever felt you ought to cut down on your drinking?

E Eye-opener: Have you ever had a drink first thing in the morning to steady your nerves or to get rid of a hangover?

The T-ACE is considered positive with a score of two or more. Affirmative answers to the A, C, and E questions are each scored one point. A reply of more than two drinks to the T question is scored two points.

Data from Chang G. Screenings and brief interventions in prenatal care settings. Alcohol Res Health 2004/2005;28:80–4; Sokol RJ, Martier SS, Ager JW et al. The T-ACE questions: practical prenatal detection of risk-drinking. Am J Obstet Gynecol 1989;160:863–71.

Table 2
Strength of evidence for recommendations

Recommendation	Grading of Recommendation	Quality of Supporting Evidence
Developmental surveillance at each health care maintenance visit	Strong	Moderate[16]
Developmental screening with standardized instrument at 9, 18, and 30 mo	Strong	Moderate[16]
Developmental evaluation for infants and toddlers identified by surveillance and screening	Strong	Moderate[16]
Early intervention for infants and toddlers with developmental delay	Strong	Moderate[16]

agencies. The social worker can interview the mother or someone who lived with her during her pregnancy. Alcohol-screening questionnaires are used in some settings. The T-ACE is recommended for use in pregnant women (**Box 3**, **Table 2**).[56,57]

Young children with FASD often present with high activity levels and disrupted sleep. A complete evaluation of these presenting symptoms includes assessment of prenatal alcohol exposure. The medical history includes a thorough behavioral assessment. A careful physical examination with attention to facial morphology follows. Affected children without the full syndrome may not have impressive dysmorphology. The University of Washington's *Diagnostic guide for fetal alcohol syndrome and related conditions: the 4-digit diagnostic code* provides a manual-based approach for assessing children for FASD.[58] New photographic software can assist in facial measurements and assist in reliable assessment.[59] Developmental assessment is warranted when FASD is diagnosed.

Children with FASD benefit from early intervention. While they often exhibit normal early-word learning, significant communication problems are common and most evident during peer interactions. Hyperactivity is also associated with learning problems and social impairment. Many children with FASD meet diagnostic criteria for ADHD. Management of children with inattention can be difficult, as it is with children with brain injury and ADHD. However, stimulant therapy is often helpful, especially for control of hyperactivity.[60] In addition, many children with FASD perform below the level predicted by their IQ scores. IQ scores in the normal range can be a barrier to accessing appropriate special education services. Some states in the United States offer special education services to children with FASD based categorically on the diagnosis.[61] While the benefit of intervention is undeniable, every effort should be made to prevent FASD.

SUMMARY

Developmental delay is common. Furthermore, indigenous children may experience higher risk for developmental delay compared with other children. Some indigenous cultures are child-focused and provide excellent care and nurturing of developmentally delayed and disabled children. Culturally specific child care practices can influence child development. Indigenous children can benefit from developmental surveillance, screening, and evaluation (see **Table 2**). Finally, early intervention is recommended for young children with developmental delay.

REFERENCES

1. Costello EJ, Edelbrock C, Costello AJ, et al. Psychopathology in pediatric primary care: the new hidden morbidity. Pediatrics 1988;82:415–24.

2. Lavigne JV, Binns HJ, Christoffel KK, et al. Behavioral and emotional problems among preschool children in pediatric primary care: prevalence and pediatricians' recognition. Pediatric Practice Research Group. Pediatrics 1993;91:649–55.
3. Diderichsen F, Evans T, Whitehead M, et al. The social basis of disparities in health. In: Diderichsen F, Evans T, Whitehead M, editors. Challenging inequities in health: from ethics to action. New York: Oxford University Press; 2001. p. 13–23.
4. Emerson E. Poverty and people with intellectual disabilities. Ment Retard Dev Disabil Res Rev 2007;13:107–13.
5. Skinner D, Weisner TS. Sociocultural studies of families of children with intellectual disabilities. Ment Retard Dev Disabil Res Rev 2007;13:302–12.
6. Emerson E, Hatton C. Poverty, socioeconomic position, social capital and the health of children and adolescents with intellectual disabilities in Britain: a replication. J Intellect Disabil Res 2007;51:866–74.
7. Panikkar B, Brugge D. The ethical issues in uranium mining research in the Navajo Nation. Account Res 2007;14:121–53.
8. Bowerman RJ. Alaska Native cancer epidemiology in the Arctic. Public Health 1998;112:7–13.
9. Martin P, Ryan B. Natural-series radionuclides in traditional aboriginal foods in tropical northern Australia: a review. Scientific World Journal 2004;4:77–95.
10. Jones CR. A United States perspective on long-term management of areas contaminated with radioactive materials. Radiat Prot Dosimetry 2004;109:75–7.
11. Van Oostdam J, Donaldson SG, Feeley M, et al. Human health implications of environmental contaminants in Arctic Canada: a review. Sci Total Environ 2005;(351–2):165–246.
12. Laduke W. Indigenous environmental perspectives: a North American primer. Akwe:kon Journal 1992;9:52–71. Available at: http://www.eric.ed.gov/ERICWebportal/custom/portlets/recordDetails/detailmini.jsp?_nfpb=true&_&ERICExtSearch_SearchValue_0=EJ460202&ERICExtSearch_SearchType_0=no&accno=EJ460202. Accessed October 19, 2009.
13. Arctic Pollution 2009. Arctic Montoring and Assessment Programme, Oslo. Available at: http://www.amap.no. Accessed July 24, 2009.
14. Saint-Amour D, Roy MS, Bastien C, et al. Alterations of visual evoked potentials in Inuit children exposed to methylmercury and polychlorinated biphenyls from a marine diet. Neurotoxicology 2006;27:567–78.
15. Fraser S, Muckle G, Despres C. The relationship between lead exposure, motor function and behavior in Inuit preschool children. Neurotoxicol Teratol 2006;28:18–27.
16. Despres C, Beuter A, Richer F, et al. Neuromotor functions in Inuit preschool children exposed to Pb, PCBs, and Hg. Neurotoxicol Teratol 2005;27:245–57.
17. Lozoff B, De Andraca I, Castillo M, et al. Behavioral and developmental effects of preventing iron-deficiency anemia in healthy full-term infants. Pediatrics 2003;112:846–54.
18. Halterman JS, Kaczorowski JM, Aligne CA, et al. Iron deficiency and cognitive achievement among school-aged children and adolescents in the United States. Pediatrics 2001;107:1381–6.
19. Christofides A, Schauer C, Zlotkin SH. Iron deficiency and anemia prevalence and associated etiologic risk factors in associated First Nations and Inuit communities in Northern Ontario and Nunavut. Can J Public Health 2005;96:304–7.
20. Li L, Drayna D, Hu D, et al. The gene for severe combined immunodeficiency disease in Athabascan-speaking Native Americans is located on chromosome 10p. Am J Hum Genet 1998;62:136–44.

21. Li L, Moshous D, Zhou Y, et al. A founder mutation in Artemis, an SNM1-like protein, causes SCID in Athabascan-speaking Native Americans. J Immunol 2002;168:6323–9.
22. Pastor-Soler NM, Schertz EM, Rafi MA, et al. Metachromatic leukodystrophy among southern Alaskan Eskimos: molecular and genetic studies. J Inherit Metab Dis 1995;18:326–32.
23. Holve S, Hu D, McCandless SE. Metachromatic leukodystrophy in the Navajo: fallout of the American-Indian wars of the nineteenth century. Am J Med Genet 2001;101:203–8.
24. Crow YJ, Black DN, Ali M, et al. Cree encephalitis is allelic with Aicardi-Goutiéres syndrome: implications for the pathogenesis of disorders of interferon alpha metabolism. J Med Genet 2003;40:183–7.
25. Milian M, Erin JN. Diversity and visual impairment: the influence of race, gender, religion, and ethnicity on the individual. New York: AFB Press; 2001.
26. Semba R, Bloem M, Piot P. Nutrition and health in developing countries. New Jersey: Humana Press; 2008. p. 114–5.
27. Huston A. Children in poverty: child development and public policy. New York: Cambridge University Press; 1994. p. 139.
28. Grantham-McGregor S, Ani C. A review of studies of the effect of iron deficiency on cognitive development in children. J Nutr 2001;131:649S–68S.
29. Klimis-Zacas D, Wolinsky I. Nutritional concerns of women. Boca Raton: CRC Press; 2003. p. 81.
30. Bradley R, Corwyn R. Socioeconomic status and child development. Annu Rev Psychol 2002;53:371–99.
31. Duncan GJ, Brooks-Gunn J. Consequences of growing up poor. New York: Russell Sage Foundation; 1997.
32. Duncan GJ, Brooks-Gunn J, Klebanov P. Economic deprivation and early-childhood development. Child Dev 1994;62:296–318.
33. Chase-Lansdale PL, Mott FL, Brooks-Gunn J, et al. Children of the National Longitudinal Survey of Youth, a unique research opportunity. Dev Psychol 1991;27:918–31.
34. Infant, Health, and Development Program. Enhancing the outcomes of low-birth weight, premature infants. JAMA 1990;263:3035–42.
35. Lee VE, Burkam DT. Inequality out of the starting gate: social background differences in achievement as children begin school. Washington, DC: Economic Policy Institute; 2002.
36. Korenman S, Miller JE, Sjaastad JE. Long-term poverty and child development; evidence from the NLSY. Child Youth Serv Rev 1995;17:127–55.
37. American Academy of Pediatrics. Identifying infants and young children with developmental disorders in the medical home: an algorithm for developmental surveillance and screening. Pediatrics 2006;118:405–20.
38. Ages and stages questionnaires. web site. Available at: http://www.agesandstages.com. Accessed July 2, 2009.
39. Parents' evaluation of developmental status. Available at: http://www.pedstest.com. Accessed July 2, 2009.
40. Modified checklist for autism in toddlers. Developmental behavioral pediatrics online. Available at: http://www.dbpeds.org/media/mchat.pdf. Accessed July 2, 2009.
41. Chisholm JS. Swaddling, cradleboards and the development of children. Early Hum Dev 1978;2:255–75.
42. Tardif T, Shatz M, Naigles L. Caregiver speech and children's use of nouns versus verbs: a comparison of English, Italian, and Mandarin. J Child Lang 1997;24:535–65.

43. Getner D, Boroditsky L. Early acquisition of nouns and verbs: evidence from Navajo. In: Mueller-Gathercole VC, editor. Routes to language. London: Psychology Press; 2009. p. 5–36.
44. Boroditsky L. How does our language shape the way we think? In: Brockman M, editor. What's next? Dispatches on the future of science. US: Vintage Books; 2009. p. 116–44.
45. Levinson SC, Wilkins DP, editors. Grammars of space: explorations in cognitive diversity. New York: Cambridge University Press; 2006.
46. Goodz N. Interactions between parents and children in bilingual families. In: Genesee F, editor. Educating second language children: the whole child, the whole curriculum, the whole community. New York: Cambridge University Press; 1994. p. ix.
47. Umbel VM, Pearson BZ, Fernandez MC, et al. Measuring bilingual children's receptive vocabularies. Child Dev 1992;63:1012–20.
48. Cummins J. The influence of bilingualism on cognitive growth: a synthesis of research findings and explanatory hypotheses. Working Papers on Bilingualism 1976;9:11–43. Available at: http://www.eric.ed.gov/ERICWebportal/custom/portlets/recordDetails/detailmini.jsp?_nfpb=true&_&ERICExtSearch_SearchValue_0=ED125311&ERICExtSearch_SearchType_0=no&accno=ED125311. Accessed October 19, 2009.
49. Diaz R. Thought and two languages: the impact of bilingualism on cognitive development. In: Gordon E, editor, Review of research in education, vol. 10. Washington, DC: American Educational Research Association; 1983. p. 23–54.
50. Glascoe FP. Parents' concerns about children's development: prescreening technique or screening test? Pediatrics 1997;99:522–8.
51. Sices L, Drotar D, Keilman A, et al. Communication about child development during well-child visits: impacts of parents' evaluation of developmental status screener with or without an informational video. Pediatrics 2008;122:e1091–9.
52. Dyches TT, Wilder LK, Sudweeks RR, et al. Multicultural issues in autism. J Autism Dev Disord 2004;34:211–22.
53. Autism Diagnostic Observation Schedule. Western psychological services. Available at: http://portal.wpspublish.com/portal/page?_pageid=53,70384&_dad=portal&_schema=PORTAL. Accessed July 24, 2009.
54. Harris KR, Bucens IK. Prevalence of fetal alcohol syndrome in the Top End of the Northern Territory. J Paediatr Child Health 2003;39:528–33.
55. Miller L, Tolliver R, Druschel C, et al. Centers for Disease Control and Prevention. Fetal alcohol syndrome—Alaska, Arizona, Colorado, and New York, 1995–1997. MMWR Morb Mortal Wkly Rep. 2002;24:433–5.
56. Chang G. Screenings and brief interventions in prenatal care settings. Alcohol Res Health 2004;28:80–4.
57. Sokol RJ, Martier SS, Ager JW, et al. The T-ACE questions: practical prenatal detection of risk-drinking. Am J Obstet Gynecol 1989;160:863–71.
58. Diagnostic guide for fetal alcohol syndrome and related conditions: the 4-digit diagnostic code. Fetal Alcohol Syndrome Diagnostic and Prevention Network. University of Washington. Available at: http://depts.washington.edu/fasdpn/pdfs/guide99.pdf. Accessed July 2, 2009.
59. Astley SJ, Clarren SK. A case definition and photographic screening tool for the facial phenotype of fetal alcohol syndrome. J Pediatr 1996;129:33–41.
60. Peadon E, Rhys-Jones B, Bower C, et al. Systematic review of interventions for children with fetal alcohol spectrum disorders. BMC Pediatr 2009;9:35.
61. Lupton C, Burd L, Harwood R. Cost of fetal alcohol spectrum disorders. Am J Med Genet C Semin Med Genet 2004;127C:42–50.

Injuries and Injury Prevention Among Indigenous Children and Young People

Lawrence R. Berger, MD, MPH[a,b,*], L.J. David Wallace, MSEH[b,c],
Nancy M. Bill, MPH, CHES[b]

KEYWORDS

- Indians • Injuries • Accidents • Prevention
- Child • Indigenous

When asked what were the 3 most important health issues facing American Indians and Alaska Natives (AI/AN), a former director of the US Indian Health Service (IHS) was said to have replied, "Injuries, injuries, and injuries." Injuries can be devastating for individuals, families, and entire communities. Injuries account for 71% of childhood deaths in AI/AN children and young people in the United States (**Fig. 1**).[1] Almost the entire disparity in overall child mortality rates between AI/AN children and US white children would disappear if their mortality from injury was equal.[2]

This article aims to raise the visibility of injuries as a leading cause of preventable mortality and morbidity among indigenous communities in the United States and internationally. The approaches to injury prevention that are likely to be most effective are discussed. Several case studies are provided to illustrate how effective strategies have been translated into successful community-based interventions by indigenous communities.

CAUSES OF MORTALITY FROM INJURY AMONG AI/AN CHILDREN AND YOUNG PEOPLE

With 560 federally recognized tribes,[3] and more than half the population residing outside tribal lands,[4] there is enormous geographic and economic diversity in AI/AN. The nature and rates of injuries faced by individuals living in such diverse communities vary. Patterns of injury also differ by age group, reflecting fundamental differences in

[a] Department of Pediatrics, University of New Mexico School of Medicine, 1 University of New Mexico, Albuquerque, NM 87106, USA
[b] Injury Prevention Program, Indian Health Service, OEHE-EHS-TMP 610, 801 Thompson Ave, Suite 120, Rockville, MD 20852, USA
[c] 1330 Saratoga Avenue, Steamboat Springs, CO 80487, USA
* Corresponding author. Department of Pediatrics, University of New Mexico School of Medicine, 1 University of New Mexico, Albuquerque, NM 87106.
E-mail address: bergerlaw@msn.com (L.R. Berger).

Pediatr Clin N Am 56 (2009) 1519–1537
doi:10.1016/j.pcl.2009.09.016
0031-3955/09/$ – see front matter © 2009 Published by Elsevier Inc.

pediatric.theclinics.com

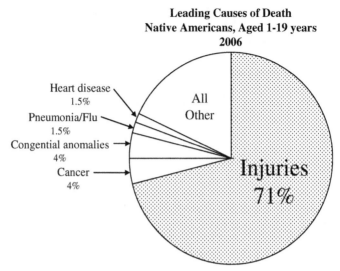

Leading Causes of Death
Native Americans, Aged 1-19 years
2006

Heart disease 1.5%
Pneumonia/Flu 1.5%
Congential anomalies 4%
Cancer 4%
All Other
Injuries 71%

Fig. 1. Leading causes of death in Native Americans, aged 1–19 years, 2006. More than two-thirds of all deaths involving American Indian and Alaska Native children and young people (aged 1–19 years) are the result of injuries and violence.

developmental circumstances (**Table 1**).[1] Of the AI/AN population, 38% are younger than 20 years, compared with 29% of the total US population.[5] The combination of a younger population profile and high rates of injuries among younger age groups results in injuries accounting for 40% of the years of potential life lost before age 65 years (more than heart disease, cancer, and diabetes combined).[6]

There has been progress toward reducing the burden of injuries among AI/AN. In a 20-year period (1982–1984 vs 2002–2004), the age-adjusted AI/AN mortality rate for unintentional injuries fell 28%, compared with a 5% decline for the United States as a whole.[1] Injuries caused by motor-vehicle accidents are the leading cause of unintentional deaths from injury among AI/AN children and young people (aged 1–19 years), accounting for two-thirds of those deaths.[1] (In Alaska, however, drowning is the leading cause of death among AI/AN children and motor vehicles are second.)

EFFECTIVE STRATEGIES FOR INJURY PREVENTION AMONG CHILDREN AND YOUNG PEOPLE

Injury prevention and control has matured to the extent that much is known about effective strategies in highly industrialized countries, numerous examples of success-ful community interventions have been reported, and excellent textbooks on injury

Table 1
Ranking and percentage of leading cause of injury death, by age group, AI/AN, 2003–2006

Rank	Infant (%)	Age 1–9 Years (%)	Age 10–19 Years (%)
1	Unintentional suffocation (44.6)	Motor vehicle traffic (36.8)	Motor vehicle traffic (44.1)
2	Homicide (20.1)	Homicide (14.2)	Suicide (24.6)
3	Motor vehicle traffic (18.0)	Drowning (11.6)	Homicide (11.0)
4	Falls (2.9)	Fires/burns (9.3)	Unintentional poisoning (4.2)
5	Drowning (2.2)	Pedestrian, nontraffic (6.3)	Drowning (2.8)

control are available.[7-12] The recently published (2007) *Handbook of injury and violence prevention*, edited by leading researchers at the Centers for Disease Control and Prevention (CDC), provides comprehensive reviews of effective and promising interventions, and sections on crosscutting issues and translating research into practice. Internationally, the importance of child injuries has been highlighted by 2 recent publications from the United Nations: *The world report on child injury prevention* and *The world report on violence against children.*[13,14]

A summary of proven and promising strategies appears in **Table 2**.[15-46] These recommended strategies are based on reviews of evidence by individual experts and collaborative groups of international stature. In injury prevention, the latter groups are represented by the Cochrane Database of Systematic Reviews[47] and the CDC's Task Force on Community Prevention Services.[48]

The Cochrane Database of Systemic Reviews is a component of the Cochrane Library. The database, which is updated every 3 months, has more than 3400 reviews. Each review involves multinational teams of experts and consumers, follows a structured format, uses a search strategy that includes unpublished and non-English studies, and assesses the quality of evidence according to predefined criteria.

The Task Force on Community Preventive Services "is an independent, nongovernmental, volunteer body of public health and prevention experts, whose members are appointed by the Director of CDC."[48] It has reviewed more than 200 interventions, including interventions to reduce injuries caused by motor vehicles, violence among children and young people, and alcohol-related injuries. Based on each systematic review, the Task Force recommends interventions for community implementation and identifies areas needing more research.

A major limitation of the "systematic review of published literature" process is that there are few, rigorously evaluated, injury-prevention interventions involving indigenous communities, especially for middle- and low-income countries, in which the nature and circumstances of injuries for indigenous communities are often different from those in highly industrialized countries. There are several important reasons for the scarcity of methodologically sound studies. Indigenous communities are often marginalized from the dominant society. Their numbers are usually small in relation to the total population of a country, their political influence minimal, and their needs often ignored because of geographic isolation, discrimination, and racism. There is often a deep distrust of outsiders that is engendered by a history of subjugation, exploitation, and loss of land, natural resources, and dignity. In the past, researchers may have published articles about sacred ceremonies or traditional practices without the consent of the Native community, or written disparagingly about the communities, making the communities reluctant to participate in any academic endeavor. Even without such a history, community leaders may be hesitant to have their communities stigmatized by open discussion of serious community problems like suicide or domestic violence. There may also be cultural barriers, such as the beliefs that speaking words like "death" or "child abuse" causes those tragedies to occur, that suicide is an immoral act that brings shame to the victim's family and community, or that loss of life through injuries is inevitable and is not preventable.

Traditional approaches to prevention and healing are especially difficult to evaluate. Traditional leaders and healers "may oppose the articulation, surveillance, regulation, and evaluation of traditional healing practices."[49] Small sample sizes, nonrandomized selection of program recipients, and variability in the nature and degree of exposure to traditional interventions present methodological challenges. Yet tribe-specific interventions, such as those aimed at "cultural restoration" or healing "spirit sickness," may have great power to transform individuals and ameliorate high-risk behaviors

Table 2
Proven and promising strategies to reduce injuries among children and young people

Mechanism/Type of Injury	Strategies (Recommended Grade)	Quality of Supporting Evidence and Key Findings	References
Motor-vehicle or bicycle injuries			
Increase use of child safety seats	Mandatory use laws (strong)	High. Laws decreased fatal injuries by 35%, but need to be enforced	15–18
	Community-wide information and enhanced enforcement campaigns such as checkpoints, saturation patrols (strong)	High. Child safety seat use increased 12% on average	15–18
	Distribution of child safety seats and education programs (strong)	High. Increased use of child safety seats by 23%	15–18
	Distribution and education programs to increase use of booster seats (strong)	High. Distribution, education, and incentive programs all were proven effective in increasing booster seat use among 4–8-year-olds	19
Increase use of safety belts	Mandatory use laws (strong)	High. Laws increased safety belt use by 33% compared with states with no law. Primary enforcement laws on average increase safety belt use by 14% compared with secondary laws	16–18,20
	Enhanced enforcement programs (strong)	High. Enhanced enforcement, such as "Click it or Ticket" campaigns increased safety belt use on average by 16%. Added benefit that they may increase detection of DUI or other offenses	16–18,20
Protect young drivers	Graduated driver licensing systems (strong)	High. Median decrease in young driver crash rates in the first year was 31%	18,21,22
	Night-time driving restriction curfews (strong)	High. Most fatal night-time crashes among young drivers occur between 9 pm and midnight. Several studies from the United States and Canada have found that ordinances that restrict unsupervised teen driving at night reduced teen driver fatalities by about 25%	21

Reduce alcohol-impaired driving	0.08% BAC laws (strong)	High. States that lowered their BAC laws from 0.1% to 0.08% saw a median decrease in alcohol-related fatal motor-vehicle crashes of 7%	16–18,23
	Zero tolerance laws for minors (strong)	High. Lower BAC limits for young and inexperienced drivers have been shown to reduce crash rates	16–18,23
	Sobriety checkpoints (strong)	High. Proven effective in reducing alcohol-related crashes and deaths by approximately 17%–25%. Recommended to be a part of all police enforcement programs	16–18,23
	School-based programs (strong)	Moderate. Sufficient evidence to recommend school programs to reduce riding with a drinking driver; insufficient evidence to determine if effective in reducing alcohol-impaired driving	17,18
	Mass media campaigns to reduce alcohol-impaired driving (strong)	High. Studies have found that robust mass media campaigns reduce alcohol-related crash rates by about 13%	17,18
	Designated driver programs (weak)	Low. Insufficient evidence to determine effectiveness	17,18
Reduce head trauma	Helmets for bicycle riders (strong)	High. Programs to promote helmet use by bicycle operators and passengers can have a substantial impact on reducing bicycle-related head injury	24,25
	Helmets for motorcyclists (strong)	High. Motorcycle helmets are 72% effective in reducing head injury. Helmet laws that cover riders of all ages increase helmet use from less than 50% to nearly 100%	26,27
Fire and burns			
Reduce residential fire deaths/injuries	Install smoke alarms (strong)	High. Researchers have found that having a working smoke alarm in the home reduced the risk of death from a house fire by as much as 71%. Research conducted in Native American homes recommended installing photoelectric alarms in place of ionization alarms to prevent nuisance alarms	28–30
	Smoke alarm distribution, and education and media campaigns (strong)	High. Fire injury rates were reduced by up to 80% after targeting high-risk neighborhoods with smoke alarm distribution combined with an education and media campaign	29,31

(continued on next page)

Table 2
(continued)

Mechanism/Type of Injury	Strategies (Recommended Grade)	Quality of Supporting Evidence and Key Findings	References
Reduce scald burns	Reduce hot water temperatures to 120°F or lower (strong)	High. Legislation and ordinances to require hot water heaters be preset at 120°F has proven to be the most effective in reducing scald burns to young children and older adults. Media campaigns and home visits are also effective in encouraging homeowners to measure and reduce hot water temperatures to 120°F. Educational campaigns alone have not been effective	32
Drowning			
Reduce drowning in natural bodies of water	Programs to promote wearing of PFDs, floatation coats (strong)	Moderate. PFD and float coat education and distribution programs have increased the use of these safety devices in Alaska Native villages	33,34
Reduce drowning in swimming pools	Install 4-sided fencing around pools (strong)	High. Installing 4-sided isolation fencing around swimming pools is a proven effective strategy in preventing drowning among children from birth to 5 years	34
Violence			
Reduce child maltreatment	Early childhood nurse home visitation programs (strong)	High. 40%–80% reduction in reported child abuse and neglect among children who received the home visit intervention compared with controls	35–38

Reduce self-destructive behaviors (suicide prevention)	Restrict access to lethal means (Strong)	High. Restricting access to lethal methods decreases suicides by those methods. Priority should be given to the most commonly used methods in each country	39,40
	School-based prevention programs to increase protective factors (eg, improve communication and problem-solving skills) and reduce risk factors (eg, identifying self-destructive behaviors) (strong)	Moderate. The Zuni Life Skills Development program has shown promising results among AI/AN young people of high-school age	40–42
	Physician education in recognizing and treating depression (strong)	High. Improved detection of depression, coupled with appropriate use of antidepressants, can be further enhanced through case management and quality improvement interventions	39
	"Gatekeeper" education: training individuals who have frequent contact with vulnerable populations to identify at-risk individuals and direct them to treatment (strong)	Moderate. Sufficient evidence of effectiveness "when gatekeeper roles are formalized and treatment options are readily available"	39,43,44
Reduce aggressive or violent behavior	Universal school-based programs (strong)	High. Universal programs teach all students in a given school or grade about violence and its prevention, or about topics such as positive social skills, problem-solving, and conflict resolution. All intervention strategies were associated with a 7% to 32% median reduction in violent behavior	45
Prevent alcohol-related injuries			
	Enhanced enforcement of laws prohibiting sale of alcohol to minors (strong)	High. Sufficient evidence of effectiveness that enhanced enforcement of laws prohibiting sale of alcohol to minors limits underage alcohol purchases	46

(continued on next page)

Table 2
(continued)

Mechanism/Type of Injury	Strategies (Recommended Grade)	Quality of Supporting Evidence and Key Findings	References
	Regulation of alcohol outlet density (strong)	High. Sufficient evidence to recommend licensing and zoning regulations to limit the density of alcohol outlets, based on the association between high density of alcohol outlets and excessive alcohol consumption and related harms	46
	Maintaining limits on days of sale (strong)	High. Strong evidence that repealing limits on sales of alcoholic beverages on weekend days contributed to excessive alcohol consumption and related harms	46
	Increasing alcohol taxes (strong)	High. Strong evidence of the effectiveness of increasing the unit price of alcohol by raising taxes to reduce excessive alcohol consumption and related harms. "Public health effects are expected to be proportional to the size of the tax increase"	46

Abbreviations: BAC, blood alcohol concentration; PFDs, personal flotation devices.

and hopelessness.[50,51] Although randomized controlled trials are the "gold standard" for clinical and public health research,[9] "some experts, particularly in the developing world, have noted the Western cultural bias found in the traditional randomized controlled trial and program evaluation approaches used in the United States and have called for the expansion of acceptable designs and types of data used in evaluations."[52]

IMPLEMENTING INJURY-PREVENTION STRATEGIES IN INDIGENOUS COMMUNITIES

In addition to being scientifically sound, effective strategies need to be developmentally appropriate. Recommendations for child passenger safety in automobiles, for example, vary according to the age, height, and weight of the child.[53] Strategies also need to be culturally appropriate. For example, window guards and stair gates are not priorities in preventing falls by children in a village in which all the dwellings are single-story with earthen floors.

The content and process of community interventions should reflect the unique cultural, political, and historical factors of each community. Interventions should:

1. Be based on demonstrated needs established through reliable data and community input;
2. Use evidence-based strategies and "best practices";
3. Employ a combination of approaches, rather than a single approach: social marketing, education, environmental modification, engineering, regulations and enforcement, traditional practices;
4. Include an evaluation component.

The process should involve a collaboration that:

1. Respects the sovereignty and dignity of tribes by obtaining tribal approvals before conducting an intervention or publishing results;
2. Involves the community at all stages of the intervention: planning, implementation, and evaluation.
3. Maximizes benefits to the community:
   a. Provides employment, training, empowerment (genuine role in decision-making), equipment, and other permanent resources;
   b. Addresses other community issues and promotes social and cultural values: eg, cultural preservation (language, values, history, stories), poverty (offer incentives for participation), literacy (children's books), social isolation (intergenerational activities)
4. Maximizes benefits to the local program staff, such as education and training opportunities, recognition, and awards;
5. Creates partnerships at the local, regional, and national levels: within the community (eg, among the highway department, police, schools, and courts) and with other tribes, nonprofit organizations, the private sector, and government agencies.

Two resources for collaborative interventions are the Web sites of The Community Toolbox[54] and the Community Anti-Drug Coalitions of America.[55]

The Injury Prevention (IP) Program of the US IHS is a model for national efforts to address injuries in indigenous communities. Promoting community-based interventions using evidence-based strategies is a cornerstone of the program. Other guiding principles are to build the capacity of tribes to design, implement, and evaluate their own injury-prevention programs, gather and analyze local data to guide decisions and evaluate interventions, and promote collaboration and partnerships to effect change.[56] A 12-member Tribal Steering Committee provides guidance to the program, serves as a liaison with tribes, and advocates for injury prevention at the area and national levels. The director and many IHS staff are enrolled tribal members.

In addition to providing injury prevention services to tribes at the local, area, and national levels, the IHS IP program conducts many training courses (week-long core courses and a year-long Fellowship in injury prevention), provides technical assistance to tribes, and funds capacity-building programs through a Tribal Injury Prevention Cooperative Agreement Program (TIPCAP).[57] Through TIPCAP, more than $13 million has been awarded to 51 tribes and tribal organizations for community-based injury-prevention programs. The IHS program has invited external evaluators to assess the comprehensiveness and quality of its activities, including collaborative relationships with tribes, resource allocation, and efforts to build tribal capacity.[58]

INTERNATIONAL ASPECTS OF INJURIES AMONG INDIGENOUS CHILDREN

The United Nations Children's Fund (UNICEF) estimates that there are 350 million indigenous people, representing roughly 5000 indigenous groups in more than 70 countries.[59] There is a growing literature concerning injuries among indigenous children living in highly industrialized countries, particularly the United States, Canada, Australia, and New Zealand. High rates of suicide, trauma caused by land transport, assaultive violence, fires, falls, poisonings, and drowning are common. Although the major types of injury are often similar for indigenous and nonindigenous children, mortality from many injuries is often higher for indigenous children.[60–63] The 2007 report of Canada's longitudinal health survey of First Nations people noted that "injury is probably the most under-recognized public health problem facing First Nations today."[64] The proportion of children less than 12 years old who experienced injuries in the previous year was 18% for First Nations children living "on reserve," compared with 10% for Canada as a whole. For young people aged 12–17 years, the proportion was 50% for First Nations young people, compared with 24% across Canada. The injury mortality (2002–2006) for Aboriginal and Torres Strait Islander Australian children aged 5–18 years was 3 times greater than for nonindigenous Australian children (33.3 vs 10.8 deaths/100,000, respectively).[65] Among the Māori of New Zealand, the injury mortality rate for children 5–14 years old is 1.7 times greater than for non-Māori children (9.8 vs 5.9/100,000).[65]

In less-industrialized countries, indigenous children share the injury risk factors of economically disadvantaged children living in similar circumstances. These risk factors include poverty, rapid motorization and industrialization, urbanization, child labor, substandard living conditions, and economic exploitation.[66] Often living in remote rural areas, indigenous children are particularly vulnerable to violence stemming from military operations. High rates of child trauma (physical and emotional) result from bombings and land mines, recruitment of child soldiers, genocidal tactics, and rape. The World Report on Violence Against Children notes that even in times of peace indigenous children are "especially vulnerable to different forms of violence" and are "especially likely to be excluded, discriminated against and bullied."[14] In rural areas, indigenous children are at risk of poisoning from highly toxic pesticides, injuries from agricultural field work with large animals and machinery, and pedestrian injuries from motor vehicles traveling at high speed on rural roads (**Fig. 2**). Living in remote areas where national governments often have a "weak presence" means that indigenous children are also subject to forced labor and debt bondage in lumber, mining, and other hazardous industries. According to a study of 19 countries in the Latin American region by the International Labor Organization (ILO), nearly 10% of the total child

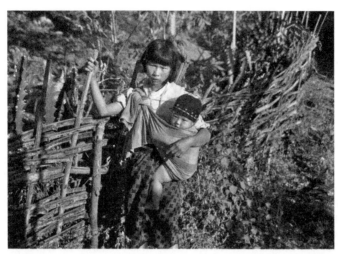

Fig. 2. For young women of the hill Tribes of Thailand, heavy agricultural work and full-time child care are routine aspects of life. Photograph by Lawrence Berger. *Courtesy of* Lawrence R. Berger, MD, MPH, Albuquerque, NM.

and adolescent population aged 5 to 17 years works in the worst forms of labor, in which violence is routine."[4] Addressing child labor and the impact of war requires national and international action. Hopeful initiatives include the United Nations' "Agenda against War" and the ILO's International Program on the Elimination of Child Labor.[67,68]

Alcohol and substance abuse is a crosscutting issue for many types of injuries, internationally, in nearly all cultures, and among all social classes. It is especially prominent in many indigenous communities in which historical trauma, poverty, unemployment, discrimination, and multigenerational abuse of alcohol play a role. Underage drinking places young people at high risk of many forms of injury, including car crashes and self-destructive behaviors. Children and young people are also affected as victims of intoxicated drivers, abusive family relationships, and assaults. The complexity of root causes (physical, emotional, historical, and spiritual) means that effective strategies include medical advances, behavioral and educational interventions, culture-specific approaches, and changes in public health systems at the community, national, and international levels.[69]

CASE STUDIES

The purpose of the following case studies is to illustrate how effective strategies have been successfully implemented in AI/AN communities. They also reveal the balance between fidelity and adaptation of interventions, especially in response to cultural practices and beliefs, financial circumstances, and administrative constraints. The descriptions of the case studies are, in large part, abstracted from their original publications. The names of specific tribes are included only if they appeared in the title and text of the source publications.

Case Study: Motor-Vehicle Occupant Safety: Tribal Codes and Enforcement

Among the Navajo in the 1980s, the death rate from motor-vehicle accidents was 5 times greater than for the overall US population. Injuries caused by motor-vehicle accidents were the second leading cause of hospitalization in IHS facilities.

Yet in 1988, only 14% of Navajo adults wore seat belts and only 7% of children rode in child safety seats.

The Navajo Nation Tribal Council modified its motor vehicle safety code in 1988 to require use of safety belts for all adult vehicle occupants and car safety seats for all children. The Navajo Office of Highway Safety then organized a comprehensive seat belt campaign to increase public awareness of the law and the benefits of restraint use. The program combined school-based education, public information, car seat loan programs, incentives (such as T-shirts, bumper stickers, and "Saved-By-The-Belt" awards), and enforcement of the restraint law. It involved cooperation among the Navajo Department of Highway Safety, police, social service programs, IHS, Bureau of Indian Affairs (BIA) Road Safety program, New Mexico Traffic Safety Bureau, local businesses (which provided incentives and financial support), and other agencies and individuals.

The campaign incorporated cultural teachings and norms, as well as contemporary public health principles. There were educational programs for elementary through high schools, presentations at community chapter houses, meetings with judges, billboards, and radio spots in Navajo and English. A Navajo Medicine Man delivered a blessing for the program on Navajo radio, which reaches an audience of 60,000 people. A Navajo chapter of the National Safe Kids child safety program was established. A coloring book, "Let's talk about traffic safety", was published featuring Navajo people, landscapes, and activities. In framing safety messages, the emphasis was on family responsibility, self-protection, and caring for children. Direct references to dangers, suffering, or mortality were avoided. The campaign was intergenerational: bilingual presentations addressed the older generation, who relayed the safety messages to school-age children, who in turn relayed them to their parents. Hundreds of community health representatives were trained to discuss car seat use during their home visits with Navajo families. The "Saved-By-The-Belt" awards were especially popular among families and the media. Individuals who were involved in crashes while using seat belts or car seats were honored and given awards such as new car safety seats. The resulting news stories depicted the honorees as positive role models for safe transportation. After the public information campaign was started, Navajo police began to enforce the restraint laws rigorously, establishing roadblocks, issuing citations, and explaining to drivers the importance of wearing seat belts and using car seats for their children. While the educational activities were valuable in raising awareness about the new law, rigorous enforcement of the law was a key component to increasing seat belt use.

After 2 years, adult seat belt use rose to more than 70% of motor-vehicle occupants. Seat belt use in tribal vehicles was consistently more than 90%. Child restraint use rose to 40%. There was a 28% reduction in the overall rate of hospitalizations caused by injuries from motor-vehicle accidents (**Fig. 3**). Among children less than 5 years of age, the mean annual hospital discharge rate fell 55% (from 62.2/100,000 in the years 1983–1988 to 28.0 in the years 1991–1995).[70,71]

Case Study: Preventing Child Maltreatment: Paraprofessional Home Visitors

"Family Spirit" (FS) is a large-scale family-strengthening program for reservation-based, teenage mothers. It incorporates home visiting, case management, and parenting education.[72] Unlike the Nurse Family Partnership home-visiting model described earlier under "Effective strategies," FS uses American Indian paraprofessionals for home-based services, rather than nontribal individuals with professional nursing degrees.

FS was developed using community-based, participatory research methods. Program services are provided from the beginning of the mother's third trimester until her baby's second birthday. The program aims for 52 total visits, each lasting about

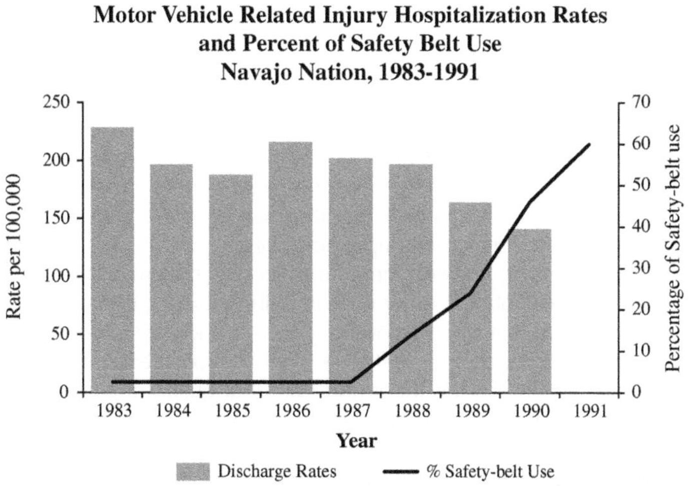

**Motor Vehicle Related Injury Hospitalization Rates
and Percent of Safety Belt Use
Navajo Nation, 1983-1991**

Discharge Rates   —— % Safety-belt Use

Fig. 3. A dramatic increase in seat belt use was associated with a 30% decline in the rate of hospital admissions from motor-vehicle injuries in the Navajo Nation.

60 minutes. The program includes parent training and education to promote the baby's physical, developmental, and emotional health; personal support and life skills training; and accessing community resources (eg, medical care, education, legal and financial support, substance abuse services). The curricular content is based on community input, child-care and parenting information from expert publications, and review of other home-visiting programs. Enrollment in FS is voluntary. Interested parents are recruited from prenatal clinics and school nurses, and by word of mouth.

The program is conducted by American Indian outreach workers (Family Health Educators [FHEs]), who are trained by public health experts from Johns Hopkins University. For several reasons FS chose to use paraprofessionals from the community, rather than non-Indian professionals, to delivery the home-based services. First, the FHEs are better able to address language and cultural barriers because they are community members who speak English and the traditional language. Second, during the project planning phase, many community members reported they would personally prefer local FHEs to non-Indian professionals to enter their homes and provide services. Third, higher salaries, and difficulty in recruiting professionals to work in rural communities, would prohibit implementation of a home-visiting model in many tribal communities. Finally, FHEs would more likely remain in the community in the long term, and assume important roles in enabling the tribe to gain full ownership of the program.

Efforts are under way to replicate FS at additional reservation-based tribes, for American Indians living in a large metropolitan area, and nationally through the IHS Head Start Program. Although preliminary studies are promising,[73,74] results of a 5-year, randomized controlled trial of FS are eagerly awaited, to see if the paraprofessional-based, home-visiting model proves effective in reducing child maltreatment.

Case Study: Alcohol-impaired Driving

The San Carlos Apache (SCA) Tribe in Arizona has 12,000 members residing on the reservation's 2812 square miles. In 2000, the death rate from injury caused by motor-vehicle accidents was nearly 8 times greater than for the United States overall (117 vs 15.5/100,000). Alcohol was a factor in at least 50% of fatal crashes. National studies had shown that about 1-fourth of all deaths from motor-vehicle accidents among children involved alcohol; and that 26% of young drivers (15–20 years old) who were killed in crashes had exceeded the legal drink-driving limit.

In December 2004, the SCA Police Department established a motor vehicle injury prevention program (MVIPP) with 4 years of funding from the CDC. The initial focus was on reducing alcohol-impaired driving. The primary strategies were to increase the number of sobriety checkpoints, support a tribal council resolution to lower the legal limit to 0.08% blood alcohol concentration, and conduct a media campaign to change behaviors regarding alcohol-impaired driving.

At a sobriety checkpoint, law enforcement officers systematically stop vehicles to assess drivers' level of alcohol or other drug impairment using behavioral tests ("field sobriety tests") and portable alcohol breathalyzers. The MVIPP developed policy and procedure manuals, educational materials, and media resources using online resources and site visits to other tribal and nontribal police departments. Between 2004 and 2006, there were 21 sobriety checkpoints involving 7536 vehicles, and 1104 arrests for "driving under the influence" (DUI). The comprehensive media campaign involved the tribe's newspaper and radio station, local casino marquee, public bulletin boards, and educational booths at public events. Focus groups were held to develop specific and culturally appropriate messages.

These efforts were associated with a 33% increase in DUI arrests, a 20% reduction in crashes involving injuries or fatalities, a 33% reduction in night-time crashes, and a 27% reduction in crashes reported by police. That the largest (33%) decline in motor-vehicle crashes occurred during night time supports the conclusion that the DUI campaign contributed to decreased drinking and driving.

Among the factors contributing to the success of the program were implementing effective strategies to address DUI; obtaining multiyear funding; housing the prevention program in the tribe's police department; establishing a separate DUI Task Force within the department; providing incentives (eg, meals, awards, news coverage) to police officers who participated in the checkpoints; recruiting an especially motivated and effective program coordinator; documenting community support through key-informant interviews, community surveys, and focus groups; and forming partnerships with community groups, other tribal departments, and state and federal agencies (eg, the IHS, CDC, BIA, multiple law enforcement agencies, and the Intertribal Council of Arizona).[75]

Case Study: Reducing Suicidal Behaviors

In 1988, the annual rate of suicide and suicide attempts (combined) for a tribal nation in the south-western United States was 15 times higher than the overall US rate. In response, a partnership among tribal leaders, community members, and IHS implemented a population-based approach to prevention. Begun as a demonstration project, the initiative evolved within 12 years into the tribe's Department of Behavioral Health, with a staff of 57 and an annual budget of more than $1 million.[76]

The tribe is rural and geographically isolated, with a population of about 3000 and a high rate of unemployment. The suicidal behavior prevention program targeted each year approximately 800 young people aged 10 to 24 years. The program sought to identify individuals and families at high risk for suicide, violence, and mental health problems; provide mental health services and implement prevention activities targeting them; and implement "a communitywide system approach to enhance community knowledge and awareness."

The community planning process involved tribal leaders, health care providers, parents, elders, young people, and clients. A major theme that emerged from the 50 community planning sessions was that "to prevent suicide, underlying issues of alcoholism, domestic violence, child abuse, and unemployment must also be confronted." The recommendations of the workgroups were summarized in a widely distributed report. They formed the basis not only for the Adolescent Suicide Prevention Project (ASPP) but also for the passage of a tribal domestic violence code, establishment of a child abuse prevention program, and initiatives addressing drug and alcohol abuse and fetal alcohol syndrome.

The ASPP incorporated screening and clinical interventions; social services, such as child and adult welfare activities; school-based prevention programs, including general life skills development; and community education for adults and young people on topics from parenting to the nature of self-destructive behaviors. Outreach activities also occurred in unconventional settings, such as outdoor venues where troubled young people and alcohol abusers congregate and at community functions such as traditional and modern dances.

The professional staff conducted case reviews on a weekly basis to coordinate services, develop treatment plans, and make referrals. They also worked as a team with "natural helpers," often providing services outside their offices, such as in cars or outdoors. The natural helpers were neighborhood volunteers chosen for peer training, program advocacy, referrals to mental health services, and lay counseling.

Sustained data collection and information gathering included clinical record reviews, lists of prevention activities, and certification of suicide completions by the state's Office of Medical Investigation. Two-thirds of all self-destructive acts, and 83% of the completions, were alcohol related; 95% of suicidal behavior occurred among people who had a significant family history of trauma (eg, family disruption, violent death of relatives, abuse, or neglect) and 86% of self-destructive individuals experienced significant individual trauma.

Between 1988 and 2002, there was a 60% decrease in total self-destructive acts (suicide completions, attempts, and gestures), from 36 to 14 annually. The decrease was a reflection of a steady decline in attempts and gestures; suicide completions remained constant at 1 to 2 per year.

Several important lessons are that a comprehensive approach to suicide prevention should focus on underlying social, psychological, and developmental conditions. High-quality, direct patient care services (including screening and treatment of depression and substance abuse) must be accessible through traditional and nontraditional settings. Program staff must be trained and supported to maintain a public health perspective. Community involvement is essential in all aspects of the program to ensure that activities are "culturally, environmentally, and clinically appropriate." Although long-term program goals remain constant, program objectives and activities need to shift according to ongoing data collection, community input, and feedback from program staff.

SUMMARY

In many aspects, the challenges of reducing child injuries among indigenous communities are daunting. The importance of addressing injury problems in all their dimensions (cultural, political, environmental, behavioral, and clinical), and the limited resources available, make the identification and implementation of effective strategies imperative. Successful interventions should mobilize the vitality and strengths of indigenous families and communities and their commitment to creating lives of beauty, harmony, and balance, recognizing the inherent worth of every individual, and improving the lives of children to the seventh generation and beyond.

REFERENCES

1. Centers for Disease Control and Prevention. WISQARS (Web-based injury statistics query and reporting system). Available at: http://www.cdc.gov/injury/wisqars. Accessed May 1, 2009.

2. Berger LR, Wallace LJD, Bill N. Reduce injuries: eliminate disparities in child mortality rates among American Indian and Alaska Native children and youth. IHS Prim Care Provid 2007;32(7):203–8.

3. Ogunwole SU. We the people: American Indians and Alaska Natives in the United States. Census 2000 special report. Washington, DC: US Census Bureau; 2006.

4. Castor ML, Smyser MS, Taualii MM. A nationwide population-based study identifying health disparities between American Indians/Alaska Natives and the general populations living in select urban counties. Am J Public Health 2006;96:1478–84.

5. US Census Bureau. American Indian, Alaska Native tables from the statistical abstract of the United States: 2004–2005. Table no. 14. resident population by race, Hispanic origin, and age: 2000 and 2003. Available at: http://www.census.gov/statab/www/sa04AI/AN.pdf. Accessed May 14, 2009.

6. Piland NF, Berger LR. The economic burden of injuries involving American Indians and Alaska Natives: a critical need for prevention. IHS Prim Care Provid 2007;32(9):269–73.

7. Doll LS, Bonzo SE, Mercy JA, et al, editors. Handbook of injury and violence prevention. New York: Springer; 2007.

8. Christoffel T, Gallagher SS. Injury prevention and public health. 2nd edition. Sudbury (MA): Jones and Bartlett Publishers; 2006.

9. Rivara FP, Cummings P, Koepsell TD, et al, editors. Randomized trials. In: Injury control: a guide to research and program evaluation. Chapter 9. Cambridge (UK): Cambridge University Pressl; 2001. p. 116–28.

10. Chalk R, King PA, editors. Violence in families: assessing prevention and treatment programs. Washington, DC: National Academy Press; 1998.

11. Widome M, editor. Injury prevention and control for children and youth. Elk Grove Village (IL): American Academy of Pediatrics; 1997.

12. Christoffel T, Teret SP. Protecting the public: legal issues in injury prevention. New York: Oxford University Press; 1994.

13. Peden M, Oyegbite K, Ozanne-Smith J, et al, editors. World report on child injury prevention. Geneva: World Health Organization; 2008. Available at: http://www.who.int/violence_injury_prevention/child/injury/world_report/en. 2008. Accessed May 19, 2009.

14. Pinheiro PS. The world report on violence against children. United Nations Secretary-General's study on violence against children. Geneva. 2006. Available at: http://www.violencestudy.org/IMG/pdf/I._World_Report_on_Violence_against_Children.pdf. Accessed May 19, 2009.

15. Zaza S, Sleet DA, Thompson RS, et al. Task force on Community Preventive Services. Reviews of evidence regarding interventions to increase use of child safety seats. Am J Prev Med 2001;21(4S):31–47.

16. Task Force on Community Preventive Services. Motor-vehicle occupant injury: strategies for increasing use of child safety seats, increasing use of safety belts, and reducing alcohol-impaired driving. MMWR Recomm Rep 2001;50(RR07):1–13.

17. Task Force on Community Preventive Services guide to community preventive services, motor vehicle occupant injury. Available at: http://www.thecommunityguide.org/mvoi/default.htm. Accessed June 5, 2009.

18. Dellinger AM, Sleet DA, Shults RA, et al. Interventions to prevent motor vehicle injuries. In: Hass EN, Doll LS, Bonzo SE, editors. Handbook of injury and violence prevention. New York: Springer; 2007. p. 55–79.

19. Ehiri JE, Ejere HOD, Magnussen L, et al. Interventions for promoting booster seat use in four to eight year olds travelling in motor vehicles. Cochrane Database Syst Rev 2006. Available at: http://www.cochrane.org/reviews/en/ab004334.html. Accessed October 12, 2009.

20. Dinn-Zarr TB, Sleet DA, Shults RA, et al. Task Force on Community Preventive Services. Reviews of evidence regarding interventions to increase use of safety belts. Am J Prev Med 2001;21(4S):48–65.

21. Rivara FP, Thompson DC, Beahler C, et al. Systematic reviews of strategies to prevent motor vehicle injuries. Am J Prev Med 1999;16(Suppl 1):1–5.

22. Hartling L, Wiebe N, Russell K, et al. Graduated driver licensing for reducing motor vehicle crashes among young drivers. Cochrane Database Syst Rev 2004. Available at: http://www.cochrane.org/reviews/en/ab003300.html. Accessed October 12, 2009.

23. Shults RA, Elder RW, Sleet DA, et al.Task Force on Community Preventive Services. Reviews of evidence regarding interventions to reduce alcohol-impaired driving. Am J Prev Med 2001;21(4S):66–88.

24. Thompson DC, Rivara FP, Thompson RS. Effectiveness of bicycle safety helmets in preventing head injuries: a case-control study. JAMA 1996;276:1968–73.

25. Injury-control recommendations: bicycle helmets. MMWR Morb Mortal Wkly Rep 1995;44(RR-1):1–18.

26. Doll LS, Bonzo SE, Mercy JA, et al. Handbook of injury and violence prevention. New York: Springer; 2007. p. 69.

27. Liu B, Ivers R, Norton R, et al. Helmets for preventing injury in motorcycle riders. Cochrane Database Syst Rev (Issue 4, Art. No. CD004333. pub2DOI:10.1001/14651858.CD004333.pubs). Chichester(UK): Wiley; 2003.

28. Runyan CW, Bangdiwala SI, Linzer MA, et al. Risk factors for fatal residential fires. N Engl J Med 1992;327(12):859–63.

29. Warda JL, Ballesteros MF. Interventions to prevent residential fire injury. In: Hass EN, Doll LS, Bonzo SE, et al, editors. Handbook of injury and violence prevention. New York: Springer; 2007. p. 97–115.

30. Kuklinski DM, Berger LR, Weaver JR. Smoke detector nuisance alarms: a field study in a Native American community. NFPA J 1996;90:65–72.

31. Mallonee S, Istre GR, Rosenburg M, et al. Surveillance and prevention of residential-fire injuries. N Engl J Med 1996;335(1):27–31.

32. Injury Prevention Policy. Tap water scalds. Available at: http://www.safetypolicy. org/pm/scald.htm. Accessed October 12, 2009.

33. Alaska Department of Health and Social Services, Injury Prevention and Emergency Medical Services. Kids Don't float program. Available at: http://www.hss.state.ak. us/dph/ipems/injury_prevention/kids_dont_float.htm. Accessed June 5, 2009.

34. Quan L, Bennett EE, Branche CM. Interventions to prevent drowning. In: Hass EN, Doll LS, Bonzo SE, et al, editors. Handbook of injury and violence prevention. New York: Springer; 2007. p. 81–96.

35. Olds DL, Henderson CR Jr, Chamberlin R, et al. Preventing child abuse and neglect: a randomized trial of nurse home visitation. Pediatrics 1986;78(1): 65–78.

36. Olds DL, Robinson J, Pettitt L, et al. Effects of home visits by paraprofessionals and by nurses: age 4 follow-up results of a randomized trial. Pediatrics 2004; 114:1560–8.

37. Hahn RA, Bilukha O, Crosby A, et al. First reports evaluating the effectiveness of strategies for preventing violence: early childhood home visitation: findings from the Task Force on Community Preventive Services. MMWR Recomm Rep 2003;52(RR-14): 11–20.
38. Task Force on Community Preventive Services guide to community preventive services, violence prevention, early childhood home visitation. Available at:. http://www.thecommunityguide.org/violence/home/index.html. Accessed June 5, 2009.
39. Mann JJ, Apter A, Bertolote J, et al. Suicide prevention strategies: a systematic review. JAMA 2005;294:2064–74.
40. Knox KL. Interventions to prevent suicidal behavior. In: Hass EN, Doll LS, Bonzo SE, et al, editors. Handbook of injury and violence prevention. New York: Springer; 2007. p. 183–201.
41. Borowsky IW, Resnick MD, Ireland M, et al. Suicide attempts among American Indian and Alaska Native youth: risk and protective factors. Arch Pediatr Adolesc Med 1999;153:573–80.
42. LaFromboise TD. The Zuni life skills development curriculum: description and evaluation of a suicide prevention program. J Couns Psychol 1995;42:479–86.
43. Knox KL, Litts DA, Talcott GW, et al. Risk of suicide and related adverse outcomes after exposure to a suicide prevention programme in the US Air Force: Cohort study. BMJ 2003;327:1376–8.
44. Walker LD, Loudon L, Walker PS, et al. Suicide prevention for American Indian and Alaska Native communities: DRAFT. Portland, Oregon: One Sky Center, Oregon Health & Science University; 2006. Available at: http://www.onesky center.org. Accessed May 11, 2009.
45. Guide to community preventive services. School-based programs to reduce violence. Available at: http://www.thecommunityguide.org/violence/schoolbased programs.html. Accessed on May 14, 2009.
46. Guide to community preventive services. Preventing excessive alcohol use. Available at: http://www.thecommunityguide.org/alcohol.html. Accessed May 12, 2009.
47. The Cochrane Collaboration. Available at: http://www.cochrane.org. Accessed June 15, 2009.
48. Guide to community preventive services. Centers for Disease Control and Prevention, Atlanta. Available at: http://www.thecommunityguide.org. Accessed June 15, 2009.
49. Leong FTL, Leach MM. Suicide among racial and ethnic minority groups: theory, research and practice. New York: Routledge; 2007. p. 192.
50. Grossman DC, Putsch RW, Inui TS. The meaning of death to adolescents in an American Indian community. Fam Med 1993;25(9):593–7.
51. Spicer P. Culture and the restoration of self among former American Indian drinkers. Soc Sci Med 2001;53(2):227–40.
52. Doll L, Bartenfeld T, Binder S. Evaluation of interventions designed to prevent and control injuries. Epidemiol Rev 2003;25:51–9.
53. American Academy of Pediatrics. Car safety seats: a guide for families. Available at: http://www.aap.org/family/Carseatguide.htm. 2009. Accessed June 15, 2009.
54. The Community Toolbox. Available at: http://www.ctb.ks. Accessed June 15, 2009.
55. Community Anti-Drug Coalitions of America. Available at: http://www.cadca.org. Accessed June 15, 2009.
56. Hicks K, Morones R, Wallace LJD, et al. Public Health Practice and the IHS Injury Prevention Program: guiding principles. IHS Prim Care Provid 2007;32(9):274–80.
57. Letourneau RJ. The role of technical assistance in the IHS Tribal Injury Prevention Cooperative Agreements Program (TIPCAP): enhancing injury prevention

capacity among tribes and tribal organizations. IHS Prim Care Provid 2007;32(7): 218–22.

58. Crump CE, Letourneau RJ. Developing a process to evaluate a national injury prevention program: the IHS Injury Prevention Program. In: Steckler A, Linnan L, editors. Process evaluation for public health interventions and research. Chapter 12. San Francisco (CA): John Wiley and Sons; 2002. p. 321–57.

59. UNICEF news note: international day of the world's indigenous people. August 8, 2008 Available at: http://www.unicef.org/media/media_45117.html. Accessed June 14, 2009.

60. Harrop AR, Brant RF, William A, et al. Injury mortality rates in Native and Non-Native children: a population-based study. Public Health Rep 2007;122:339–46.

61. Langley J. Injury to Maori. Inj Prev 1998;4:322.

62. Australian Institute of Health and Welfare. A picture of Australia's children. Cat. no. PHE 58. Canberra: AIHW; 2005.

63. Bernard SJ, Paulozzi LJ, Wallace DL. Fatal injuries among children by race and ethnicity—United States, 1999–2002. MMWR Surveill Summ 2007;56(5):1–16.

64. RHS National Team. First Nations Regional Longitudinal Health Survey 2002/2003. Assembly of First Nations/First Nations Information Governance Committee. Ottawa, Ontario. 2007.

65. Smylie J, Adomako P. Indigenous children's health report: health assessment in action. Toronto (ON): Janet Smylie, Kennan Research Center; 2009.

66. Berger LR, Mohan D. Injury control: a global view. New Delhi: Oxford University Press; 1996.

67. UNICEF. The State of the World's Children 1996. Agenda against War. Available at: http://www.unicef.org/sowc96/antiwar.htm. Accessed on June 15, 2009.

68. ILO: International program on the elimination of child labor. Available at: http://www.ilo.org/ipec/lang–en/index.htm. Accessed June 15, 2009.

69. Trimble JE, Beauvais F. Health promotion and substance abuse prevention among American Indian and Alaska Native communities: issues in cultural competence. Series 9. Washington, DC: Center for Substance Abuse Prevention Cultural Competence; 2001.

70. Bill N, Buonviri G, Bohan P, et al. Safety-belt use and motor-vehicle-related injuries—Navajo Nation, 1988–1991. MMWR Morb Mortal Wkly Rep 1992;41(38):705–8.

71. Phelan KJ, Khoury J, Grossman D, et al. Pediatric motor vehicle related injuries in the Navajo Nation: the impact of the 1988 child occupant restraint laws. Inj Prev 2002;8:216–20.

72. Center for American Indian Health, Johns Hopkins School of Public Health: family spirit project. Available at: http://www.jhsph.edu/caih/Service_Projects/Behavioral_Health_Research_and_Service_Projects.html#Family_Spirit. Accessed June 3, 2009.

73. Walkup JT, Barlow A, Mullany BC, et al. Randomized controlled trial of a parapro-fessional-delivered in-home intervention for young reservation-based American Indian mothers. J Am Acad Child Adolesc Psychiatry 2009;48(6):591–601.

74. Barlow A, Varipatis-Baker E, Speakman K, et al. Home-visiting intervention to improve child care among American Indian adolescent mothers: a randomized trial. Arch Pediatr Adolesc Med 2006;160:1101–7.

75. Reede C, Piontkowski SP, Tsatoke G. Using evidence-based strategies to reduce motor vehicle injuries on the San Carlos Apache reservation. IHS Prim Care Provid 2007;32(7):209–12.

76. May PA, Serna P, Hurt L, et al. Outcome evaluation of a public health approach to suicide prevention in an American Indian tribal nation. Am J Public Health 2005; 95(7):1238–44.

History, Law, and Policy as a Foundation for Health Care Delivery for American Indian and Alaska Native Children

Judith Thierry, DO, MPH, FAAP[a],*, George Brenneman, MD[b],
Everett Rhoades, MD[c], Lance Chilton, MD[d,e]

KEYWORDS

- Legislation • American Indian Alaska Native
- Health policy • Indian child welfare
- Indian Health Service • Public law treaties

Most American Indian and Alaska Native Children (AIAN) receive health care that is based on the unique historical legacy of tribal treaty obligations and a trust relationship of sovereign nation to sovereign nation. From colonial America to the early 21st century, the wellbeing of AIAN children has been impacted as federal laws were crafted for the health, education and wellbeing of its AIAN citizens. Important public laws are addressed in this article, highlighting the development of the Indian Health Service (IHS), a federal agency designed to provide comprehensive clinical and public health services to citizens of federally recognized tribes. The context during which various acts were made into law are described to note the times during which the policy making process took place. Policies internal and external to the IHS are

[a] Office of Clinical and Preventive Services, Indian Health Service, 801 Thompson Avenue, Suite 300, Room 313, Rockville, MD 20852, USA
[b] 719 Maiden Choice Lane, BR 441, Catonsville, MD 21228, USA
[c] University of Oklahoma, College of Public Health, Room 532, Rogers Building, 800 Northeast 15th Street, Oklahoma City, OK 73104, USA
[d] Department of Pediatrics, Young Children's Health Center, University of New Mexico, 306A San Pablo Southeast, Albuquerque, NM 87108, USA
[e] 2604 Candelaria Road Northwest, Albuquerque, NM 87107, USA
* Corresponding author.
E-mail address: Judith.thierry@ihs.gov (J. Thierry).

Pediatr Clin N Am 56 (2009) 1539–1559
doi:10.1016/j.pcl.2009.09.018
0031-3955/09/$ – see front matter. Published by Elsevier Inc.

pediatric.theclinics.com

summarized, widening the lens spanning the past 200 years and into the future of these first nations' youngest members.

COLONIAL PERIOD TO 1921

As the United States emerged a young, independent nation, policies with respect to its relationship with Indian tribes began to formulate. Many of the nation's founders, including Benjamin Franklin, Thomas Jefferson, and George Washington, had close interaction with Indian leaders and were acquainted with Indian concepts of social organization and government. The importance of this cross-fertilization influenced early Indian policy and received Congressional recognition in 1988 by joint resolution of the US House of Representatives and US Senate.[1]

Article I, Section 8 of the United States Constitution, which states "Congress shall have power … To regulate Commerce with foreign nations, and among the several States, and with the Indian Tribes,"[2] is referenced commonly as the basis for recognition of tribal sovereignty and established a basis for future federal Indian health policy including Indian children. Federal policy often was codified through treaties between Indian tribes and the US government. Until 1871, when treaty making with Indian tribes ended, 389 treaties and agreements had been made between the US government and various Indian tribes.[3]

Following exposure to European contagious diseases, frightening epidemics of smallpox, measles, cholera, and tuberculosis threatened the very existence of Indian tribes and health of non-Indian communities also. These epidemics continued into the late 1800s and early 1900s.[4] Without known curative treatments or effective prevention in the early 1800s, one could do little more than be afraid and watch the waves come and go leaving behind heavy consequences of mortality and morbidity. Smallpox vaccination, tested and used by Jenner around 1800, became available. As its acceptance and use increased in the general population, early government policy addressed limited use among Indians.

One important health issue that received considerable policy attention through most of the 1800s, from some Indian leaders and government, was the particularly serious adverse health and social effects of alcohol use among Indians. Restriction of access seemed to be the only intervention available.

An early example of this occurred in 1753 around the time the Carlisle Treaty. Deliberations leading to the Carlisle Treaty focused primarily on ensuring a mutual defense against the French through collaboration between the provincial government of Pennsylvania and members of the Six Nations. In discussions before the treaty's signing on Nov. 1, 1753, Scarrooyady, an Iroquois leader, complained to Franklin and others responsible to the provincial government, about the distribution of rum among Indians and stated that the chiefs wanted the practices stopped.

"Your traders now bring us scarce any Thing but Rum and Flour. They bring us little Powder and Lead, or other valuable Goods. The rum ruins us. We beg you would prevent its coming in such Quantities, by regulating the Traders. We desire it be forbidden, and none sold in the Indian Country. Those wicked Whiskey Sellers, when they have once got the Indians in Liquor, make them sell their very Clothes from their Backs."

This request was taken seriously, and Franklin's opposition to liquor trade among Indians became stronger when he later observed many Indians who had participated in the treaty discussions become disorderly and intoxicated.[5]

Policies authorizing and supporting medical services to Indians emerged slowly through the 1800s. Early evidence of this occurred when President Jefferson made efforts to address smallpox among Indians. He developed an interest in protecting American Indians from smallpox and persuaded a visiting delegation of Indian chiefs to be vaccinated with Kinepox (Kinepox, the smallpox vaccine used in early 19th century and developed by Jenner in the late 1790s, was used and promoted by Jefferson.) during the winter of 1801 to 1802. On a later occasion, Jefferson, aware of smallpox epidemics along the Missouri River, issued special instructions in his instructions (June 20, 1803) to Meriwether Lewis:

"Carry with you some matter of the Kinepox; inform those of them with whom you may be, of it['s] efficacy as a preservative from the small-pox; & instruct & incour-age [sic] them in the use of it. This may be especially done wherever you winter."[6]

Because of lack of refrigeration at the time, the vaccine unfortunately became inac-tive and not useable to vaccinate Indians on the Missouri expedition, as Jefferson had hoped.

Adverse health and social effects of alcohol consumption among Indians remained a focus as shown in numerous treaties, administrative reports, and legislative acts. The Trade and Intercourse Act of March 30, 1802, authorized President Jefferson "to take such measures…to prevent or restrain the vending or distribution of spirituous liquors among…Indian tribes."[7] On December 31, 1808, Jefferson wrote to governors of the states and territories regarding access Indians had to "liquors." In his commu-nication, Jefferson requested submission of the matter to "your Legislature … that they should pass effectual laws to restrain their citizens from vending and distributing spirituous liquors to the Indians."[7]

In 1824, the War Department created an Indian office, Bureau of Indian Affairs (BIA),[7] and, 8 years later, in 1832 Congress authorized the first commissioner of Indian Affairs and located him in the War Department. Section 4 of this authorizing act stated, "that no ardent spirits shall be hereafter introduced, under any pretense, into the Indian country."[7] In 1834, the final codification of the Trade and Intercourse Act autho-rized sharp fines for illegal distribution of alcohol to and among Indians.[7] In President Andrew Jackson's annual message to Congress in 1835 on "Indian Removal," his words about Indians and alcohol re-emphasized policy, "Summary authority has been given by law to destroy all ardent spirits from their [Indian] country."[7] On March 3, 1847, Congress enacted an amendment to the Trade and Intercourse Act that added strength, including imprisonment up to 2 years, if one was convicted of providing alcohol to Indians.[7] On March 15, 1854, in the Treaty with Oto and Missouri Indians, the tribes desired to have "ardent spirits" excluded from "their country," and any tribal member who "brings liquor into their country or drinks liquor" could have their annuities withheld.[7] In his 1874 annual report, the commissioner of Indian Affairs addressed the emerging issue of Indian citizenship and alluded to failure of policies that tried to control the supply of rum and gunpowder to Indians.[7]

Administration of Indian affairs continued in the War Department until March 1849, when Congress enacted legislation for transfer of the administration of Indian affairs to the Department of Interior (DOI). While still under the War Department, Indians living near forts received limited, unorganized care, including smallpox vaccinations, from military physicians. The public health importance was clear and received support of $12,000 from Congress.[8] A treaty with the Sioux in September 1837, authorized an annual expenditure "for the benefit of Sioux Indians" of $8,250 for "the purchase of medicines, agricultural implements and stock, and for the support of a physician, farmers, and blacksmiths and for beneficial objects."[9]

The move of Indian affairs to the DOI in 1849 and creation of an Indian Peace Commission in 1867 signaled increasing interest in broader welfare issues of Indians and their communities and the need to deal with increasing complexity of the government's interaction and relationship with Indian nations. Organizations outside of government in support of Indians emerged and strong advocacy recognized the intolerable situations and injustices for many Indian tribes. The federal relationship with Indian tribes sought to reduce hostility and military confrontations and to find ways to meet social, educational, and health needs of Indian families and communities. Congressional enactment of The Indian Peace Commission was to establish peace with certain "Hostile Indian Tribes," with an approach to identify and confront the causes for hostilities in a peaceful manner.[7] The Jan. 7, 1868, report from this Commission was very critical of the harsh, unjust treatment to Indians and found that this maltreatment was the root cause of hostilities. These two congressional actions certainly had important influence in opening the door to a foundation for more thoughtful and supportive future policy.[7]

Policy began to show more specific government support. In a treaty with the Ottoe and Missouri Indians in 1854, the government agreed to pay to the Indians sums of money "for such beneficial objects...that will advance them in civilization..." and "for medical purposes."[7] The Fort Laramie Treaty of April 29, 1868, included up to $3,000 for "a residence for the physician" and "to furnish annually to the Indians the physician..."[7] In 1880, the DOI was administering four hospitals and employing 77 physicians.[10] In an "unratified" agreement written and signed, 1882 to 1883, with "Sioux of Various Tribes," the government agreed to "furnish to each reservation, herein made and described, a physician, miller, engineer, farmer, and blacksmith for a period of 10 years from the date of this agreement."[11] A further development in the late 1880s was building Indian hospitals in association with Indian boarding schools. Deaths caused by tuberculosis and other epidemic diseases of students alarmed authorities and prompted action that led to provision of inpatient services for boarding students.[12]

In his 1910 annual report, Commissioner of Indian Affairs Robert Valentine recognized the severe health needs of Indians and articulated the need to apply modern (at that time) interventions. He emphasized the importance of interventions and services that were "scientifically developed along lines which have already been successfully tried out by modern preventive medicine." He alluded to the use of "new" health education technology with the use of "stereopticon slides and moving pictures." Words in his report, still applicable today, reflected a major step forward in 1910 in a government effort to improve the health status of Indian families. Three points Valentine emphasized:

> "(1) An intensive attack upon two diseases that most seriously menace the health of Indians—trachoma and tuberculosis; (2) preventive work on a large scale, by means of popular education along health lines and more effective sanitary inspection; (3) increased attention to the physical welfare of the children in schools, so that the physical stamina of the coming generation may be conserved and increased..."[7]

The content of Valentine's report served to indicate government policy on Indian health was turning toward more constructive and rational approaches based on public health, disease prevention, and health promotion. Valentine's report represents an important turning point in health policy and vanguard to important to later legislation embodied in the Snyder Act of 1921,[7] an act that set future direction on government policy supporting needs of Indian health programs that has continued to the present.

THE SNYDER ACT AS THE FOUNDATION FOR INDIAN HEALTH POLICY, 1921

Overall Indian policy following passage of the General Allotment Act of 1887 (24 Statute 384; 25 U.S.C. Section 331–58) until the 1934 Indian Reorganization Act (48 Statute 984; 25 U.S.C. Section 451 ff.) is commonly referred to as the period of allotment and assimilation.[13] During this time, relatively little change in overall Indian health policy occurred; rather, efforts were made to strengthen existing programs as noted in the report of Commissioner Valentine. Near the end of this period, however, two events profoundly affected subsequent Indian health policy: The Snyder Act of 1921 (P. L. 67–85, 42 Statute 208) and the Meriam Report of 1928.[14] The latter has been cited in many publications and will be discussed. The Snyder Act, the formal authorization for Indian health services, established features peculiar to Indian health care that have remained in effect for more than 80 years. The language in the Act (P.L. 67–85, 42 Statute 208) relating to Indian health is extremely brief:

> *"The Bureau of Indian Affairs shall expend such moneys as the Congress from time to time may appropriate ... for the benefit, care and assistance of Indians throughout the United States ... for the relief of distress and conservation of health ... and for the employment of physicians..."*

As a result of the language, "... shall expend such moneys as the Congress from time to time may appropriate ...", Indian health services are discretionary, rather than entitlement, in nature. That is, the BIA could expend only the funds appropriated by the Congress (in effect operating under a funding cap). This distinguishes the IHS from entitlement programs such as Medicare, Medicaid, and State Child Health Insurance Program (SCHIP) and forces strict attention to priorities in the planning for health programs.

The language, "... of Indians throughout the United States ..." is notable for the absence of clear definition of those Indians eligible for federal health services. The Congress, through the Snyder Act, provided authorization for care of Indians, otherwise not defined, regardless of location of residence. The present limitation of services to certain Indians, such as those residing in metropolitan locations, is the result of limited resources, not Congressional definition of eligibility. Funding limitations have dictated the long-standing IHS policy of giving first priority to Indians residing on, or near, reservations. These priorities are an excellent example of the molding of policy by funding levels.

The language "... for the relief of distress and conservation of health ..." is likewise of major importance. In this clause, Congress laid the foundation for a health program fundamentally unlike other programs for the civilian population. The term "relief of distress" reflects language contained in certain treaties and certain previous appropriations acts.[15] For example, after 1911, Congress appropriated funds under the heading "relief of distress and prevention of contagious diseases," and following the Snyder Act, appropriation legislation often contained language that included funds for "conservation of health" (Snyder Act of 1921 [P.L. 67-85, 42 Statute 208]).

Based upon this language, subsequent programs included emphasis on health promotion and wellness, including such programs as attention to health conditions on the reservation, prevention of diseases, making home visits when necessary, reporting communicable diseases, inspection of water supplies, examination of students at the beginning of the school year, duties of field nurses, and others.[14]

The Snyder Act not only provided authorization for the expenditure of appropriated funds, it established the character of subsequent Indian health programs. Its emphasis on conservation of health antedated by decades subsequent public policy. What followed was a comprehensive, community-based health system in which preventive and environmental programs were integral parts.[16]

THE TRANSFER ACT, 1954

On August 5, 1954, vitally important legislation (Public Law 83–568) was enacted to transfer Indian health services out of the DOI to the Department of Health, Education, and Welfare (DHEW) (now the Department of Health and Human Services (DHHS)). Implementation of this legislation in July, 1955, represented major change in Indian health policy and involved transfer of all facilities, programs, and responsibilities maintained and operated by the Commissioner of Indian Affairs of the BIA to be administered by the surgeon general of the United States Public Health Service (USPHS).[7] At the time of transfer, there were 13 school infirmaries.

This transfer was the culmination of discussion and debate over many years. As early as 1919, transfer of Indian health programs to the USPHS had been discussed. A proposal made by the House Committee on Indian Affairs[17] went nowhere in the face of objections made by the BIA and the USPHS. Again in 1943, the Committee on Indian Affairs wanted Congress to consider transfer of Indian health to the USPHS, but Congress had its hands too full with World War II.[18]

Heightened awareness and concern emerged when two very important reports, the Meriam Survey, 1928,[19] and the Parran Survey, 1954,[20] were released. They described serious morbidity and mortality among American Indians and Alaska Natives (AIAN) and insufficient health programs and health care services. To heighten the urgency for action, BIA Indian services reported 100 physician and 188 nurse vacancies in 1944. To help cover these vacancies, more than 50 physicians and dentists in the USPHS Commissioned Corps were detailed to the BIA.[18,21] A bill, introduced in 1947, called for a transfer of Indian health services to the DHEW.[18] Strong support backing the bill came from the 1949 Hoover Commission's task force on public welfare,[22] and national organizations including the American Public Health Association, National Tuberculosis Association, the American Medical Association, and the Association of State and Territorial Health Officers. Some Indian tribes were also supportive. Initial opposition from the two involved government departments, DHEW and DOI, later was changed to positions of support.[18]

Rationale on the transfer seemed to follow two threads with incongruent endpoints, but ultimately resulted in improved health services for AIAN. The time of discussion leading to transfer occurred at a time of heightened implementation of the government's "termination policy," and, voiced by some, the transfer would be a step toward unloading government responsibility by "freeing" Indians from the supervision of the BIA.[23] It is notable that termination of over 100 tribes occurred around the time that transfer was debated and enacted. The other thread was strong support, beginning in the early 1900s, for much-needed effective public health programs and health services for Indian communities. In the words of Sen. Edward Thye of Minnesota, who introduced the bill in the Senate, the purposes of the transfer were "to improve health services to our Indian people; to coordinate our public health program; to further our long-range objective of integration of our Indian people in our common life."[24]

Final passage of The Transfer Act P.L. 83–568 on August 5, 1954, and its implementation in 1955 resulted in an infusion of health personnel, additional funding, and stronger public health programs for Indian communities. Immediately, the first director of the Division of Indian Health (later the IHS) appointed a maternal and child health specialist to ensure that vulnerable Indian maternal, infant, and child populations had focused programs and services. Clearly the results were positive; health status trends soon demonstrated improvements in the health status of AIANs.[25]

INDIAN SANITATION FACILITIES CONSTRUCTION ACT, 1959

Efforts by the newly appointed IHS director and the surgeon general soon after the transfer resulted in the 1959 Indian Sanitation Facilities Construction Act (P.L. 86–121; 73 Statute 267, July 31, 1959). This act, which amended The Transfer Act, established one of the most important programs relating to Indian health, especially that of infants and children: the availability of safe water and sewage disposal.[26] Prior to implementation of this act, acute gastroenteritis was responsible for many deaths, especially among infants and children. **Fig. 1** contrasts sanitation efforts with declining gastroenteric and postneonatal mortality rates during the same time period. Although this demonstrates an intriguing comparison ,cause and effect are impossible to prove. Indeed many hospitals had wards devoted to care for infants and children suffering from acute gastroenteritis. It generally is acknowledged that programs authorized by this act have improved Indian health as much as, if not more than, any other single factor.

The act did more, however. Section C of the act states: "the Surgeon General shall consult with, and encourage the participation of, the Indians concerned, States and political subdivisions thereof, in carrying out the provisions of this section." This section implicitly[27] resulted in two subsequent policies of major importance.

The first is that the IHS would not begin a local program until it first had received a formal tribal request. This brought the tribes to the table and created a situation in which tribes could begin partnerships with the IHS. Further, operation of the water treatment facilities was the responsibility of tribes themselves (with technical assistance provided by the IHS when requested). It is fair to say that these policies, along with preferential employment of local Indians, were significant precursors to Indian self-determination.

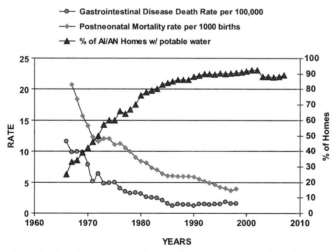

Fig. 1. Gastrointestinal and postneonatal mortality rates compared with percent of homes with sanitation facilities for American Indians and Alaska Natives 1960–2000. (*Adapted from* Ludington J. Home Safety Assessments/Interventions in American Indian Homes: A Role for IHS Engineering Staff. IHS Trends 2000–2001; with permission.) Safe Water and Waste Disposal Facilities. IHS Fact. Sheet June 2009. Available at: http://info.ihs.gov/SafeWater.asp.

Second, this act, along with the stimulus of the Indian Health Care Improvement Act (IHCIA) in 1976, resulted in an environmental program that now extends far beyond the provision of safe water and sewage, encompassing many programs directed specifically towards children and youth. Equally significant, the importance of the "integration of environmental health services into the overall IHS program" cannot be underestimated. This integration of various environmental and other programs into a national clinical system is one of the distinguishing characteristics of the IHS.[28]

INDIAN SELF-DETERMINATION AND EDUCATIONAL ASSISTANCE ACT OF 1975

The movement toward self-determination had its roots in reaction to federal tendencies toward assimilation and termination, which peaked in the 1950s and 1960s. AIAN tribes sought to walk the narrow line between maintaining the federal government's responsibility to its trust and treaty obligations to the tribes and asserting their autonomy as sovereign nations.[29] In addition, many senators and representatives pressed the administration to consider the prevalence of reservation poverty as an appropriate and necessary battleground in the war on poverty begun during the administration of Lyndon B. Johnson.[30]

Assimilation of Indian tribal members into a majority culture was an underlying current in Indian policy during the late 19th and early 20th centuries. Its manifestations were many, perhaps most vividly and perniciously expressed in reservation and off-reservation boarding schools during that period. "Kill the Indian in him, and save the man," Capt. Richard H. Pratt wrote in 1892, referring to efforts made at the Carlisle (Pennsylvania) Indian School, which he had founded, and elsewhere to inculcate mainstream culture and language in place of students' tribal cultures and languages.[31]

Termination became a congressionally sanctioned technique for assimilation after World War II; it contemplated "giving the full rights of citizenship" to Native Americans while ending federal recognition and support for tribes. During its heyday, from about 1950 until the practice was officially ended by President Johnson in 1964, some 109 Indian bands and tribes were terminated. Individual members of the tribes were to be given title to their lands in exchange for an end to federal support, including health care. In many cases, notably with the Menominee (Wisconsin) and Klamath (Oregon) tribes, the results were disastrous, with loss of tribal lands to speculators and wealthy non-natives.

Because no one ever seriously contemplated making the Indian treaties moot by returning Native Americans' lands to them, it was clearly impossible to return to the status quo ante. Thus by the late 1960s, abrogation of the trust and treaty obligations of the government came to be recognized as equally unpalatable. The unlikely pair of President Richard Nixon and Senator Henry (Scoop) Jackson of Washington combined to draft and ready for passage a number of forward-looking laws affecting Native American groups in the early 1970s. Both had participated in more hurtful policies in the 1950s, Nixon as vice-president during the termination period, and Jackson, as sponsor of termination legislation with respect to tribes within his own state. Bergman and colleagues[32] credit Nixon's conversion to his earlier admiration for his Native American football coach at Whittier College. Jackson's conversion is noted to have occurred after his appointment to the Senate Interior Committee in 1971, and his contact with committee staff member Forrest Gerard, himself a member of the Blackfeet tribe. The Gerard-Jackson partnership, with the patronage of President Nixon, resulted in the passage of several important bills, including the Alaska Native Claims Settlement Act (1971), the Indian Health Care Improvement Act (1976), and the Indian Self-Determination and Education Assistance Act (1971).

The preamble to Indian Self-Determination and Educational Assistance Act (ISDEAA) indicates its break with policies of the past:

"The Congress... finds that (1) the prolonged Federal domination of Indian service programs has served to retard rather than enhance the progress of Indian people and their communities by depriving Indians of the full opportunity to develop leadership skills crucial to the realization of self-government, and has denied to the Indian people an effective voice in the planning and implementation of programs for the benefit of Indians which are responsive to the true needs of Indian communities; and (2) the Indian people will never surrender their desire to control their relationships both among themselves and with non-Indian governments, organizations, and persons."[33,34]

The act specified an orderly transition of many programs from the control of federal agencies, largely the BIA and the IHS, to tribal control. The concepts were simple; tribes could petition the BIA and/or the IHS to operate programs that those agencies ran in Indian country. Federal supervision of the quality of the programs would continue. Tribes could request that their shares of all levels of administration, from the BIA or IHS headquarters to the area offices to the local service units be paid to them, and that they would also be eligible for contract support costs, funds to pay the costs incurred by tribes in preparation and administration of their programs.

Although the concepts may have been simple, application of those concepts to transfer of government processes has been difficult. Rosser[29] made the point that tribes assuming programs also would have to assume the possibility of failure without being able to blame the federal government for that failure. Failure, if it came, might make tribal governments liable to blame from their constituents. Although the tribes would get both monetary and advisory support for the transition, they would have to put in place all the personnel and business systems previously available through the BIA and the IHS. They would need to integrate tribally hired personnel with ISP Personnel and Public Health Service Commissioned Corps officers, and they would need to learn the arcane skills associated with billing both private insurers and also the major federal payers, Medicare and Medicaid.

A series of subsequent congressional acts have modified ISDEAA, generally in the direction of making the process easier and less directive. Indian self-governance legislation passed in 1994 and 2000[35,36] moved the process more toward the autonomy end of the maintenance of trust responsibility $\leftarrow \rightarrow$ autonomy continuum. Thus some tribes operate their compacted health programs with more autonomy under Title V of the 2000 PL 106–260, while others operate their contracts under closer federal direction under Title I of PL 93–638. In the popular parlance, both sets of tribal programs are called "638-ed," a numerical verb unfamiliar to many outside the sphere of federal Native American programs. Direct Service Tribes (DST) or federally maintained programs became known as I. Tribally run programs became known as T, and urban Indian programs as U, creating the collective I/T/U.

By 2001, most Indian health programs were being operated by tribal entities under Title I contracts or Title V compacts (540 of the 749 total programs [72%, **Table 1**]).[37] The penetration of "638ing" into the 12 IHS areas varied from the entire programs in the California and Alaska areas, to no tribally operated facilities in 2001 in the Tucson, Arizona, and Aberdeen IHS areas. As one can see from **Table 1**, tribes were more likely to assume responsibility for ambulatory care facilities (80%, includes health centers, school health centers, Alaska village clinics, and health stations) than hospitals (27%). Similar statistics regarding transition of responsibility for BIA programs are beyond the scope of this article.

Facilities	Hospitals	Health Centers	Alaska Village Clinics	Health Stations	School Health Centers	Youth Regional Treatment Centers
IHS	31	61	N/A	30	2	2
Tribal	14	227	166	102	13	10

Table 1
Progress in self-determination and self governance by 2001

Data from Indian Health Services Fact Sheets. Available at http://info.ihs.gov/Profile09.asp. Accessed May 27, 2009.

Tribes have been able to choose which aspects of their health care program are most appropriate to maintain in a climate of fiscal constraint. For example, some tribal programs have removed over-the-counter medications from their formularies, or have increased funding for vision and dental services.

"No one argues with the overall goal of the 638 legislation to give control to tribes. At an implementation level there have been concerns that tribes would not have the expertise or sophistication to run a complex health system or that the system would become embroiled in local tribal politics. In general these fears have been unfounded." (Holve S, Chief Clinical Consultant for Pediatrics, personal communication, 2009)

On isolated occasions, tribes have relinquished control of health programs back to the IHS. Most, however, have maintained a high level of service to tribal members. Some commentators feel that Native American self-determination and self-governance have been a source of pride and renewal for Native American communities.

Swimmer,[38] former principal chief of the Cherokee Tribe and highly placed official in the DOI of two administrations, notes some of the unintended consequences of the self-determination process. He cites some loss of the economies of scale conveyed by a unitary IHS, noting that this is important, because the IHS is and has always been underfunded:

"[In 1995], grossly inadequate funding is an intractable impediment to meaningful progress for the health of the Indian nations. The government spends $ 5000 per capita every year for health care for the general population, $ 3803 for federal prisoners, and yet only $ 1914 per capita for Indian health care... Although many commentators agree that IHS does an impressive job given their limited resources, IHS facilities are nevertheless overcrowded and underfunded."

Some tribes, Swimmer indicates, have been concerned that the movement toward self-determination would end the federal government's trust obligation to Native Americans. "Some tribes fear that self-determination and self-governance will lead to the dissolution of the IHS and, with it, dissolution of federal responsibility for Indian health care."[39] Indeed, as tribal shares have been withdrawn from the IHS, tribes remaining within the IHS structure have had their shares of the total reduced. Small tribes have hesitated to withdraw their own shares, but have had their services squeezed as larger tribes have compacted or contracted services. Some small area services cannot be subdivided and have disappeared as tribal shares have been removed. For example, in the Albuquerque, New Mexico, area, area-wide services and direct service programs in the metropolitan area have been reduced as larger tribes have taken their shares. Similar cutbacks at IHS headquarters also have led to decreases in program activities. Many of these negative consequences would be ameliorated if the IHS were to be funded at a level comparable to other US health care programs.

Despite these tempering observations, Washburn summarizes the generally positive results of self-determination as follows:

"As a result [of obtaining the right to contract federal services to be provided by the tribes themselves], tribal governments developed in an extraordinary fashion and Indian reservations are very different places today than they were in the 1960s. Today, on many Indian reservations, tribal governments are the primary providers of all government services."[30]

INDIAN HEALTH CARE IMPROVEMENT ACT, PUBLIC LAW 94—437, 1976

The Indian Health Care Improvement Act, Public Law 94–437 (IHCIA) was the authorizing legislation upon which the 94th US Congress set into motion for the appropriation of funds for the IHS from 1976 to 2001. Enacted Sept. 30, 1976, President Gerald R, Ford in his signing statement the next day, said:

"I AM [sic] signing S. 522, the Indian Health Care Improvement Act. This bill is not without its faults, but after personal review I have decided that the well-documented needs for improvement in Indian health manpower, services, and facilities outweigh the defects in the bill. While spending for Indian Health Service activities has grown from $128 million in FY 1970 to $425 million in FY 1977, Indian people still lag behind the American people as a whole in achieving and maintaining good health. I am signing this bill because of my own conviction that our first Americans should not be last in opportunity."[40]

The preamble text presages the IHS mission with the statement,

"The major national goal of the United States is to provide the quantity and quality of health services which will permit the health of Indians to be raised to the highest possible level and to encourage the maximum participation of Indians in the planning and management of those services."[41]

Findings in 1976 showed alarming health disparities for Indian people as compared with the general population. Issues to be addressed ran the gamut of adherence to building codes, increasing hospital accreditation, closing the gap on community sanitation needs, meeting the severe housing shortages, and attending to the workforce vacancy rates. The Declaration of Policy is unequivocal in its language.

"Sec. 3. The Congress hereby declares that it is the policy of this Nation, in fulfillment of its special responsibilities and legal obligation to the American Indian People, to meet the national goal of providing the highest possible health status to Indians and to provide existing Indian health services with all resources necessary to effect that policy."[40,41]

The IHCIA and its reauthorizations provided for funding for the IHS until 2001. Annual attempts since that time to reauthorize the act have not met with success. As recently as March 2009, Rachel A. Joseph, cochair of the National Steering Committee to Reauthorize the IHCIA stated

"… the majority of illnesses and deaths from disease in Indian country could be prevented if the needed funding and contemporary programs for healthcare were available to American Indians and Alaska Natives."

She went on to say, "Passage of the Indian Health Care Improvement Act reauthorization is a vital component of any healthcare reform."[42]

Beyond published testimony in subsequent attempts at reauthorization, surprisingly little has been published on the IHCIA by way of policy analysis and despite its being the cornerstone legislation for health care delivery for federally-recognized tribes. The Secretary of DHEW, in his 1997 Report to Congress outlined advancements as were also found in a 1978 Progress Report to the National Congress of American Indians (NCAI) during Emery Johnson's tenure as IHS director. The act's impact on workforce, takes on substance and dimension. It noted that "P.L. 94–437 authorized 612 positions and $208,797,000 for F.Y. 1978," while appropriations actually provided for 477 positions and a lesser sum of money.[43]

Title I or Indian Health Manpower addresses access to care through the Health Professions Recruitment Program for Indians, the Health Professions Scholarship Program for Indians, Indian Health Service Summer Extern Program, and Continuing Education Allowances. Threads of early treaty language on education, along with findings from the 1910 Valentine Report on public health and education and the Snyder Act's stated purpose emphasizing "general support and civilization, including education" renew their presence in IHCIA authorizing language under Title I. Accordingly, the IHS mission statement is as follows: "Our mission... to raise the physical, mental, social, and spiritual health of American Indians and Alaska Natives to the highest level."[44] Linkages between education, manpower, and delivery of health care are set forth in Title VI, which supports a feasibility study of an American Indian School of Medicine.

Title II or Health Services authorized additional resources by way of annual increases to address the backlog and unmet needs in both direct patient care settings and across broader service delivery issues. Mirroring the problems seen today, the health disparities spanned "patient care, field health, dental health, mental health, alcoholism, and facility maintenance and repair."[41] Phasing in of the Model Dormitory Mental Health Project and Therapeutic and Residential Treatment Center (for Indian children) were early steps taken to address the unmet needs of child and youth. Health Facilities (Title III) would have implications for nurseries, delivery units, clinic space for well child, prenatal and family services, as well as inpatient wards for the infectious diseases so prevalent in childhood. Access to Health Services (Title IV) contained Medicare and Medicaid reimbursement language that allowed for the expanded capacity to improve services and assure the upgrade of services through consultation with the Joint Commission on the Accreditation of Health Organizations (JCAHO/JCO). Achieving accreditation brought about improved collections. Early Periodic Screening, Diagnosis and Treatment (EPSDT) for children 0 to 19 years of age as specified in P.L. 437 was a means to assure comprehensive well child care to Indian children. Reauthorization language as recent as 2008 develops substantial sections to SCHIP, which was reauthorized and expanded as the Children's Health Insurance Program Reauthorization Act of 2009 (CHIPRA). Title V of P.L. 94–437 is devoted to health services for urban Indians, giving specific importance to issues of child abuse and neglect, youth mental health, alcohol/substance abuse treatment, and preventive services. Such mandates became tokenism and restrictive when appropriations failed to follow, leaving urban Indian programs little with which to implement despite an over 60% urban AIAN population.

By the 1992, the third and most recent reauthorization saw the original P.L. 94–437's 16 pages expand to well over 60. Sixty-one health objectives span coronary heart disease, overweight, adolescent suicide, child/infant blood lead level screening, teen pregnancy, and fetal deaths.[45] One objective seeking to "reduce the infant mortality rate (IMR) to no more than 8.5 per 1000 live births" was reached 8 years later when the IMR was 8.3 per 1000 live births for AIAN infants. This rate is again on the increase and also is not adjusted for race and ethnicity miscoding. The AIAN rate remains 20% higher than the US all-races rate, and exhibits a disproportionate postneonatal IMR.[46]

The July 2003 report by the US Commission on Civil Rights, *A Quiet Crisis Federal Funding and Unmet Needs in Indian Country,* noted the gap in services to AIAN populations that preventive health, a mainstay of pediatrics, is among equally pressing needs of health care, education, public safety, housing, and rural development, echoing the Snyder Act's listing of socioeconomic needs. The Commission goes on to state for the HHS, US Department of Housing and Urban Development (HUD), Department of Education (DOE), BIA, Department of Justice (DOJ), and US Department of Agriculture (USDA) that while they

> *"... are responsible ... inadequate funding, overall and within specific program area's, has rendered doing so impossible. ...conditions in Indian Country could be greatly relieved if the federal government honored its commitment to funding. Unfortunately, Native Americans living on tribal lands do not have access to the same services and programs available to other Americans, even though the government has a binding trust obligation to provide them. The trust responsibility makes the provision of services to Native Americans a legal entitlement, not just a moral, social or economic one."[47]*

The constraints of inadequate annual appropriations coupled with an expired P.L. 94–437 signal a breach in policy making, part of this quiet crisis. Health, safety, housing and education, indispensable requirements in the welfare of AIAN children and youth, will continue to reverberate beyond this expired legislation.

INDIAN CHILD WELFARE ACT, 1978

By the latter part of the 1970s, Congress had turned decisively away from an earlier generation's assimilation policy toward AIAN. The importance to the tribes of the first two bills, the ISDEAA and the IHCIA, cannot be overestimated. To ensure that Indian children grow and mature within their kinship and culture remained a high priority. Tribal autonomy and survival remained at stake as long as states could remove children from Native American families and place them with families unacquainted with tribal traditions and cultures, however well-meaning these majority culture families might be. Children thus removed were assimilated into that majority culture regardless of their tribe's interests.

In the years leading up to the Indian Child Welfare Act (ICWA), a remarkably high proportion of Native American children were removed from their families and placed, usually with white American families. The extent of the problem was elucidated in a report made by the Association on American Indian Affairs[48] and was largely supported by a study done by the Children's Bureau of the then-Department of Health, Education, and Welfare.[49] The investigators found, for example, that more than 25% of Minnesota Indian children were in out-of-home placements. Native American children were being removed from their families' homes at a rate as great as 19 times that for non-Native children. At times, these out-of-home placements were made because substance abuse had decreased parents' ability to be effective with their children, or because of perceived child abuse or neglect. The definition of neglect, however, was often overly broad; in some jurisdictions, children were removed from their homes primarily because of parental poverty, which was considered neglect in and of itself.

In its preamble, the ICWA states its reason for being:

> *"There is no resource that is more vital to the continued existence and integrity of American Indian tribes than their children ... and that an alarmingly high percentage*

of such children are placed in non-Indian foster and adoptive homes and institutions. The states ... have often failed to recognize the essential tribal relations of Indian people and the culture and social standards prevailing in Indian communities and families. It is the policy of this Nation to protect the best interests of Indian children and to promote the stability and security of Indian tribes and families..."[50]

ICWA covers all children who are or are eligible to be members of federally recognized tribes. States must establish "beyond a reasonable doubt" that out-of-home placement is needed, and indigent Native American parents are to be provided with legal representation. Tribal input is to be sought in any instance of need for children of Native American heritage needing to be placed out of their own homes, whether temporarily in foster care, or permanently in adoption. Tribes can petition for the removal of court proceedings from state courts to tribal courts whenever children had been living on federal reservations. Active efforts must be made by states to provide remediation of problems found in Native parental homes before placement outside those homes is to be considered. Where as many as 85% to 90% of Native American children removed from their homes had been placed in non-Native homes prior to passage of ICWA, the law specified that such placements are to be considered only in the last resort, after placement with relatives, with members of the same tribe, and members of other tribes. Two years later, Congress passed a more widely applicable adoption law, P.L. 96–242, the Adoption Assistance and Child Welfare Act, which extended many of ICWA's provisions, including parental notice requirements, to all US children.[51]

Several studies have looked at the effectiveness of ICWA in meeting the act's stated goals. Plantz and colleagues[52] studied four widely scattered states' compliance with the ICWA in 1989. The group found mixed success in complying with key features of the ICWA. In particular, they found that states had not worked hard to remediate conditions within Native American children's birth homes prior to initiating removal proceedings.

MacEachron and colleagues[53] 1996 study of data from before and after passage indicated that adoption of Native children decreased 93% from 1975 to 1986, and that foster placement decreased by 31%. The study concluded that tribes had gained substantial control over the placement of their children, and that the adoption rate of Native American children had declined to be only slightly above the rate for other US children.

In a 2002 study published by the National Indian Child Welfare Association, Brown and colleagues[54] noted substantial compliance by the State of Arizona with the provisions of ICWA. Tribal notification of state proceedings was taking place regularly, if not always in the ways specified by the act. In general, children removed from families were being placed according to the priorities specified in ICWA. Tribes were intervening in cases in state courts, and generally found the courts attentive to tribal priorities and to ICWA requirements. Jones and colleagues[55] in 2000 found less compliance in an extensive study of North Dakota cases, with ICWA requirements for tribal notification, transfer of cases to tribal courts, and preference for placement being followed in a minority of cases.

Rep. Don Young of Alaska noted on the 25th anniversary of ICWA's passage that ICWA's effects had

"been remarkable. Tribes have acted forcefully to help keep families intact. Because of the ICWA, many tribes and states have developed significant cooperative relationships aimed at eliminating state child welfare policies and implementing practices targeted at maintaining the integrity of American Indian and Alaska Native AIAN families and tribes. As a result, ICWA's promise to benefit the welfare

of American Indian and Alaska Native AIAN children has benefited many thousands of these children, enabling them to mature into functioning and contributing citizens of their tribes and of the Nation."[56]

Young introduced a bill to amend ICWA, which would have corrected several loopholes in the original 1978 act, the most important being the "existing Indian family" exception that had been cited by some courts to bypass ICWA's provisions by finding that the child in question had not maintained a "social or cultural relationship with an Indian tribe."[57] As of the time of writing, this legislation had not yet been passed.

THE OMNIBUS DRUG ACT OF 1986

The Omnibus Drug Act of 1986 provided language authorizing residential substance abuse treatment programs for Indian youth in each of the IHS Areas.[58] One of several analyses by Novins and colleagues[59] sought to understand the mental health needs and program delivery to the residents in one of nine residential programs. Using a medical record review, they looked at substance use and comorbid psychiatric symptoms stratified by gender. They identified the need for better understanding of residential treatment program design, gender differences, and both the mental health intake and treatment plan as part of substance abuse treatment for children and adolescents.

THE FUTURE OF AMERICAN INDIAN HEALTH POLICY

C. Everett Koop, MD, SC.D, surgeon general of the US Public Health Service in his 1987 address "Beyond Survival" at the First National Conference on Health Promotion Disease Prevention for American Indians and Alaska Natives begins,

> *"I am most pleased to be here today since this conference is the first public event that I am aware of which exposes one of the best kept secrets in the public health services: The Indian Health Service, I say best kept secret because the Indian Health Service has quietly and without much fanfare established itself as a leader in health services planning and delivery..."*

Foremost, Koop noted the Indian leadership in health care delivery of a comprehensive system of care, the notable reductions in infant mortality, achievements in sanitation, advancements in obstetric care, and numerous community-based education efforts.[60]

As described previously, Indian health policy has been a dynamic process extending to the earliest days of the United States, and it has been influenced by multiple sources, both governmental and nongovernmental. There is no reason to believe that this evolution has reached a point of stability. On the contrary, there is good reason to believe that quite substantial changes are pending, again from various sources. To the best of the authors' knowledge, relatively few publications directly address future changes in Indian health policy.[61–63] As in the past, anticipated policies are likely to be the result of changes internal to the IHS and changes external to it. By far the most significant external change is establishment of some form of covered access to health care for all citizens of the United States.[64,65]

Future changes in Indian health policy will involve focus on tribal self-governance and its ramifications. A recent evolution flowing from this policy has been the creation of three distinct and separate Indian health services as prefaced and collectively referred to as the I/T/U programs. Some of the consequences flowing from this development have been discussed already. It is likely that efforts to ameliorate some of the untoward consequences experienced by the direct service tribes (DST) will ensue. The fundamental question will be the extent to which tribes choose to enter into self-governance or choose to receive services directly from the IHS. Assuring comprehensive public health services and age-appropriate evidence-based medical care for Indian children across the I/T/U programs has its challenges. It will require attention to the input of standardized documentation of clinical care and the output of regional and nationally aggregated reporting of data in a climate where medical information systems and their infrastructure continue to develop. Data are required to provide a clear picture to policy makers, of the services rendered, trends in health disparities, and community interventions designed for Indian children and their families.

A policy change that impacted the directorship of the IHS was a 1992 amendment to the IHCIA (P.L. 94–437), which made the director an appointee of the president. It is reasonable to expect that the politicization of that position will influence future Indian health policy. Efforts have been underway for the past several years to make the position an assistant secretary for Indian health. It is unclear how AIAN issues and consequently Indian child health issues will be impacted.

For some time, the IHS has struggled with the need for improved definition of the population for which it is responsible; that is, a clearer definition of those Indians who are eligible to receive care through the IHS. While this need has largely resulted from inadequate levels of funding, it is likely to continue to be a problem that will be addressed in the future. Its impact on Indian children is unknown.

The most dominant external force acting on future Indian health policy will be health care reform with possibly a publicly funded option in which the federal government will underwrite the major costs. Obviously, such a development will have profound effects on subsequent Indian health policy, just as the Medicare, Medicaid, and state CHIP programs already have done. Such funding policies are basic to access to care and the comprehensive services for Indian children both within the Indian Health Care System or I/T/U and in the private sector. Intake, enrollment, and maintenance of enrolled status for eligible Indian children into these programs are crucial. Portability of coverage for boarding school and residential treatment for participating youth is necessary. Two concerns will dominate future considerations relating to Indian health policy in the era of health care reform:

1. The sovereignty of the tribes and the respective government-to-government relationship between federally recognized tribes and the federal government
2. The dual entitlement possessed by members of federally recognized tribes arising from their relationship to the federal government and which accrue to them by virtue of being US citizens

Indian tribes will object to any perceived threat to their sovereignty, to the existing government-to-government relationship; or perceived effort to abrogate existing treaty responsibilities of the federal government. Indians presently receive federal health care as a result of a prepaid health program paid for through cessation of lands and therefore will resist any programs that will require them to pay additionally for health services. Will Indian people resist the likely establishment of "means testing" to determine levels of health care coverage? Congress is likely to undertake a thorough examination of any duplication of services that could arise from continuation of some, if not all, of the I/T/U programs. Lastly, as citizens of states, AIANs are eligible for a host of programs, including the Maternal and Child Health

Bureau Title V services, most notably the Children with Special Health Care Needs (CSHCN) program. DOE programs are also examples of federal funding to states that merits further assessment of their impact on tribes and Indian children's education status.

The IHS, as a provider of comprehensive community services, engages in a range of services such as environmental programs, preventive programs, the community health representatives program, and several special-emphasis programs such as diabetes and alcohol and drug abuse. Will continuation of such programs, including school-based health services be provided for, and if so, how? One of the greatest challenges that has faced the IHS in recent decades is how to pay for Contract Health Services (CHS) provided through contracts with private providers. The major characteristic of the CHS is the grossly inadequate level of funds available to pay for necessary and oftentimes more complex care, with the resultant necessity of establishing priorities for payment of such services. One possibility is that this frustrating burden might be taken over completely under health care reform while leaving the basic I/T/U infrastructure in place to provide comprehensive culturally sensitive clinical and public health services in community, primary care, and hospital settings.

It is not possible to predict which of these elements will be affected or in what way, but one must assume that some will be affected. It is also safe to say that they will be the subject of intense debate. Certainly given the complexity of the many aspects of Indian health delivery, of which tribal sovereignty is only one element, one would be well-advised to proceed with great caution and deliberation in establishing Indian health policy under any version of health care reform.

Leaving aside considerations of health care reform, many other factors will continue to affect Indian health policy. One of these is the influence of disease change itself[66,67]; that is, demographic changes and alterations in disease patterns that themselves influence policy and are likely to continue to do so in the future. Changing pediatric morbidities, trends in childhood obesity, and mental health in a demographically young population are two issues that will press upon existing allocations. The unique position of children in society requires that adults by proxy carry the responsibility of advocates as evidenced in the history, law, and policy presented previously.

According to Taylor,[68] US Indian policy varies between two polar positions. The first, expressed in the Indian Reorganization Act of 1934 (48 Statute 984) emphasized the federal–Indian relationship, trust responsibility for Indian resources, development of tribal government, and the goal of tribal economic self-sufficiency. On the other hand, a competing view holds that "Indians as American citizens, should be assisted in adjusting to the basic US governmental structure, which of course includes the states, and be served by the same governments that serve other citizens as well as paying the same taxes."[61] It is almost certain that all future policy will entail efforts to resolve these fundamentally different approaches.

According to Taylor, Indian individuals, tribal governments, Indian interest groups, state governments, and the federal government all will be involved in the formulation and application of Indian policy in the future.[61] There is no question but that the tribes themselves, along with Indian individuals, have a much greater participation in policy formulation than was formerly the case.

One might well speculate that a review of American Indian health policy, its evolution, and its various permutations would well serve policy makers planning and implementing health care reform.

REFERENCES

1. Select Committee on Indian Affairs. S Con. Res. 331. Washington, DC: US GPO; 1988. 100th Congr, 2nd Session. Available at: http://catalog.wrlc.org/cgi-bin/Pwebrecon.cgi?BBID=1813609. Accessed April 10, 2009.
2. US Constitution. Article 1, section 8. § 8, cl.?. Available at: http://www.usconstitution.net/xconst_A1Sec8.html. Accessed April 10, 2009.
3. Kappler CJ. Indian affairs: laws and treaties, volume 2 (treaties 1778–1883). Washington DC Government Printing Office; 1904. Digitalization produced by Oklahoma State University library 1999–2000. Available at: http://digital.Library.OKstate.edu/kappler. Accessed April 11, 2009.
4. Crosby AW. Virgin soil epidemics as a factor in aboriginal depopulation in America. William Mary Q 1976;33(3):289–99.
5. Johnson BE. Such a union. In: Forgotten founders. Ipswich (MA): Gambit Incorporated; 1982. p. 56–76.
6. Ford P. The writings of Thomas Jefferson, vol. 3. New York: G.P. Putnam's Sons; 1897. p. 194–9. Available at: http://www.library.csi.cuny.edu/dept/history/lavender/jefflett.html. Accessed April 15, 2009.
7. Prucha FP. Documents of United States Indian policy. 2nd edition. Expanded. Lincoln: University of Nebraska Press; 1975.
8. Johnson EA, Rhoades ER. The history and organization of Indian Health Services and systems. In: Rhoades ER, editor. American Indian health. Baltimore (MD): The Johns Hopkins University Press; 2000. p. 74–92.
9. Treaty with the Sioux. Sept. 29, 1837. Proclamation, June 15, 1838. 7 Statute 538. Available at: http://puffin.creighton.edu. Accessed April 15, 2009.
10. Shelton BL. Legal and historical roots of health care for American Indians and Alaska Natives in the United States. Prepared for the Henry J. Kaiser Family Foundation. 2004; p. 6.
11. Agreement with the Sioux of various tribes. October 17, 1882 to January 3, 1883. Unratified. House Resolution Executive Document 68. 47th Congr, 2nd Session. Available at: http://puffin.creighton.edu. Accessed April 10, 2009.
12. National Institutes of Health. Indian school hospital under the Office of Indian Affairs (c. 1883–c. 1916). From an online series, "If you knew the conditions.": health care to Native Americans. US National Library of Medicine. Available at: http://www.nlm.nih.gov/exhibition/if_you_knew/if_you_knew.05.html. Accessed April 20, 1998.
13. Pevar SL. The rights of Indians and tribes. New York: Bantam Books; 1983.
14. Meriam L. The problem of Indian administration. Baltimore (MD): Johns Hopkins University Press; 1928.
15. Felix S. Cohen's handbook of federal Indian law. Washington, DC: Government Printing Office; 1942.
16. Code of federal regulations, title 25, sections 84 and 85. Washington, DC: US Government Printing Office; 1949. p. 95ff.
17. Schamel CE, Rephlo M, Ross R, et al. Records of the committee on interior and insular affairs and its predecessors. Guide to the records of the United States House of Representatives at the National Archives, 1789–1989. Bicentennial edition, document no. 100–245. Washington, DC: National Archives and Records Administration, 1989. Available at: http://www.archives.gov/legislative/guide/house/chapter-13-indian-affairs.html. Accessed May 2, 2009.
18. Dejong DH. "If you knew the conditions." A chronicle of the Indian medical service and American Indian healthcare 1908–1955. Lanham (MD): Rowman & Littlefield; 2008.

19. Meriam L, Brown RA, Cloud HR, et al. The problem of Indian administration: report of a survey made at the request of honorable Hubert Work, secretary of the interior, and submitted to him, February 21, 1928. Baltimore (MD): The Johns Hopkins Press; 1928.
20. Parran T, Ciocco A, Crabtree JA, et al. Alaska's health: a survey report to United States department of interior, 1954. Pittsburgh (PA): The Graduate School of Public Health, University of Pittsburgh; 1954.
21. Vogel L. Planning, evaluation and research, IHS: health planning in Indian health service, trends and issues, part I. American Public Health Association Newsletter; Winter. 2007. Available at: http://www.apha.org/membergroups/newsletters/sectionnewsletters/comm/winter07/vogelarticle.htm. Accessed April 5, 2009.
22. Prucha FP. The great white father: the United States government and the American Indians. Lincoln: University of Nebraska Press; 1995.
23. Shelton BL. Legal and historical roots of health care for American Indians and Alaska Natives in the United States. An issue brief for the Henry J. Kaiser family foundation. February 2004.
24. Kunitz SJ. The history and politics of US health policy for American Indians and Alaska Natives. Am J Public Health 1996;86(10):1464–73.
25. Brenneman GR. Maternal, child, and youth health. In: Rhoades ER, editor. American Indian health. Baltimore (MD): The Johns Hopkins University Press; 2000. p. 138–49.
26. Public Law. Indian Sanitation Facilities Construction Act. 1959. Pub. L. No. 86–121. 73 Statute 267(1959). Available at: http://www.lexisnexis.com/us/lnacademic. Accessed May 2; 2009.
27. Falcone D. Health policy analysis: some reflections on the state of the art. In: Straetz RA, Lieberman M, Sardell A, editors. Critical issues in health policy. Lexington (MA): Lexington Books; 1981. p. 5.
28. Public Law. 86–121 Annual report for 2001. Indian Health Service Sanitation Facilities Construction Program. Indian Health Services, Rockville (MD). Available at: http://www.dsfc.ihs.gov. Accessed April 7, 2009.
29. Rosser E. The trade-off between self-determination and the trust doctrine: tribal government and the possibility of failure. Ark L Rev 2003;58:291.
30. Washburn KK. Tribal self-determination at the crossroads. Conn L Rev 2006;38:777.
31. Richard HP. The advantages of mingling Indians with whites. Americanizing the American Indians: writings by the "Friends of the Indian" 1880–1900. Cambridge (MA): Harvard University Press; 1973.
32. Bergman AB, Grossman DC, Erdrich AM, et al. A political history of the Indian Health Service. Milbank Q 1999;77:571–604.
33. 25 United States Code Service 540a–n.
34. P.L. 93–638. Subchapter II—Indian self-determination and education assistance. Available at: http://www.tribal-institute.org/lists/pl93-638.htm. Accessed April 12, 2009.
35. Public Law. No. 106–260. 114 Statute 711 (2000).
36. Public Law. No. 103–413, 108 Statute 4250 (1994).
37. Regional differences in Indian health, 2000–2001. Rockville (MD): Indian Health Service; 2002.
38. Swimmer R. Modern tribal government: social and economic realities and opportunities. St. Thomas L Rev 1995;7:479.
39. Swimmer R. 2000 Native American law symposium: contract support funding and the federal policy of Indian tribal self-determination. Tulsa Law J 2000;36:349.
40. Woolley JT, Peters G. The American Presidency Project [online]. Santa Barbara (CA): University of California (hosted) Gerhard Peter (database). Available at: http://www.presidency.ucsb.edu/ws/?pid=6399. Accessed April 12, 2009.

41. Public Law. Indian Health Care Improvement Act. 1976. Pub. L. No. 94–437. 90 Statute 1400 (1976). Accessed March 28, 2009.

42. Basu S. Leaders call for reauthorization of Indian health care improvement act. US Medicine. Available at: http://www.usmedicine.com/article.cfm?articleID=1878& issueID=121. Accessed April 19, 2009.

43. Indian Health Service. Annual meeting of the National Congress of American Indians. Progress report—the implementation of the Indian Health Care Improvement Act P.L. 94–437. September 18–22, 1978, Rapid City, South Dakota.

44. Available at: http://www.ihs.gov/PublicInfo/PublicAffairs/Welcome_Info/IHSintro. asp. Accessed July 18, 2009.

45. Public Law 102–573—October. 29, 1992.

46. Mathews TJ, MacDorman MF. Infant mortality statistics from the 2003 period linked birth/infant death data set. National vital statistics reports, vol. 54, number 16. Hyattsville (MD); National Center for Health Statistics; 2006.

47. United States Commission on Civil Rights. A quiet crisis: federal funding and unmet needs in Indian country, pursuant to public law 103–419 [report]. July 2003.

48. Unger S, editor. The destruction of American Indian families. New York: Association on American Indian Affairs; 1977. p. 1–90.

49. Sudia C. Impact of the 1978 Indian Child Welfare Act and the 1980 Adoption Assistance and Child Welfare Act on the out-of-home placement of American Indian children [report]. Washington, DC: Children's Bureau, Administration on Children, Youth, and Families; 1987. Available at: http://www.narf.org/icwa/ federal/index.htm. Accessed May 6, 2009.

50. 25 United States Code Service 1901, 1902.

51. P.L. 96–272. Available at: http://thomas.loc.gov/cgi-bin/bdquery/z?d096:HR03434: @@@DTOM:/bss/d096query.html. Accessed May 26, 2009.

52. Plantz M, Hubbell R, Barrett B, et al. Indian child welfare: a status report. Child Today 1989;18(1):24–9.

53. MacEachron AE, Gustavsson NS, Cross S, et al. The effectiveness of the Indian Child Welfare Act of 1978. Social Service Review 1996;70(3):451–63.

54. Brown EF, Limb GE, Chance T, et al. The Indian Child Welfare Act: an examination of state compliance in Arizona. St. Louis (MO): Washington University, National Indian Child Welfare Association. 2002.

55. Jones BJ, Gillette J, Painte D, et al. Indian Child Welfare Act: a pilot study of compliance in North Dakota. Seattle (WA): Casey Family Programs; 2000.

56. Congressional Record. 25 Anniversary of Enactment of Indian Child Welfare Act. Hon. Don Young of Alaska in the House of Representative Friday, November 7, 2003. E2282-3 Congress Session. Available at: http://www.narf.org/icwa/ federal/lh/cr110703.pdf. Accessed April 29, 2009.

57. ICWA Implementation Problems addressed by H.R. 2750. National Indian Child Welfare Association. Available at: http://www.nicwa.org/legislation/ HR27500. Accessed April 29, 2009.

58. Omnibus Drug Supplemental Appropriations Act of 1987 Pub. L. 99–500, title II, October 18, 1986, 100 Statute 1783–353, and Pub. L. 99-591, title II, Oct. 30, 1986, 100 Statute 3341.

59. Novins DK, Beals J, Manson SM, et al. The substance abuse treatment of American Indian adolescents: comorbid symptomatology, gender differences, and treatment patterns. J Am Acad Child Adolesc Psychiatry 1996;35: 1593–601. Available at: http://aianp.uchsc.edu/ncaianmhr/research/k20_novins. htm Accessed May 5, 2009.

60. Koop EC. Address to participants of the first National Conference on Health Promotion and Disease Prevention for American Indians and Alaska Natives "Beyond Survival" health challenges in American Indian and Alaska Native communities. Washington, DC: June 19, 1987.

61. Dixon M, Roubideaux Y, editors. Promises to keep: public health policy for American Indians & Alaska Natives in the 21st Century. Washington, DC: American Public Health Association; 2001. p. 311.

62. Johnson EA, Rhoades ER. The future of Indian health. In: Rhoades ER, editor. American Indian health: innovations in health care, promotion, and policy. Baltimore (MD): Johns Hopkins University Press; 2000. p. 434.

63. Report on Indian health, Task Force Six: Indian Health. Final report to the American Indian policy review commission. Washington, DC: US Government Printing Office; 1976.

64. Iglehart JK. The struggle for reform—challenges and hopes for comprehensive health care legislation. N Engl J Med. Available at: http://www.nejm.org. Accessed April 1, 2009 (10.1056/NEJMp0902651).

65. Baucus M. Call to action: health reform 2009. Available at: http://www.finance. senate.gov. Accessed March 30, 2009.

66. Kunitz SJ. Disease change and the role of medicine. Berkeley (CA): University of California Press; 1983.

67. Rhoades ER. Changing paradigms and their effect on American Indian and Alaska Native health [editorial]. Ann Epidemiol 1997;7:227–8.

68. Taylor R. American Indian policy. Mount Airy (MD): Lomond Publications Incorporated; 1983. p. 230.

History, Law, and Policy as a Foundation for Health Care Delivery for Australian Indigenous Children

Ngiare Brown, BM, MPHTM, FRACGP

KEYWORDS

- Aboriginal • Child health • Indigenous people • Australia

Aboriginal and Torres Strait Islander social and cultural imperatives cannot be fully understood or respected if an attempt is made to detail contemporary child health status and health policy issues without appropriate consideration of the historical, political, legislative, and policy contexts that have not only shaped Indigenous affairs in Australia but continue to affect Aboriginal child health and social justice.

This article does not attempt an exhaustive compendium of Aboriginal child health policy, rather it aims to identify significant historical and contemporary issues, programs, and progress to better understand the current policy in Australia relating to Aboriginal child health and well-being.

A legislative perspective is included to give context to contemporary issues based on legally sanctioned historical practices specifically designed to make Aboriginal peoples disappear, particularly through the control and assimilation of Indigenous children.

CONTEXT

Exploration of the literature on Aboriginal child health policy reveals a disjointed, poorly coordinated approach to policy addressing Aboriginal child health and well-being, despite recent initiatives directed at a more comprehensive national approach (**Box 1**). There is a paucity of in-depth policy analysis, despite the increasing focus on evidence-based health planning and management.

Historically, legislation and policy relating to Aboriginal and Torres Strait Islander peoples have focused on power and control, as shown by the ideology and practices of determining all aspects of Indigenous existence.[a] Even the move to embrace the language of self-determination was conceived without infrastructure, capacity

Bullana, the Poche Centre for Indigenous Health, Edward Ford Building A27, The University of Sydney, NSW 2006, Australia
E-mail address: n.brown@usyd.edu.au

[a] Specific policy eras in Australia identified as segregation and protection; assimilation; and self-determination.

Pediatr Clin N Am 56 (2009) 1561–1576
doi:10.1016/j.pcl.2009.10.002
0031-3955/09/$ – see front matter © 2009 Elsevier Inc. All rights reserved.

Box 1
National reform initiatives to improve early childhood outcomes

- National Partnership Agreements on Early Childhood Education to achieve universal access to quality early childhood education for all children in the year before school by 2013

- National Partnership Agreement on Indigenous Early Childhood Development to establish 35 new children and family centers and increase access to antenatal care, teenage sexual and reproductive health, and family health services for Indigenous children and families

- Six-year national Partnership Agreement on Preventive Health, with a focus on strategies to prevent chronic diseases that commence in early childhood

- A national quality agenda for early childhood education and care that includes stronger standards, streamlined regulatory approaches, a rating system, and an Early Years Learning Framework

- National workforce initiatives to improve the quality and supply of the early childhood education and care workforce

- The Closing the Gap initiative, which includes ambitious targets for Indigenous children related to infant mortality, literacy, and numeracy, and participation in quality early childhood education

- A National Framework for Protecting Australia's Children

- The Melbourne Declaration on Education Goals for Young Australians

- A National Family Support Program, which brings together 8 Commonwealth programs for children, families, and parenting

- Paid parental leave arrangements

- A National Plan to Reduce Violence against Women and Children

- Development of an Early Intervention and Prevention Framework under the National Disability Agreement

- A National Partnership Agreement on Homelessness, with a focus on intervening for children and their families at risk of homelessness.

Investing in the early years – A National Early Childhood Development strategy. An initiative of the Council of Australian Governments, July 2009. Commonwealth of Australia 2009. Attorney-General's Department, Canberra, ACT, 2600.

---

development, and resourcing commitments to ensure initiatives in Aboriginal affairs were viable and sustainable. The construct of self-determination is still often referred to as a "failed experiment", and the hollow promise of Indigenous equality reinforced by disappointments and challenges in the public arena such as lack of high level Indigenous political representation and the demise of the Aboriginal and Torres Strait Islander Commission.[b–d]

Discriminatory legislation, policy, and practices are responsible for ongoing intergenerational health problems and political and social barriers to more timely progress in improving outcomes. Persistent, and in some instances increasing, disparities[1,2] between Aboriginal and non-Aboriginal child outcomes require prompt but considered

---

[b] Neville Bonner was the first Aboriginal Member of Parliament, an elected Liberal party. representative.
[c] Aden Ridgeway was the second Aboriginal Member of Parliament and NSW senator 1999–2005.
[d] The Aboriginal and Torres Strait Islander Commission was established under the Labour Government in 1990 and abolished under the Coalition Government in 2005.

action in partnership with Aboriginal communities and representative organizations, focusing on access to primary care and improved housing and environmental infrastructure. "The assessment of contemporary policies to reduce social and economic disadvantage experienced by Aboriginal families is vital".[3]

Developments in the Northern Territory demonstrate that governments are still willing to exercise strict and punitive controls over Aboriginal individuals and communities. The Little Children are Sacred Report[4] identified a broad and inclusive set of recommendations addressing Aboriginal child sexual abuse in the Northern Territory; the report was informed by a consultative community process and was evidence based. In response the Commonwealth Government announced the Northern Territory Emergency Response,[5] or the Intervention, a set of measures including income management, child health checks, and the compulsory acquisition of Aboriginal land. These measures were not informed by evidence, nor linked to mechanisms for evaluation or accountability.

The ever-changing landscape of Indigenous affairs, in which innovation is constrained by political and financial cycles, further demonstrates that State and Commonwealth departments are still unsure about how best to deliver comprehensive and sustainable social services and infrastructure to address priority issues in a coordinated, respectful, and culturally appropriate manner, despite decades of evidence and best practice guidelines.[6,7]

Aboriginal child health policy benefits from being a politically and socially attractive issue and a priority in health for all populations. Persistent disparities in life expectancy and perinatal and infant health outcomes ARACY[2] have improved in the past 30 years in jurisdictions in which identifying data are routinely collected for analysis and action.[8] This is the result of the application of mainstream approaches and best practice standards to maternal and infant health, such as routine antenatal care and childhood immunization. There have also been successful programs specifically developed for Aboriginal and Torres Strait Islander mothers and babies and delivered by community-controlled health services, including the "Strong Women Strong Babies Strong Culture" initiative in the Northern Territory and Townsville Mums and Bubs program.

LEGISLATION AND POLICY

Since colonization, legislation has had a significant influence on Aboriginal and Torres Strait Islander policy and control, reflected in "case law, treaties and other legal and political documents which have affected Indigenous peoples' rights in Australia."[9] For nearly 2 centuries the Aboriginal policy environment was defined by legally sanctioned approaches to segregation, protection, assimilation, and self-determination.

Segregation and Protection

Protection Acts shaped the practices of government departments and other relevant authorities from the 1830s to the 1930s. There were extensive controls of where Aboriginal people could live and work[e,f]; with whom they could associate or marry[g];

---

[e] The Aboriginal protection and restriction of the sale of Opium Act 1897 (QLD) allowed superintendents to determine where Aboriginal people would live.

[f] Aborigines Act 1905 (WA) prohibited cohabitation between Aboriginal people and others.

[g] The Aboriginal Ordinance Act 1918 (NT) "ensured that Aboriginal people could not drink or possess or supply alcohol or methylated spirits, could not come within two chains of licensed premises, have firearms, marry non-Aboriginal people without permission or have sex across the colour line".

the function and performance of cultural responsibilities; where they could travel[h]; and the teaching and practice of Aboriginal languages.

In part, the protectorate system was based on the belief that Aboriginal peoples would develop agricultural communities and not interfere with land claims of colonists; however, during the middle of the nineteenth century the survival of Aboriginal people was questioned. Contemporary analysis determined that the Aboriginal race was doomed and the best option would be to "smooth the dying pillow".

Reserves were created on annexed land, and Aboriginal family groups were shifted to strictly controlled communities, in which welfare was the responsibility of a Chief Protector or a Protection Board, sanctioned by protectionist legislation. Through various Protection Acts, Chief Protectors, Guardians, and Reserve Superintendents were appointed and responsible for the implementation and oversight of legislative requirements determining the daily activities of Aboriginal people.

In some states, the Chief Protector was the legal guardian of all Aboriginal children, given powers negating the rights of parents to raise children in Aboriginal family and community environments.[i,j] The New South Wales (NSW) Protection Act[10] allowed the removal of mixed heritage or lighter skinned children, the movement of entire communities, and the placement of Aboriginal children in training homes to learn domestic duties, and remained in force until 1969.

Protectionist legislation was passed to legitimize the removal of Aboriginal children by government officials from families and communities without the same strict application of due process or duty of care.

Motives underpinning these actions included to "inculcate European values and work habits in children, who would then be employed in service to the colonial settlers"[11] and the conversion of Aboriginal children to Christianity. This policy was effective in distancing Aboriginal children from their families and Aboriginal cultural practices,[k] and inhibiting early childhood development, socialization, and learning opportunities.

There was legislation to control sexual relations between Aboriginal and non-Aboriginal men and women.[l,12]

In January 1901, at Federation, the 6 self-governing colonies become the States of the Commonwealth of Australia. The Australian Constitution[13] made only 2 references to Aboriginal and Torres Strait Islander peoples:

- Section 51 (xxvi) left the power to legislate regarding Aboriginal people (the so-called race power) to the States "The Parliament shall, subject to this Constitution, have power to make laws for the peace, order and good government of the Commonwealth with respect to: the people of any race, other than the Aboriginal race...");

---

[h] Native Welfare Act 1954 (WA) 'natives' not to travel without a valid reason.

[i] Northern Territory Aborigines Act 1910 (NT) chief protector appointed legal guardian of all Aboriginal people.

[j] Aborigines (Training for Children) Act 1923 (SA) made the chief protector legal guardian of all half-caste children and allowed the removal of children from families to be sent to non-Indigenous homes and institutions until 21 years of age.

[k] Foundation Act 1934 (SA) – appointed a protector of aborigines to "make them friendly to the settlers, induce them to labour, lead them to civilisation and religion".

[l] Aboriginals protection and restriction of the sale of Opium Amendment Act 1934 (Qld) made intercourse between Aboriginal women and non-Aboriginal men illegal.

- Chapter 12, Section 127 excluded "Aborigines" from the collection of census information: "in reckoning the numbers of people...Aboriginal natives shall not be counted".

A Royal Commission in Western Australia (WA) in 1904[14] identified extensive abuses of the rights of Aboriginal people in WA, but recommended greater protection through more extensive control. These additional controls would focus on children, and efforts directed at the eradication of the "Aboriginal problem" through initiatives to erase collective memory of identity and disconnect children from their cultural bonds and merge them into the non-Indigenous community.

The Aborigines Act 1905 (WA) created a new office of the Chief Protector, who was granted legal guardianship for all Aboriginal and "half-caste" children less than 16 years of age. Similarly, the Aborigines Protection Act 1909 (NSW) established the Board of Protection of Aborigines. The Board was responsible for the custody, maintenance, and education of children, and its powers included the ability to make it illegal for any "half-caste" to live on a reserve. Amendments to the Act[15] gave the Board of Protection greater powers, including the authority to remove Aboriginal children from their families and to assume full control of any Aboriginal child if they considered the "moral or physical welfare of the child unsatisfactory", without the same strict application of legal requirements. In some jurisdictions, government debate centered on the ideal age for the forcible removal of Aboriginal children (from birth to 2 years, according to South Australian authorities).[16]

Assimilation and Integration

...unlike white children who came into the state's control far greater care was taken to ensure that [Aboriginal children] never saw their parents or families again[11]

Legislation determined who was or was not Aboriginal.[m] Aboriginality was defined according to skin color and blood quantum, and was related to welfare entitlements, such as who would live on missions, receive rations, or be eligible for employment or education. Skin color was the key to policy and practice: lighter skinned children were considered more likely to be accepted by the non-Indigenous population, to be absorbed into the wider community, and eventually lose their Indigenous identity.

In 1937 the Commonwealth Governments convened a 'Conference of Commonwealth and State Authorities'[17] to address Aboriginal welfare. The official recommendation of the conference was that Aboriginal people of mixed descent should be assimilated into the broader, white community, that those not living "tribally" should be educated, and all others should remain on reserves.

...the destiny of the natives of aboriginal origin, but not the full blood, lies in their ultimate absorption by the people of the Commonwealth, and it therefore recommends that all efforts be directed to that end ...with a view to their taking their place in the in the white community on an equal footing with the whites[18]

The forced removal of Aboriginal children was conducted according to the regulations of assimilation policies. Implicit in assimilation policies was the belief that there was nothing of value in Aboriginal and Torres Strait Islander culture, that

---

[m] The Aborigines Act Amendment Act 1936 (WA) like many of the State legal instruments gave a definition of "native".

non-Indigenous models of child rearing were superior, and that poverty was considered synonymous with neglect.

> We have the power under the act to take any child from its mother at any stage of its life...Are we going to have a population of one million blacks in the Commonwealth or are we going to merge them into our white community and eventually forget that there were ever any Aborigines in Australia? (A O Neville, Chief Protector of Aborigines, WA Native Welfare Conference, 1937).

In 1951 the Commonwealth convened the Australian Conference for Native Welfare, at which the policy of assimilation was "officially" adopted. However, by this time most States already sanctioned assimilationist policies, enforced by law.

Under amendments to the Aboriginal Protection Act in NSW[19] an Aborigines' Welfare Board replaced the Board of Protection. The duties of the Welfare Board included promoting and assisting Aboriginal assimilation into the non-Aboriginal community. Similarly, in Victoria[20] an Aborigines Welfare Board was established to promote assimilation.

The Bringing Them Home Report documents the experiences and effects on individuals and families who have lived through and live with the effects of these policies and practices.

Bringing Them Home

A "National Inquiry into the Separation of Aboriginal and Torres Strait Islander Children from their Families" was conducted in 1995 by the Australian Human Rights Commission (AHRC), and the Report of the Inquiry was published in 1997; it is known as the "Bringing Them Home Report of the Stolen Generation".

> The questions this history raises for us to contemplate today, at the very least, is what the implications are for relations between Aboriginal and white Australians, and what traces of that systematic attempt at social and biologic engineering remain in current child welfare practices and institutions. (van Krieken, 1991, p 144, Bringing Them Home Report).

Since colonization Aboriginal children have been separated from their families, kidnapped, and exploited. A national survey of Indigenous health in 1989 found that 47% of Aboriginal respondents had been separated from both parents during childhood, compared with 7% of non-Aboriginal respondents.

> ...we were a very lonely, lost and sad displaced group of people...neither black nor white...simply a lost generation of children.[21]
> ...the consistent theme for post-removal memories is the lack of love, the strict, often cruel, treatment by adults, the constantly disparaging remarks about Aboriginality – and the fact that the child should be showing more gratitude for having been taken from all that – and of course, the terrible loneliness and longing to return to family and community.(Bringing Them Home Report, chapter 10, Part 3).

The intended and unintended negative impacts of assimilationist approaches were compounded by ongoing practices consistent with segregation until the 1960s, including separate sections in public places and hospitals, and refusing to enroll Aboriginal children in school.

Self-determination

The 1960s saw a significant social and political shift in the approach to Aboriginal and Torres Strait Islander affairs. The Aboriginal Affairs Act 1962 (Southern Australia [SA]) saw the establishment of the Department of Aboriginal Affairs and the Aboriginal Affairs Board. The Commonwealth Electoral Act 1962 (Commonwealth [Cth]) granted Aboriginal people the right to vote at the federal level without having the right at state level.

The Adoption of Children 1964 (Queensland) promoted changes to child placement principles, with preferential consideration given to Aboriginal child placement with Aboriginal family members, extended family members, or other Aboriginal community members. The Social Welfare Ordinance 1964 (Northern Territory) abolished the assimilation program.

In the 1967 Commonwealth Referendum[22] 91% of the voting public supported the propositions pertaining to Constitutional change regarding the rights and recognition of Aboriginal people. The Referendum amended s51 (xxvi) of the Constitution and repealed s127, giving power to the Commonwealth to make laws in regards to Aboriginal people and to count them in the census.

1968 saw the establishment of the Commonwealth Office of Aboriginal Affairs, which was to become the Department of Aboriginal Affairs. In 1969 the Aborigines Welfare Board in NSW was abolished and all states had repealed legislation allowing the removal of Aboriginal children according to protection policies.

The Aborigines Act 1969 (NSW) established the Aboriginal Advisory Council, with Aboriginal membership providing advice directly to the Minister. The Department of Child Welfare became responsible for Aboriginal children across the state.

In 1972 the Whitlam Government was instated, and the Commonwealth Government pursued policies of self-determination to "restore Aboriginal people of Australia their lost power of self-determination in economic, social and political affairs."[23]

The Community Welfare At 1972 (SA) promotes Aboriginal language and culture. The Racial Discrimination Act 1975 is 1 of only 2 pieces of legislation (the other is the Sex Discrimination Act) that applies international human rights treaty norms and standards to domestic legal frameworks. There are several other international human rights instruments with particular relevance to Aboriginal children, their health and well-being, but although Australia is a signatory to most (including the Convention on the Rights of the Child,[24] but excluding the United Nations Declaration on the Rights of Indigenous People)[25] there has been limited application and interpretation of responsibilities into domestic legislation or statutory interpretation in case law.

The last 40 years have seen the development of the community-controlled sector across health and Aboriginal legal services, and legislative changes to child protection principles[26] and child placement.[27,28] In Kruger, Bray v Commonwealth (1997)[29] 146 ALR 126 the High Court of Australia decided that the Aboriginal Ordinance 1918 (Cth), which authorized the removal of Aboriginal children, was not constitutionally valid.

CHALLENGES
Resourcing and Coordination

Aboriginal children and their communities continue to experience the effects of nearly 2 centuries of oppressive and discriminatory legislation and policy, yet benefit from only 1 to 2 generations of the social and political shift toward self-determination, participation, and control. Programs implemented using this approach, however, seem most often to be under-resourced, poorly planned, short term, and with limited mechanisms for accountability.[7,30,31] Evidence has been inconsistently applied, programs and policy fragmented and uncoordinated across jurisdictions and levels of government. In addition to insufficient health expenditure to eliminate excess morbidity and mortality,[32] there is an undersupply and maldistribution of the health workforce to meet Aboriginal child health needs.

Data and Data Sources

There is a persistent underidentification of Aboriginal and Torres Strait Islander status in records of births and deaths. The National Perinatal Data Collection, for example, is a national data set that includes all Australian births. The Aboriginal or Torres Strait Islander status of the mother is collected, but not that of the father or baby.

The Commonwealth publishes a regular report on the health of Australia's Indigenous peoples[33]; however, there is a paucity of national and nationally representative data relating to Aboriginal child health outcomes and significant deficiencies in existing data availability and completeness.[34]

"The Northern Territory is the only jurisdiction in which Indigenous identification in mortality has been of sufficient and sustained quality to allow time series analysis"[35] and few data collections are specific to the health of Aboriginal and Torres Strait Islander children.[36,37]

Ongoing Effects

Health professionals and policy-makers should not underestimate the effect of unresolved, intergenerational trauma of 200 years of policy and legislation that sanctioned behaviors specifically designed to make Aboriginal and Torres Strait Islander peoples disappear.

Professor Helen Milroy,[n] an Aboriginal psychiatrist who specializes in child and adolescent mental health, works extensively with Aboriginal young people, dealing with the effects of unresolved intergenerational grief and trauma. In the Western Australian Aboriginal Child Health Survey Professor Milroy refers to a psychological analysis of historical events and effects as "the denial of humanity, the denial of existence, the denial of identity" and argues that this manifests as mental illness, physical morbidity and mortality, and social dysfunction. Further, poor mental health status and impaired social and emotional well-being for children and young people result from the unresolved effects on previous generations of historical and contemporary social, political, economic, and educational policies and practices. Socioeconomic status, poverty, chronic stress, lack of control over life circumstances, and lack of choice all affect outcomes.

Evidence demonstrates that strong cultural links and practices (eg, extended family, access to traditional land, use of traditional dialects and languages) are protective factors and improve resilience against emotional and behavioral problems.[38]

CURRENT POLITICAL AND POLICY INITIATIVES
The AHRC "Close the Gap" Campaign

In February 2006, the Australian Human Rights and Equal Opportunity Commission (HREOC), now the AHRC, published the Social Justice Report 2005.[39] The report proposed that a human rights based approach should be applied to Aboriginal and Torres Strait Islander health inequality and be used to develop a framework for addressing and overcoming disparities in health and social justice. The report recommended an evidence-based approach to policy and service delivery to drive the elimination of disparities within a generation.[40] The Social Justice Commissioner, Tom Calma, provided leadership in bringing together Aboriginal and Torres Strait

---

[n] Prof Helen Milroy is the senior clinical academic at the University of Western Australia, School of Medicine and Dental Health.

Program	Domain	Target	Comments	Time
Table 1 **Maternal and child health**				
To achieve parity in perinatal and infant mortality rates within 10 years				
Mothers and babies	Access	All Aboriginal women and children have access to appropriate mother and baby programs		5–10 y
	Antenatal care	50% reduction in premature births and low birth weight babies		5–10 y
	Acute respiratory infection prevention	50% reduction in community and hospital rates of acute respiratory infections	Immunizations, nutrition, serious, disabling injuries requiring hospitalization	5–10 y
	Acute respiratory infection treatment	>90% of children diagnosed with acute respiratory infections receive full treatment and appropriate follow-up		
	Gastro prevention	50% reduction in community and hospital rates of gastroenteritis	Immunizations, nutrition, serious, disabling injuries requiring hospitalization	5–10 y

Health Targets for Maternal and Child Health Equality, as presented by the Health Targets Subcommittee; Human Rights and Equal Opportunity Commission "Closing the Gap" Summit, Canberra, March 2008.

Islander organizations[o] to work in partnership on the development and dissemination of targets, benchmarks, and timelines to achieve health equality.

Specific targets regarding Aboriginal child health were developed, addressing areas in which greatest disparities persisted and in which greatest gains could be made with appropriate service access and utilization and clinical best practice. The targets identified other actions required to achieve health equality across jurisdictions, levels of governments, government departments, and nongovernment stakeholders (**Table 1**).[41]

Other subcommittees developed targets addressing primary care, infrastructure, and workforce, with further targets under development on the social and cultural determinants of Aboriginal health. This initiative has been successful in shaping the language and content of recent government policy, services, and budgetary commitments.[42]

---

[o] Including the Australian Indigenous Doctors' Association, the Congress of Aboriginal and Torres Strait Islander Nurses, the National Aboriginal Community Controlled Health Organisation, and other institutions and advocates in Aboriginal health and human rights.

Council of Australian Governments: Closing the Gap and Overcoming Indigenous Disadvantage

In 2002 the Council of Australian Governments (COAG) made a collective commitment to overcome Indigenous disadvantage, with progress against identified targets and indicators to be documented and published regularly.

In 2003 the heads of Australian Governments committed to reporting against key indicators of Aboriginal and Torres Strait Islander disadvantage, including accountability to improving outcomes, in regular "Overcoming Indigenous Disadvantage: Key Indicators" reports. The framework for these reports is based on best available evidence on the underlying determinants of disadvantage to assist the development of child health policy that focuses on prevention and determine where policies will have the greatest impact.

"Further, the COAG Indigenous Reform process has established 7 working groups to advance reforms in policy…these working groups have explicit terms of reference relating to social inclusion and outcomes for Aboriginal and Torres Strait Islander peoples."[43] Child and maternal health has been identified as a priority reform area.

In December 2007 COAG reaffirmed its commitment to partnerships across all levels of government to work with Aboriginal and Torres Strait Islander communities to address "closing the gap" on Indigenous disadvantage. Six "Closing the Gap" targets have been set by COAG to complement headline indicators previously identified by a COAG Steering Committee in consultation with Aboriginal community members, services, and researchers.[44] The COAG child-focused targets are

- Life expectancy at birth: closing the life expectancy gap within a generation
- Young child mortality: halving the gap in mortality rates for Indigenous children less than 5 years old within a decade
- Early childhood education: ensuring all 4 year olds in remote communities have access to early childhood education within 5 years
- Reading, writing, and numeracy: halving the gap for Indigenous students in reading, writing, and numeracy within a decade
- Year 12 attainment: halving the gap for Indigenous students in year 12 attainment rates by 2020
- Employment

The Working Group on Indigenous Reform has responsibility for integrating improved outcomes into national agreements to achieve the COAG targets.

Healthy for Life

Early childhood is 1 of 3 identified priority areas in government arrangements for Indigenous affairs. The Healthy for Life initiative aims to improve the health of Aboriginal and Torres Strait Islander mothers, infants, and children and those affected by chronic disease. The initiative adopts a whole-of-life approach to address the developmental and early childhood antecedents of disease later in life, particularly chronic conditions such as cardiovascular disease, renal disease, and diabetes. Associated programs focus on improving the capacity of primary care services in maternal and child health, and chronic disease prevention, screening, and management.

In 2005 the Commonwealth developed a new Aboriginal and Torres Strait Islander Child Health Check item supported by Medicare. All Indigenous children from birth to 14 years of age are entitled to an annual health check under Medicare, to support and complement Healthy for Life initiatives.

The Longitudinal Study of Indigenous Children: Footprints in Time

"Footprints in Time" is a longitudinal study of Aboriginal and Torres Strait Islander children that will track 2 age group cohorts: 0 to 12 months and 4- to 5-year-olds.[p] The study aims to identify risks and protective factors that influence the development of a strong cultural identity and positive health and social outcomes. It is anticipated that the findings will inform communities, governments, and other departments about improved and appropriate approaches to health, education, relationships, infrastructure, housing, and cultural development initiatives.[45]

Indigenous Family Violence and Child Abuse

The Prime Minister convened a "round-table" meeting with Aboriginal and Torres Strait Islander leadership in 2003. A working group was given the task of developing a strategy for COAG: the National Framework for Preventing Family Violence and Child Abuse in Indigenous Communities, endorsed in June 2004.[46] The Framework focused on prevention as a national priority, the development of bilateral agreements, approaches to safety, partnerships, support mechanisms, strong and resilient families, local solutions, and addressing the cause. An action strategy was developed in 2006, with commitments to customary law, law enforcement, Indigenous leadership, protection of victims, drug and alcohol rehabilitation services, health and well-being of children, and compulsory school attendance, addressed in bilateral, jointly funded initiatives.[47]

Indigenous Early Childhood Development National Partnership

In July 2008 COAG agreed to the development of an integrated policy framework that would be used as the foundation for reform and investment across all levels of government for Indigenous early childhood development.[48] The vehicle for this framework is the Indigenous Early Childhood Development National Partnership Agreement, which commits each State and Territory to action, linked to funding. The Partnership Agreements have 3 elements

- The development of Children and Family Centers across Australia in areas where there are high numbers of Aboriginal and Torres Strait Islander residents and identified disadvantage
- Increasing accessibility to services for Indigenous youth for teenage sexual and reproductive health programs and antenatal care
- Increasing access and use of maternal and child health services by Aboriginal and Torres Strait Islander families

National Early Childhood Development Strategy

The National Early Childhood Development Strategy represents a collaborative relationship between Commonwealth and State and Territory Governments to "ensure that by 2020 all children have the best start in life to create a better future for themselves and the nation."

The principles of the strategy focus on the whole child, from the antenatal period through to 8 years of age, and is inclusive of all children, with additional support provided to reduce social inequalities, enhance positive factors, and reduce risks. The strategy promotes a whole-of-service system approach, including universal and targeted support and services across all levels of

---

[p] "Footprints in time" will run from 2008 to 2011 in 11 sites (regional, urban, and remote) across Australia.

government and nongovernment agencies, respect for diversity and difference as a strength, and helping children develop a positive sense of self and culture (see **Box 1**).

Aboriginal and Torres Strait Islander Health Performance Framework Reports

These reports provide feedback against the Health Performance Framework, developed under the auspice of the Australian Health Minister's Advisory Council (AHMAC) to summarize Aboriginal and Torres Strait Islander health status and measure the impact of policy on Indigenous health outcomes. Child health and early childhood development are priority areas, and measures relating to child health outcomes include infant mortality, low birth weight, smoking (during pregnancy and around children), oral health, hearing loss, and pneumonia.[49]

The Australian Early Development Index

The Australian Early Development Index (AEDI) is a population level measure of early childhood development and has been adapted from the Canadian Early Development Instrument, trialed and validated for use in Australia against the Longitudinal Study of Australian Children. The AEDI was piloted in 60 communities across Australia, except the Northern Territory, between 2004 and 2007. More than 3000 teachers from 1400 schools (representing around 56,000 children) have completed the AEDI checklists.[50] The Indigenous AEDI (I-AEDI) Adaptation Study is being undertaken by the Telethon Institute for Child Health Research, through the Kulunga Research Network and the Center for Developmental Health, Curtin University, Perth, Western Australia. The project will

- Evaluate how the AEDI is working for Aboriginal and Torres Strait Islander children
- Ensure the AEDI can identify and collect information on culturally relevant ways in which Indigenous children learn and behave
- Develop tools and resources to assist in capacity building in Indigenous communities and communities with Aboriginal and Torres Strait Islander peoples[51]

National Health and Hospital Reform Commission

"A Healthier Future for All Australians" is the final report of the National Health and Hospital Reform Commission (NHHRC), which aims to inform the governments of Australia with a practical approach to national health reform. There are 3 reform goals[52]

1. Tackling major access and equity that affect health outcomes for people now
2. Redesigning our health system so that it is better positioned to respond to emerging challenges
3. Creating an agile and self-improving health system for long-term sustainability

There are 5 identified priorities for improving access and equity in Australia. The first priority of the NHHRC is to address Aboriginal and Torres Strait Islander health disparities through changes to funding, accountability and responsibility, and quality services. Specific initiatives will address workforce, nutrition, and strengthening primary care, with a focus on families and communities.

Home Visit Program

A new home visit program was announced early in 2008. The program is based on the Nurse Family Partnership initiative pioneered in the United States by Professor Olds, the Director of the Prevention Research Center for Family and Child Health at the University of Colorado.

It is designed to engage and support first-time, financially disadvantaged mothers. In the original program, home visits by health staff began in the antenatal care period and continued through the first 2 years of life of the infant. In Australia visits will continue through to 8 years of age. Evidence from more than 2 decades of experience in the United States demonstrates short-term and long-term benefits such as improved birth weights, cognitive ability, and school readiness; and mothers smoking less, developing improved parenting skills, and using community services more readily and effectively.

The program is aimed at giving Indigenous children a healthier start in life through ongoing home visits, and several services have been identified as pilot sites, including 2 or 3 Aboriginal communities. The initiative has not been trialed previously in Indigenous communities, regional, rural, or remote areas, or with other health professionals such as Aboriginal health workers.

A Healthy Start to Life

The Commonwealth announced future research priorities in December 2002. The National Health and Medical Research Council (NHMRC) is the agency responsible for the implementation of Australia's research agenda around Promoting and Maintaining Good Health and the 4 subpriority areas:

- A Healthy Start to Life
- Ageing Well, Ageing Productively
- Promoting Health and Preventing Disease
- Strengthening Australia's Social and Economic Fabric

Aboriginal and Torres Strait Islander health issues are prioritized across these areas, and in particular "research into child developmental health and wellbeing, maternal health – including the intra-uterine environment – and the early years of a child's life are critical periods. Programs which intervene during these periods are more successful at improving core developmental outcomes than later interventions."[53] The agenda also recognizes that determinants of health lie beyond the health sector specifically, and culture, identity, community function, and cohesiveness are critical antecedents for improved health outcomes for Aboriginal and Torres Strait Islander peoples.

Healthy Start to Life focuses on initiatives and factors that promote resilience and well-being during pregnancy, infancy, childhood, and adolescence.

WAYS FORWARD

Although progress has been made in some areas of child health and development, such as infant mortality,[54] several areas require additional investment to drive significant and timely improvements in health and social justice.

Health indicators are designed to focus policy attention on priority issues for children's health, development, and well-being through comparison across jurisdictions and from subpopulations. Indicators provide a mechanism to assist policy and planning and measure progress.[55] The development of indicators that are specific to Aboriginal and Torres Strait Islander children and are cognizant of the cultural and social determinants of health is an essential step in providing policy direction and measuring progress against identified targets, which should necessarily be developed in partnership with Aboriginal leadership and professional expertise.

Monitoring, evaluation, and reporting of progress require a robust and comprehensive system for data collection and analysis. A consistent national approach to reporting methods, data sources, clinical details, case definitions, and data quality is essential and should be supported by appropriate Indigenous status identification processes at service points of contact, and birth and mortality recording. This in turn contributes to the evidence base that should ideally inform policy.

Any reform in Aboriginal child health requires a sustained commitment and investment in linking levels of government and other jurisdictions, particularly education. A focus on the developmental antecedents of health and the development of chronic disease is important for understanding intergenerational effects of policy, infant health, and early childhood development, bringing together a whole-of-life approach to child health and development.

Investment also extends to financial and workforce support to enable effective implementation, data collection, monitoring, and analysis of policy and service delivery. Policy effect assessments should be considered before the implementation of all new initiatives.

SUMMARY

It is impossible to understand the current status of Aboriginal and Torres Strait Islander child health without an introduction to colonization, historical policies, intergenerational trauma, and contemporary effects.

To move forward the key pillars need to be addressed of policy consistency and coordination across State, Territory and Commonwealth jurisdictions and across all levels of government; an evidence-based approach to policy development and implementation; appropriate resourcing, including financial, infrastructure, and workforce investment; and more comprehensive data collection and analysis.

Improvements in Aboriginal and Torres Strait Islander child health and development will also be reliant on the promotion of a national identity respectful of Indigenous existence, strong Aboriginal leadership, high level political commitment, and a broader social commitment to Indigenous social inclusion and social justice.

REFERENCES

1. Australian Research Alliance for Children and Youth (ARACY) report card on the wellbeing of young Australians 2008. Available at: www.aracy.org.au/reportcard. Accessed June, 2009.
2. ARACY report card on the wellbeing of young Australians: technical report. Available at: www.aracy.org.au/reportcard. Accessed June, 2009.
3. Freemantle C, Read A, de Clerk N, et al. Patterns, trends and increasing disparities in mortality for Aboriginal and non-Aboriginal infants born in Western Australia, 1980–2001: population database study. Lancet 2009;367(9524):1758–66.
4. Ampe akelyernemane meke mekarle "Little children are sacred": report of the Northern Territory Board of Inquiry into the Protection of Aboriginal Children from Sexual Abuse. Darwin: Northern Territory Government; 2007.
5. Brough M. (Minister for Families, Community Services and Indigenous Affairs), National emergency response to protect children in the NT, media release, June 21 2007.
6. Brown A, Brown NJ. The Northern Territory Intervention: voices from the centre of the fringe [editorial]. Med J Aust 2007;187(11/12):621–3.

7. Ring I, Brown N. Indigenous health: chronically inadequate responses to damning statistics. Med J Aust 2002;177.
8. Overcoming indigenous disadvantage: key indicators 2009.
9. Austlii Indigenous Law Resources. Available at: www.austlii.edu.au. Accessed April, 2009.
10. Aborigines Protection Act 1909 (NSW).
11. Bringing them home: report of the national inquiry into the separation of Aboriginal and Torres Strait Islander children from their families, April 1997. Human Rights and Equal Opportunity Commission, Commonwealth of Australia; 1997.
12. Aboriginal Act Amendment Act 1939 (SA).
13. Commonwealth of Australia Constitution Act.
14. Royal Commission into the Condition of the Natives 1904 (WA).
15. Aborigines Protection Amending Act 1915 (NSW).
16. Royal Commission 1913 (SA).
17. Aboriginal welfare – Initial Conference of Commonwealth and State Aboriginal Authorities. Canberra, April 21–23, 1937.
18. From the minutes of the conference; National Library of Australia archives online. Available at: http://nla.gov.au/nla.aus-vn118931. Accessed September, 2009.
19. Aborigines Protection (Amendment) Act 1940 (NSW).
20. Aborigines Act 1957 (Victoria).
21. Confidential submission 167 Bringing them home report.
22. Constitutional alteration (Aboriginals) 1967 (Cth) Referendum.
23. Timeline of legislation affecting Aboriginal people. Available at: www.aboriginaleducation.sa.edu.au. Accessed May, 2009.
24. Convention on the Rights of the Child.
25. United Nations Declaration on the Rights of Indigenous People.
26. Children's Protection Act 1993 (SA).
27. Adoption Act 1993 (Australian Central Territory).
28. Family Law Reform Act 1995 (Cth).
29. Kruger, Bray v Commonwealth (1997) 146 ALR 126.
30. Ring I, Brown N. Achieving sustainable improvements in Aboriginal and Torres Strait Islander health. Isos Internet Conference. Available at: www.isosconference.org.au. Accessed May, 2009.
31. Ring I, Brown N. Aboriginal and Torres Strait Islander Health: implementation, not more policies. In: Gunstone, editor. History, politics and knowledge: essays in Australian indigenous studies. Victoria: Australian Scholarly Publishing Pty Ltd; 2008. p. 2–17.
32. Freemantle J, McAullay D. Health of Aboriginal and Torres Strait Islander children in Australia. In: Smylie J, editor. Health of indigenous children: health assessment in action. 2009.
33. The health and welfare of Australia's Aboriginal and Torres Strait Islander peoples. Australian Bureau of Statistics, Australian Institute of Health and Welfare. 2008.
34. Freemantle E, Zurynski YA, Deepika M, et al. Indigenous child health: urgent need for improved data to underpin better health outcomes. Med J Aust 2008; 188(10):588–91.
35. Overcoming indigenous disadvantage: key indicators 2008. p. 75.
36. National Aboriginal and Torres Strait Islander Health Survey.
37. National Aboriginal and Torres Strait Islander Social Survey.
38. Zubrick SR, Lawrence DM, Silburn SR, et al. The Western Australian Aboriginal Child Health Survey: the health of Aboriginal children and young people. Perth: Telethon Institute for Child Health Research; 2004.

39. Social justice report 2005. Aboriginal and Torres Strait Islander Social Justice Commissioner, HREOC, Sydney NSW.
40. Achieving Aboriginal and Torres Strait Islander health equality within a generation: a human rights based approach. Aboriginal and Torres Strait Islander Social Justice Commissioner. Sydney: Human Rights and Equal Opportunity Commission; 2006.
41. Closing the gap: national Indigenous health equality targets. Outcomes from the National Indigenous Health Equality Summit, Canberra March 18–20, 2008; Aboriginal and Torres Strait Islander Social Justice Commissioner and the steering committee for Indigenous Health Equality. Sydney: Human Rights and Equal Opportunity Commission; 2008.
42. Macklin J, Minister for Families, Housing, Community Services and Indigenous Affairs. Closing the gap in the Northern Territory, media release 12 May 2009.
43. Aboriginal and Torres Strait Islander health performance framework report 2008.
44. Overcoming indigenous disadvantage: key indicators 2008 report.
45. Available at: www.health.gov.au/internet/main/publishing.nsf/content/phd-child-health-index. Accessed August, 2009.
46. COAG Communiqué June 25, 2004.
47. Social justice report 2007, Aboriginal and Torres Strait Islander Social Justice Commissioner. Sydney: Human Rights and Equal Opportunity Commission; 2008.
48. Hon Jenny Macklin. Minister for Families, Housing, Community Services and Indigenous Affairs. Available at: http://www.jennymacklin.fahcsia.gov.au/internet/jennymacklin.nsf/print/closing_gap_nt. Media release. Accessed May 12, 2009.
49. Australian Health Ministers' Advisory Council. Aboriginal and Torres Strait Islander health performance framework report 2008 summary. Canberra: AHMAC; 2008.
50. Australian Early Development Index – 2009–2011. National implementation data protocol [final draft]. Canberra: Australian Government Department of Education, Employment and Workplace Relations; 2009.
51. Building better communities for children: community preparation and implementation guide. A partnership between the Centre for Community Child Health, The Royal Children's Hospital Melbourne, and the Telethon Institute for Child Health Research. Perth.
52. Australian Government, NHHRC. A healthier future for all Australians: final report June 2009. Commonwealth of Australia; 2009.
53. Australian Government NHMRC. Aboriginal and Torres Strait Islander research. A healthy start to life. Policy Framework; 2003.
54. Overcoming indigenous disadvantage: key indicators. report. Canberra: Steering Committee for the Review of Government Service Provision; 2009.
55. Australian Health Ministers' Conference, Community and Disability Services Ministers' Conference, National Headlines indicators for children's health, development and wellbeing, update June 2008.

Index

Note: Page numbers of article titles are in **boldface** type.

doi:10.1016/S0031-3955(09)00158-8
0031-3955/09/$ – see front matter © 2009 Elsevier Inc. All rights reserved.
pediatric.theclinics.com

Moving?

Make sure your subscription moves with you!

To notify us of your new address, find your **Clinics Account Number** (located on your mailing label above your name), and contact customer service at:

Email: journalscustomerservice-usa@elsevier.com

800-654-2452 (subscribers in the U.S. & Canada)
314-447-8871 (subscribers outside of the U.S. & Canada)

Fax number: 314-447-8029

Elsevier Health Sciences Division
Subscription Customer Service
3251 Riverport Lane
Maryland Heights, MO 63043

*To ensure uninterrupted delivery of your subscription, please notify us at least 4 weeks in advance of move.

Printed and bound by CPI Group (UK) Ltd, Croydon, CR0 4YY

03/10/2024

01040450-0012